Register Now for Online Access to Your Book!

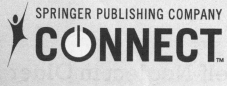

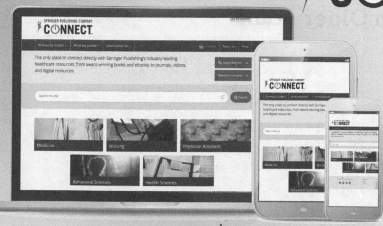

Your print purchase of *Self-Neglect in Older Adults,* **includes online access to the contents of your book**—increasing accessibility, portability, and searchability!

Access today at:

**http://connect.springerpub.com/content/book/978-0-8261-4083-8
or scan the QR code at the right with your smartphone
and enter the access code below.**

HN1H72J0

*Scan here for
quick access.*

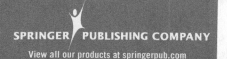

SPRINGER PUBLISHING COMPANY

View all our products at springerpub.com

T0171930

Self-Neglect in Older Adults

Mary Rose Day, DN, MA, PHN, RPHN, RM, RGN, is a nurse consultant in public health nursing and older adult care. Prior to this, she was a lecturer at the Catherine McAuley School of Nursing and Midwifery, University College Cork (UCC), Cork, Ireland. She has also held a range of nursing and management posts in acute care, long-term care, and community settings. She has DN, MA, and BSc degrees in nursing from UCC; a certificate in teaching from Harvard University; and a diploma in management from the Royal College of Surgeons, Dublin, Ireland. She has authored several journal articles, book chapters, and reports, and she continually contributes to nursing/social care and medical publications. Dr. Day has contributed to conferences and symposia on older people and community nursing nationally and internationally. She is a member of the Institute of Community Health Nursing and coordinated the Ageing Research Cluster of the Institute for Social Sciences in the 21st Century from April 2014 to January 2015 and is a committee member of the All Ireland Gerontological Nurses Association.

Geraldine McCarthy, PhD, MSN, MEd, RNT, RGN, Fellow RCSI, is emeritus professor at the Catherine McAuley School of Nursing and Midwifery, University County Cork (UCC), Cork, Ireland, and chair of the South/South West Hospital Group, which comprises nine hospitals in the South of Ireland. Prior to this, she held positions as founding professor and dean of the Nursing and Midwifery School at UCC, and head of the College of Medicine and Health, providing strategic leadership in research and education programs in medicine, dentistry, therapies, pharmacy, and nursing and midwifery. Dr. McCarthy holds an MEd degree from Trinity College, Dublin, and MSN and PhD degrees in nursing from Case Western Reserve University, Cleveland, Ohio. She has held a number of health care posts in Ireland, the United Kingdom, the United States, and Canada, and has been a member of a number of national and international bodies, including the Fulbright Commission. She has been an editor/author of a number of books and continually contributes to nursing publications.

Joyce J. Fitzpatrick, PhD, MBA, RN, FAAN, FNAP, is Elizabeth Brooks Ford Professor of Nursing, Frances Payne Bolton School of Nursing, Case Western Reserve University (CWRU) in Cleveland, Ohio, where she was dean from 1982 through 1997. She is also an adjunct professor, Department of Geriatrics, Ichan School of Medicine, Mount Sinai Hospital, New York, New York. With more than 300 publications, Dr. Fitzpatrick's work is widely published in nursing and health care literature, including more than 80 authored/edited books. She served as a coeditor of the *Annual Review of Nursing Research* series, volumes 1 to 26, and she currently edits the journals *Applied Nursing Research*, *Archives of Psychiatric Nursing*, and *Nursing Education Perspectives*, the official journal of the National League for Nursing.

Self-Neglect in Older Adults

A Global, Evidence-Based Resource for Nurses and Other Health Care Providers

Mary Rose Day, DN, MA, PHN, RPHN, RM, RGN

Geraldine McCarthy, PhD, MSN, MEd, RNT, RGN, Fellow RCSI

Joyce J. Fitzpatrick, PhD, MBA, RN, FAAN, FNAP

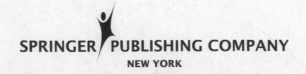

SPRINGER PUBLISHING COMPANY

NEW YORK

Springer Publishing Company, LLC
11 West 42nd Street
New York, NY 10036
www.springerpub.com

Acquisitions Editor: Elizabeth Nieginski
Compositor: S4Carlisle Publishing Services

ISBN: 978-0-8261-4082-1
ebook ISBN: 978-0-8261-4083-8

17 18 19 20 21/5 4 3 2 1

The author and the publisher of this Work have made every effort to use sources believed to be reliable to provide information that is accurate and compatible with the standards generally accepted at the time of publication. Because medical science is continually advancing, our knowledge base continues to expand. Therefore, as new information becomes available, changes in procedures become necessary. We recommend that the reader always consult current research and specific institutional policies before performing any clinical procedure. The author and publisher shall not be liable for any special, consequential, or exemplary damages resulting, in whole or in part, from the readers' use of, or reliance on, the information contained in this book. The publisher has no responsibility for the persistence or accuracy of URLs for external or third-party Internet websites referred to in this publication and does not guarantee that any content on such websites is, or will remain, accurate or appropriate.

Library of Congress Cataloging-in-Publication Data
CIP data is available from the Library of Congress.

Names: Day, Mary Rose, editor. | McCarthy, Geraldine, 1950- editor. |
  Fitzpatrick, Joyce J., 1944- editor.
Title: Self-neglect in older adults : a global, evidence-based resource for
  nurses and other health care providers / [edited by] Mary Rose Day,
  Geraldine McCarthy, Joyce J. Fitzpatrick.
Description: New York : Springer Publishing Company, [2018] | Includes
  bibliographical references and index.
Identifiers: LCCN 2017020894| ISBN 9780826140821 | ISBN 9780826140838 (e-book)
Subjects: | MESH: Self-Injurious Behavior | Aged | Self Care--psychology |
  Activities of Daily Living--psychology | Health Services for the Aged |
  Evidence-Based Medicine
Classification: LCC RA777.6 | NLM WM 165 | DDC 613/.0438—dc23 LC record available at
https://lccn.loc.gov/2017020894

Contact us to receive discount rates on bulk purchases.
We can also customize our books to meet your needs.
For more information please contact: sales@springerpub.com

Printed in the United States of America by McNaughton & Gunn.

CONTENTS

---

* Pseudonym.

CONTRIBUTORS

Sharon Abada, BS Research Assistant, School of Public Health, University of Texas, Houston, Texas

Julie Bach, PhD, MSG, MSW, LCSW Assistant Professor, Coordinator of the Gerontology Certificate, Graduate School of Social Work, Dominican University, River Forest, Illinois

Toya Band-Winterstein, PhD Senior Lecturer and Fellow, Center for Research and Study of Aging, Department of Gerontology, Faculty of Social Welfare and Health Sciences, University of Haifa, Haifa, Israel

Eleanor Bantry White, DPhil (Oxon), MPhil (Oxon), MSW (NUI), BSocSc (NUI), PCTLHE (NUI) College Lecturer in Social Work, School of Applied Social Studies, University College Cork, Cork, Ireland

Suzy Braye, BA, CQSW, MSc Independent Consultant and Emerita Professor of Social Work, School of Education and Social Work, University of Sussex, Brighton, United Kingdom

Jason Burnett, PhD Assistant Professor, Houston-McGovern Medical School, University of Texas and Texas Elder Abuse and Mistreatment Institute (TEAM), Houston, Texas

Leslie E. Clark, BSN Research Nurse, Houston-McGovern Medical School, University of Texas and Texas Elder Abuse and Mistreatment Institute (TEAM), Houston, Texas

Barbara Cohen, PhD, JD, RN Professor, Health Services Management, Berkeley College, New York, New York; Section Instructor, Nursing Simmons, Simmons College, Boston, Massachusetts

Mary Rose Day, DN, MA, RPHN, RM, RGN Nurse Consultant/College Lecturer, Catherine McAuley School of Nursing and Midwifery, University College Cork, Cork, Ireland

Catherine Devitt, MSocSc, MScEP Researcher, School of Architecture, Planning and Environmental Policy, University College Dublin, Dublin, Ireland

Israel Doron, PhD, LLM, LLB Head of the Department of Gerontology, Faculty of Welfare and Health Sciences, University of Haifa, Haifa, Israel

Paul Dowling, MSW Director of Social Services, Chicago Irish Immigrant Support, Chicago, Illinois

Joyce J. Fitzpatrick, PhD, MBA, RN, FAAN, FNAP Elizabeth Brooks Ford Professor of Nursing, Frances Payne Bolton School of Nursing, Case Western Reserve University, Cleveland, Ohio

Renee J. Flores, MD Assistant Professor, Houston–McGovern Medical School, University of Texas, Houston, Texas

Josephine P. Gomes, MD Assistant Professor of Geriatric Medicine, Department of Family and Geriatric Medicine, University of Louisville School of Medicine, Louisville, Kentucky

Graeme Halliday, BMed, FRANZCP Senior Staff Specialist Psychogeriatrician, Sydney Local Health District, Concord Hospital, New South Wales, Australia

Alison Hanlon, PhD, MSc Associate Professor, School of Veterinary Medicine, University College Dublin, Dublin, Ireland

Madelyn A. Iris, PhD Adjunct Associate Professor, Department of Medicine, Feinberg School of Medicine, Northwestern University, Chicago, Illinois

Yvonne O. Johnson, PhD, RN Associate Dean of Health Sciences, Surry Community College, Dobson, North Carolina

Patricia Leahy-Warren, PhD, Msc (Research), RGN, RM, RPHN Senior Lecturer, Catherine McAuley School of Nursing and Midwifery, University College Cork, Cork, Ireland

Jessica L. Lee, MD, MS Division of Geriatric and Palliative Medicine, McGovern Medical School, University of Texas Health Science Center, Houston, Texas

May Luu, BA (Hons) Master of Arts Student, Clinical Psychology, Member of the Centre for Collaborative Research on Hoarding, Department of Psychology, University of British Columbia, Vancouver, Canada

David McCann, BA (Hons) Social Care Worker, Rainbow Community Services, Smithstown Lodge, Julianstown, County Meath, Ireland

Geraldine McCarthy, PhD, MSN, MEd, RNT, RGN, Fellow RCSI Emeritus Professor, Catherine McAuley School of Nursing and Midwifery, University College Cork, Cork, Ireland

Joan McCarthy, PhD, MA, BA   Lecturer, Healthcare Ethics, Catherine McAuley School of Nursing and Midwifery, University College Cork, Cork, Ireland

Graham J. McDougall, PhD, RN, FAAN, FGSA   Martha Saxon Endowed Chair and Professor, Capstone College of Nursing, University of Alabama, Tuscaloosa, Alabama

Kelly Melekis, PhD, MSW   Assistant Professor, Department of Social Work, Skidmore College, Saratoga Springs, New York

Whitney L. Mills, PhD   Assistant Professor, Department of Medicine—Section of Health Services Research, Baylor College of Medicine; Investigator, Center for Quality, Effectiveness, and Safety, Michael E. DeBakey Veterans Affairs Medical Center, Houston, Texas

Helen Mulcahy, DN, Msc (Research), RGN, RM, RPHN   Catherine McAuley School of Nursing and Midwifery, University College Cork, Cork, Ireland

Aanand D. Naik, MD   Associate Professor, Department of Medicine—Section of Health Services Research, Baylor College of Medicine; Investigator, Center for Quality, Effectiveness, and Safety, Michael E. DeBakey Veterans Affairs Medical Center, Houston, Texas

Sigal Naim, MA   Doctoral Student, Department of Communication Studies, Ben Gurion University of the Negev, Be'er-Sheva, Israel; Lecturer, Department of Human Services, Max Stern Yezreel Valley Academic College, Jezreel, Israel

James G. O'Brien, MD, FRCPI   Professor Emeritus, Geriatrics Institute Scholar, University of Louisville, Louisville, Kentucky

Kieran A. O'Connor, MSc, MB, FRCPI   Consultant Physician in Geriatric Medicine, Mercy University Hospital, Cork, Ireland

Joan O'Leary[1]

David Orr, PhD, MSc   Lecturer in Social Work, School of Education and Social Work, University of Sussex, Brighton, United Kingdom

Kathleen Pace-Murphy, PhD   Assistant Professor in the Division of Geriatric and Palliative Medicine, Houston–McGovern Medical School, University of Texas, Houston, Texas; Medical and Regulatory Affairs, Novartis Pharmaceutical Corporation, East Hanover, New Jersey

Kimberlee Parker, MPH   Research Assistant, School of Public Health, University of Texas, Houston, Texas

---

[1] Pseudonym.

Michael Preston-Shoot, PhD, CQSW, PGDip SW, PGDip Psychot Professor of Social Work and Executive Dean, Faculty of Health and Social Sciences, University of Bedfordshire, Luton, United Kingdom

Katharine Slover, MNM Director of Community Outreach Services, Marillac St. Vincent Family Services, Chicago, Illinois

John Snowdon, MD, MPhil, FRANZCP, FRCPsych, FRACP Clinical Professor of Psychiatry, Sydney Medical School, Old Age Psychiatrist, Sydney Local Health District, Concord Hospital, New South Wales, Australia

Marietta P. Stanton, PhD, RN, FAAN Professor of Nursing, Capstone College of Nursing, University of Alabama, Tuscaloosa, Alabama

Bronwen Williams, MSc, BSc, PGCHE (NMC Teacher), RMN Mental Health Training Team Leader, 2gether NHS Foundation Trust, Collingwood House, Collingwood House Education and Training Centre, Horton Road, Gloucester, Gloucestershire, United Kingdom

Sheila R. Woody, PhD, RPsych Professor and Associate Head, Graduate Affairs/ Professor of Psychology, Department of Psychology, University of British Columbia, Vancouver, Canada

FOREWORD

One of the greatest success stories of the 20th century is the extension of human life expectancy. At the turn of the previous century, the average life expectancy was about 47 years of age. Today, that number is much closer to 80 years of age. Certainly, there is some variation around the globe, but, in general, owing to extraordinary strides in public health, nutrition, and health care, we can expect to live long and productive lives. However, with the advent of longer lives comes the responsibility for societies to ensure that their members live longer lives of high quality. This book underscores all the ways in which longer lives can, in fact, become entangled with a number of serious and potentially fatal situations and conditions, such as self-neglect. Congratulations to Drs. Day, McCarthy, and Fitzpatrick for taking on this momentous project, which will help provide evidence-based guidance for all of us who are struggling with enhancing the quality of life and care for older individuals in the context of self-neglect. It makes great sense that nurses have taken a lead with this book. Although its content is certainly not specific solely to the practice of nursing, we are all reminded that 90% or more of health care provided globally is provided by nurses.

When we think about the continuum of nursing practice from home care to critical care to hospice care, it is evident that the profession is well positioned to assess and intervene when there is evidence of self-neglect. The process of ensuring that effective, person-centered interventions are in place to reverse and ameliorate the tragic sequelae that go with this phenomenon is crucial. My career has been dedicated to the eradication of elder mistreatment of all types, and certainly self-neglect is a leading subtype within the broader continuum of elder mistreatment. I am so excited about the momentum building in the field, particularly the contributions of nursing and of this important textbook. This book is unique. It is the first global, evidence-based resource that targets self-neglect and the important evidence-based interventions available to help older people in need.

All of us are aware that older people have the right to self-determination and, if they make a conscious decision to be in the state of self-neglect, that is their right; none of us should use our power or paternalism to intervene in ways we would never intervene with younger individuals. I am reminded of an older patient I cared for who lived under a bridge—that was his home. When he turned 65, it was suggested that adult protective services be called in to have him institutionalized, which, in fact, happened. He protested and died shortly after. The lesson is that there is no one approach to care for those who are in a state of self-neglect, which is made clear in the pages that follow.

This book is a road map for all clinicians and health care providers who come upon the complex and often heartbreaking phenomenon of self-neglect. There is hope; there is action; and this textbook provides a guiding light.

Terry Fulmer, PhD, RN, FAAN
President
The John A. Hartford
Foundation
New York, New York

PREFACE

Self-neglect is a global phenomenon and a serious public health issue. It is a poorly defined concept, which leads to challenges in identifiying self-neglecting individuals as well as practical challenges in implementing interventions among health professionals, family members, and friends. Self-neglect can be intentional or unintentional and the difference depends on the individual's mental capacity.

This book is the first to deal exclusively with the subject of self-neglect. It is divided into six sections: Practical and Theoretical Perspectives, Issues Concerning the Self-Neglecting Individual, The Service Responds, Research Evidence, Assessment and Measurement of Self-Neglect, and Ethical and Educational Issues. The authors are from six countries: Australia, Canada, Israel, Ireland, the United Kingdom, and the United States. Many chapters include case studies or vignettes detailing what it is like to live with individuals who self-neglect or to work with them as health care professionals. Each chapter ends with a section on implications for practice and research.

Chapter 1 begins with a daughter profiling the progression of her mother's condition over time to self-neglect from personal, social, and environmental perspectives. The burden and challenges placed on all family members and the difficulty in trying to intervene and to obtain help from social and health care professionals are detailed. The frustration felt by family members who perceive that help is necessary while the mother refuses help is explained. In Chapter 2, Day describes self-neglect as the person's inability or unwillingness to provide goods and services necessary to care for life's needs. She asserts that there is no common understanding of the term and no overarching self-neglect theory and suggests that continued research and theory development are required so that professionals have a common understanding of the phenomenon.

In Section II, the singular or multiple issues that either lead to or are a consequence of self-neglect are presented. Cohen (Chapter 3) informs us of the mental health issues that may be present. McDougall and Stanton (Chapter 4) explain how delirium may sometimes be attributed to self-neglect without an understanding of the causes of the delirium itself and the relationship between delirium and impaired cognitive functioning. Hoarding is profiled in three chapters. Luu and Woody (Chapter 5) describe features, assessment, and intervention strategies that may be used in hoarding situations. Williams (Chapter 6) maintains that animal hoarding is poorly understood and underrecognized. This type of hoarding creates a risk to adults and the animals themselves and to those who try to deal with the issue. Devitt and Hanlon (Chapter 7) describe neglect issues found in farm animals and farmers themselves. The authors explore the relationship between human problems and farm animal neglect.

Snowdon and Halliday (Chapter 8) write about environmental neglect or the personal behavior and failure to protect one's environment. The authors discuss how best to assess and intervene in such cases and focus attention on the rights of individuals, their capacity to attend to their own welfare, and the rights of others in their environment. This section of the book ends with Lee writing on self-neglect and decision making (Chapter 9). In this chapter, the results of 19 studies are described. Included is a section on assessment of decision-making capacity and a case study in which the client is referred for capacity evaluation.

Section III details the response by health and social care professionals and agencies. It discusses self-neglect as a health care and environmental issue and outlines the fact that self-neglect is often brought to the attention of health care professionals by members of the public. However, self-neglect can be identified initially in acute care settings. O'Connor (Chapter 10) explains the paucity of research evidence for managing self-neglect of individuals who often present with complex medical, social, and psychological conditions. Case vignettes in acute hospital settings illustrate the types of issues encountered. Gomes and O'Brien present a medical perspective on self-neglect (Chapter 11). They address mental health, cognition, and social issues within the medical cases encountered. They present a case study and note that medical care has become so specialized that the services have been diversified. As a result, difficulties and confusion arise for individuals who need a more comprehensive interdisciplinary program for assessment and continuing management. In Chapter 12, Johnson reports on an investigation of home care nurses' perceptions of elder self-neglect in the United States. Facilitators, such as engaging family members on the health care team, specific focused education, protecting client choice, and lack of resources, are discussed. In a related study, Mulcahy and colleagues (Chapter 13) explore the perceptions of Irish public health nurses, community nurses, and social workers regarding self-neglect. Findings reveal the complexity of and personal responses to self-neglect, and challenges in managing cases. Recommendations include knowing and understanding the client, relationship-building skills, a multidisciplinary team approach, support, and training.

Lessons learned from England are profiled by Braye and colleagues (Chapter 14). These researchers draw on two studies conducted in the English context, including serious case reviews and interviews with managers, practitioners, and service users. They identify approaches that produced positive outcomes. Relationships built around the lived experience of self-neglect, together with the integration of knowledge and professional judgment regarding risk taking, are recommended as best practice.

In Chapter 15, Band-Winterstein and colleagues explore the meaning attributed to elder self-neglect by social workers in Israel using in-depth semistructured interviews. They report on intervention strategies developed by social workers that recognize individual autonomy without compromising client safety. Dowling and Slover (Chapter 16) explain how the city of Chicago addresses the issue of self-neglect among seniors. These authors describe a city-wide approach to addressing the issue through the Intensive Case Advocacy and Support Program (ICAS), outlining the historical development of the program together with research on outcomes.

In Section IV, three chapters profile research evidence and delineate many lessons for health care professionals. These chapters are different in relation to evidence for practice, and they profile perspectives from three different countries and from service providers. Melekis (Chapter 17) describes research that used a mixed-methods design to investigate service providers' perspective on their experience regarding existing resources and service needs in Vermont. Study findings point to the need for innovative, interprofessional, and interagency community responses addressing the challenging experiences, particularly as there is no formal accepted definition of self-neglect in Vermont. Chapter 18 is focused on research conducted by Burnett and colleagues regarding medication use and polypharmacy and the effects on self-neglect. Using a case study that profiles multiple comorbidities and polypharmacy, the authors conclude that a comprehensive review of medications is necessary in cases of individuals deemed as self-neglecting. In Chapter 19, McCann reports on research that was inspired through his student placement on a social care degree program in a community organization in Ireland. He studied health and social care professionals' perspectives on self-neglect and found, among other things, that self-neglect was considered with respect to prevalence and contributing factors, referral pathways and service interventions, and professional challenges and outcomes.

In Section V, methods of collecting and managing data on neglect and associated factors are presented. These deal with the construction of instruments for use by health and social care professionals and researchers to identify, measure, and potentially respond to self-neglect. In Chapter 20, Iris describes the development of the Short-Form Elder Self-Neglect Assessment Instrument. This includes 12 indicators related to physical and psychosocial aspects and 13 relating to environmental and personal living conditions. The findings of research based on the use of the instruments by practitioners are also presented. In Chapter 21, Mills and Naik contend that few tools exist to help health and social care professionals screen for everyday competence. They describe a screening tool, titled Making and Executing Decisions for Safe and Independent Living (MEDSAIL), which they developed. Furthermore, they review the literature on assessment and competence in self-neglect and describe the development, validation, and refinement of MEDSAIL. They also provide case vignettes demonstrating how the tool can be used in practice. In Chapter 22, Day and McCarthy describe the development and evaluation of a self-neglect measurement instrument (SN-37). Generation of the item pool, validity and reliability, and factor analysis are presented. Environment, social networks, emotional and behavioral liability, health avoidance, and self-determination are the factors that emerged from the factor analysis. Overall, these three chapters provide options for practitioners regarding the use of instruments for screening purposes. Chapter 22 also provides information for researchers embarking on studies of self-neglect.

Section VI comprises two chapters. Bantry White and Bach (Chapter 23) outline the pedagogical demands placed on professional educators by the complex nature of self-neglect. Specific attention is paid to reflective models of teaching and learning that center on active experiential approaches. Day and McCarthy (Chapter 24) apply an ethical decision-making tool to a self-neglecting case. This provides a step-by-step framework of actions and responsibilities to help critically reflect on and respond to an ethically challenging self-neglecting individual.

In Chapter 25, the authors summarize the major components of the text. In addition, they draw conclusions regarding implications for practice and research. We expect that all readers will find this work informative and that many new clinical and organizational changes and initiatives and research projects will emerge as a result of this publication.

Mary Rose Day
Geraldine McCarthy
Joyce J. Fitzpatrick

PRACTICAL AND THEORETICAL PERSPECTIVES

CHAPTER 1

MY MOTHER'S LIFE AND SELF-NEGLECT

Joan O'Leary[1]

This is the story of one woman's self-neglecting behavior told from a daughter's perspective. The physical, social, and environmental effects of the woman's self-neglecting behavior are described, as are the several efforts the family members have made to intervene. The story is sad because of what it means to be both the person who self-neglects and the family and friends of that individual. Thus far, no health or social service interventions have been accepted by the self-neglecting mother.

I am the daughter of a mother who self-neglects from a personal, social, and environmental perspective. This is my personal story and what I know and understand about my mother's life and what has shaped her life to the present day. Reflecting on the things that have shaped her life, I will take you through her early years, growing up, marriage, and divorce. From what I can ascertain, my mother's vulnerability was identified at an early age by her parents. Her behavior has had a considerable impact on my father, my brothers, her grandchildren, and other family members, as well as her friends. I hope that sharing my story will help others to understand the impact and consequences of self-neglecting behavior on families.

MOTHER'S EARLY YEARS

My mother is 73 years of age and was the second of five children. Her father was a solicitor, so they were comfortable financially, and by all accounts she had a normal childhood typical of the 1940s and 1950s in Ireland. Her bedroom was a large room shared with her three sisters, and her "corner" was always the tidiest of the four. According to her older sister (a retired solicitor), things began to change when both she and my mother were sent to boarding school for a year at the ages of 9 and 8, respectively. They were sent there to learn Irish as this was a requirement to register and enroll in university back then, and their school was not very good at teaching Irish. My aunt wonders whether their time away from their mother was a turning point in my mother's life as she really needed her mother and a 4-hour drive away meant that seeing her regularly was completely out of the question. It was almost like this separation was the first loss my mother had experienced.

---

[1]Pseudonym.

At around the same time, an older male cousin in his teens touched my mother and her sister "down there" when he was staying with them one night. From discussions I've had with my mother (and separately with my aunt), it happened about four times, more than enough to permanently mark my mother. She said to my aunt 50 years later that it "ruined my whole life." Strangely enough, she has selective empathy for others who have been abused, in that she will deem some worthy of empathy but not others, as she considered them to be clearly exaggerating or even lying (even though her abuse was, in the greater scheme of things, relatively mild).

All of the children, including my mother, worked in their uncle's pharmacy throughout their childhood. She says that she started taking prescription medication at the age of 10 and that this dependence continued, and expanded to alcohol, until she stopped in her late 30s. She was always the character in the family, the wild, outrageous one—bleaching her hair, wearing very modern shoes, sneaking out of the house, and so forth. Not exactly earth shattering now, but practically criminal offenses for middle-class Ireland back then. Whether it was the drugs or her personality that drove this wildness is anyone's guess, but she was most definitely the "bold" one. In secondary school, she says, she did very little other than draw, so her parents were advised to send her to boarding school as it would be much more disciplined for her. She says that she cried her eyes out for days when she got there and then cried her eyes out for days when she left years later. This was not unusual for my mother. As her brother-in-law describes her, "The only predictable thing about your mother is her unpredictability!"

While all of her siblings studied law, my mother trained to be a medical doctor and qualified in the late 1960s. She met my father when he was in his final year studying law. After moving to London for work, they got married, and my mother recalls that her father asked her on her wedding day whether she was sure about getting married. Her interpretation of this is that he did not trust my father and thought it was not a good match. My aunt's interpretation is that their father thought that my mother was not mature enough, or probably not well enough, to get married. Her father also told my father (according to my father) on the morning of the wedding to take care of my mother. Almost 50 years later, my father feels that he's broken that promise. From other comments that her siblings have made about her over the years, and their memories of their parents' reactions to my mother, it would seem that she was always a bit different to them and always thought of as vulnerable.

My parents' time before they had children was one of parties, wigs, fake eyelashes, lots of alcohol, and (for my mother) anything she could get on prescription. She tells the story of collapsing unconscious at their home in London and the ambulance being called. While the emergency medical technicians were frantically asking what she'd taken to get into this state, her friend, who was staying with them for a few days, and my father tore the house apart wondering where her stash was only to find it in the toe of her boot. She was rushed to the emergency room and had her stomach pumped. She was back at work after 2 days, telling colleagues that she'd had the flu. She also tells a story about driving back in their Porsche from a party they had been to in Brighton. My mother was again passed out from alcohol and drugs, and she did not even wake up when my father drove straight over a humped roundabout (he'd left his glasses on the beach).

MARRIED YEARS

I was born in London when my mother was 27; my brother was born 18 months later, and my second brother 18 months after that. My mother never went back to work after we were born, and because my father had done very well financially, he decided to retire. They decided to bring the children up in the small town in Ireland where he grew up—the idyllic childhood. We moved to a large, old house in the middle of the town, and then recession hit both Ireland and the United Kingdom, forcing my father to go back to work. He started commuting to London, which I think was incredibly difficult for my mother—staying alone with three very small children in a small town, knowing nobody. We went through a succession of au pairs for years, but I have a feeling we were all too wild for them, as they never lasted long.

I was 6 when my third brother was born. I remember that my mother was in bed a lot when she was pregnant with him (there was a chance she'd lose the baby) and people were very good to her at the time, which she acknowledges but still suspects that they were just interfering busybodies. Although most people would be grateful for help (with looking after children, bringing food, school runs, etc.), my mother believes that people have an agenda, are doing it for their own purposes, and are interfering and judging, rather than simply trying to help. Sadly, the baby died of a cot death when he was 3 months old.

My father started having an affair around this time (I'm not entirely sure of timescales), and I do remember at one stage that when he came back every second weekend from London, he would stay in a flat and come to see us. We spent one Christmas at our cousin's without him, and he threatened to leave permanently and take us with him unless my mother got it together (I was never sure whether this was about her drinking or the messy house). Regardless, they ambled on for the sake of the children. Divorce was not possible in Ireland until the early 2000s, so there was no option other than to plod along (my parents are now divorced).

My fourth brother was born about 2 years later—he was utterly adored, particularly by my mother and me. He was completely and utterly indulged and spoiled (despite the spoiling, he's turned out to be a fantastic adult).

My mother finally stopped drinking when I was 10 years old, and she went to dry out for 6 weeks. She has been off alcohol and drugs ever since with no relapses. She often says that she stopped drinking because she thought that she was going to lose us children to the authorities.

MOTHER'S SELF-NEGLECTING BEHAVIORS

Regarding my mother and her "messiness," I cannot remember her being any other way. I would always say to friends who came to the house that we were still unpacking (I was 3 when we moved to Ireland), which would explain the "mess." I used that excuse right up to my teens— I have no idea how I thought I'd get away with it! The house was big, and about half the rooms were never really used. My mother's classic line was "I'm a doctor, not a housewife," which always absolved her of any domestic duties—they were beneath her, and anyway, nobody had ever shown her how to do anything. She thought that I learned everything from 3 years of home economics at school and a science degree at college. She had cleaners in over the years, but invariably they would tidy things away that she then could not find, and she would accuse them of stealing whatever it was. This was a recurring theme.

DAUGHTER'S PERSPECTIVE

From a very young age, I would clean and tidy as I abhorred mess and was absolutely mortified when people called. I vividly remember drawing up a family timetable of jobs for me and my next two brothers—it never occurred to me to include my mother's name on the timetable. It had everything covered, from opening and closing shutters to hoovering, mopping, cleaning windows, picking clothes up, and tidying. It was all-consuming for me, and I even collapsed from exhaustion at about the age of 8 and was sent to bed for a week by the family physician (who was a friend of the family and who, I assume, knew the situation). My whole life was about cleaning and tidying. The most stressful bit was preparing for my father's home visits every second week, which meant I would have to clean the kitchen until the counter was gleaming, otherwise the fights would be terrifying. A messy house when my father walked in the door after 10 days would be catastrophic. The responsibility on me was huge.

MOTHER AS A COLLECTOR

My mother has never ever been able to throw something out! From orange nets to receipts for a chocolate bar, from old hoovers to windsurfing boards. Paint pots, full and empty, from the 1970s are still stacked in the house along with number plates from old cars. We have over the years tried to help her tidy up, but it is clear that she just finds it too stressful. She becomes highly panicked and agitated (and more often than not verbally abusive) when there is rubbish to be thrown out, and she insists on going through the bag before it's finally allowed out of the house. Sometimes a bag can sit there for months before she has picked through it with a fine-tooth comb.

IMPACT OF BEHAVIOR ON FAMILY

The repercussions for a family are sad, more than anything else. Of the four siblings, three of us emigrated for university and then stayed away from home working. I came back a few years ago (with three children) after almost 20 years. The brother who stayed home has two children, and another brother in America has two children as well. Our youngest brother is still single with no children. The most upsetting thing is that none of us with children ever stayed with my mother when we could come back home to visit as the house was truly in a shocking state and certainly not one that you would bring babies or small children into. Cat litter box left unemptied, dried out dog feces, compost from repotting plants, sinks that are never cleaned, newspaper piles, professional journals stacked up and not opened in 20 years but never to be thrown out. Staying with other relatives or friends when we came back pained my mother, and we usually said that it was to avoid putting her out as she was on her own and it was a lot for her to cope with. We couldn't admit that it was because of the state of the house because she would get very offended and upset and then go on the attack ("You're just all perfect"). Our youngest brother does stay with her, but he comes home at most once a year and only for a few days. He occasionally brings a girlfriend home, but they are warned of the situation well in advance so he feels that he's thoroughly armed then, and we all tend to make a big joke out of it because, of course, it's so outrageously embarrassing.

INTERVENTIONS

On two occasions, we've tried to have a big clear-out: once, when my mother went away for a month, my brother took three skips of rubbish out of the house. She was in her mid-50s then. Mum displayed a combination of relief and hysteria. The second occasion was when she was in her mid-60s, and again, she was out of the country. There was a leak in her house, and my brother and I spent about 3 days emptying anything water damaged and also using it as an opportunity to do another clear-out and rubbish and clutter filled a few skips that we hired. She seemed accepting initially, when she came back, only to end up absolutely furious after a few days (even though she couldn't identify anything in particular that she missed).

She has always been particularly vicious with me, and we wonder whether that is because my being the only girl triggers a direct comparison of our "housekeeping skills." An added reason is that I was the only one who ever did anything to tidy up, which isn't unusual in a house full of boys. She has openly admitted that whenever I help, it makes her feel like a failure and that she's probably jealous. Her bitterness and anger toward me have escalated over the years to the extent that I have promised not even to wipe a surface down anymore and I don't make any comments on the state of the house as it's become far too stressful for everyone. I do understand that she perceives as interfering and insulting what I think is being helpful. My brother who lives locally does a lot for my mother around the house on the "do it yourself" front. He also cuts the grass for her, but he has not been able to actually enter the house for a few years now because it depresses and upsets him so much.

The situation has gotten progressively worse with time, and very few people come to visit her—whether that's because she can be difficult or because of the state of the house, I don't know. Also, she sleeps a lot and is normally not out of bed until lunchtime; nor does she respond well to people just popping in, as she feels that there has to be a prior invitation (although she'll call on people unannounced herself). I try to call to her about two to three times a week and bring my younger two children with me, although they hate it and have asked why granny's house is so messy and dirty and there's nowhere for them to sit down. Unfortunately, they're not very fond of her personally because she can be quite nasty to them, shouting at them when she thinks they haven't answered her, for example. They have, but she hasn't heard them. It means that they, in turn, are angry with her, so it becomes a vicious circle. Again, whether this is part of her condition or just personality traits all of her own I don't know, but it's very sad and upsetting that they have no time for her but adore their other granny. My mother can be a great character, but really only one on one; she is not good in groups. The reality is that my children feel deeply uncomfortable in her house, which does nothing to make them feel welcome by their grandmother.

NEED FOR HEALTH AND SOCIAL CARE INTERVENTION

Our main concern now is her physical health. She's had a number of falls over the years, only a few of which she's admitted to. But a year ago, she fell backward into a tree when she sat on a plastic garden chair that was broken (and that she wouldn't throw out, of course). She got stuck in the hedge and was there for at least an hour when I just called to see her with my father. We pulled her out of the hedge and a few days later took her to hospital as her lower back was black from bruising, as was her face, and her right wrist was badly swollen, as was her right knee. To this day we still can't understand how she sustained bruising on her front when she fell backward, so we think that maybe she fell in the house either just before or just after the hedge incident. She swears she didn't, but we wonder whether she either doesn't remember or is too embarrassed to admit that she tripped in the house because of the mess (we've all tripped there because of the cluttered floors).

Her sister came to visit her during this time, and my mother was beyond furious as my aunt and I went to see my mother's general practitioner (GP) to tell her how my mother was living, show her photos, and see what could be done to help her. Clearly, she didn't want our help or feel that she needed any help. Instead of realizing that we were trying to help, my mother exploded with fury: "How dare you go behind my back, interfere in my life"! All absolutely understandable comments but unfounded as her sister told her we were going to the GP. This is a recurring theme and we (all her children, her sister, and my father) think it is stoked by her male "friend" of 20 years, Paul. Her friend is an old colleague whom she met again at Alcoholics Anonymous (AA; which they both attend), after 20 years of not having seen each other. Of the same age as my mother and an ex-alcoholic with psychiatric problems (bipolar disorder), he is on his own, having left his wife and two small children many years ago. An example of how he goads my mother is provided by an incident in which she first saw my aunt (who had traveled over 300 miles to see her after her fall) and was delighted, but when she called Paul and then hung up the phone was apoplectic with rage. Paul is exceptionally suspicious of people's motives, and he invariably plants the seeds of cynicism in my mother, which is very difficult to deal with. This happens again and again, and we're not sure whether she's just easily led as a person or if it's all part of her condition and she is being effectively provoked by a stronger person for whatever reasons, subconscious or otherwise. During this time, when my aunt was staying for a few days, my mother also made a vicious verbal attacked on my brother's 20-year-old daughter (her granddaughter). Again, we wonder whether the whole episode involving her fall and my aunt who visited thereafter and the GP was just all too much for her, provoking her to lash out.

Another concern, apart from the hazards created by physical obstacles, is her food hygiene. She wouldn't throw even a cornflake out, and her fridge has unidentifiable foodstuffs covered with green mold. We're not sure what exactly she eats and wouldn't dare ask her as the verbal abuse is not worth it. My brother and I try to give her a few dinners a week so at least we know she's eating something decent and that it won't kill her. We've asked her to come to our house for her dinners, but she says she does not want to interfere in our lives.

We're also concerned about her personal hygiene, as we're fairly certain that she rarely showers or bathes. She does wash her hair every few days, but we think that's the extent of it. She swims in the sea most days, and she says it cleans her. Like a lot of women her age who've had a number of children, she's got bladder problems that she takes tablets for, but she does occasionally leak or have accidents. The awful thing is that I have had to say to her a few times that she smells of urine, which is very embarrassing for both of us. Also, because her house is very big and impossible to heat, she wears a lot of layers, typically tracksuits and fleeces. Because she has very little concern for her personal appearance, these can be filthy and have holes in them, either from wear or from mice or moths. She has gone to the village wearing odd shoes. My brother, who is well known in the village, is frequently embarrassed by her "bag lady" appearance. And this is the woman who was at the height of fashion in her heyday.

With regard to the house, she's permanently tied to it and gets uncomfortable and agitated if she's away from it for more than a few hours as she always has "things to do." She constantly feels that she should be there tidying but will end up, for example, finding a newspaper hidden under something and reading it for the afternoon; she gets totally side-tracked and then is no further forward.

When broaching the topic of the house with my mother, we've all tried every angle we could think of, from outright rudeness about the state of the house to expressing concern about her, and from pleading and begging to offering to pay for psychological help or cleaners. Our youngest brother works for charities, and he's even stooped low enough to tell my mother that poverty-stricken families in the third-world countries he's worked in have cleaner tin shacks and mud huts than our mother's house. For a few weeks, I was going in once a week for a few hours and we did two rooms together, but it was just too stressful for her and for me trying to hold my tongue. All in vain, as those rooms are back to the way they were.

In a nutshell, how my mother lives is a major topic of daily conversation among all of her children, her ex-husband, and her own siblings. We're all constantly worried about her physical safety and her emotional and psychological well-being as her suspicious and paranoid nature has driven good friends away (including her fantastic AA sponsor whom my mother accused of stealing from her). I also hate that every single one of her grandchildren prefers their other grannies—it's heartbreaking. Finally, I'm dreading the day we have to empty the house out for the last time because, sadly, most of it will go straight to the dump in a long parade of skips. Everything she's worried about binning for many years will just be thrown out with enormous relief by her children. How terribly sad—all that angst for naught.

CONCLUSION

This story depicts self-neglecting behavior physically, socially, and environmentally. It illustrates vulnerability, multiple losses, loneliness, addiction, and attachment to objects, and refusal of interventions. The story also describes the impact my mother's behavior has had on our extended family. People, like my mum, who self-neglect often do not want help to change, yet are putting themselves and others at risk. As a family, we have many concerns about our mum's physical health, safety, and well-being. We have intervened on occasions, but this has provoked severe rage and fury. There is no simple, quick-fix solution. My mum was assessed as having the capacity to make decisions, so it is her choice, and all we can do at this time is to help reduce health and safety concerns in a respectful way, as far as we can.

IMPLICATIONS FOR RESEARCH AND PRACTICE

- Self-neglect represents a major public health issue that can have a considerable impact on children and the extended family.
- Family members' perceptions or insight into self-neglect and hoarding disorder is important.
- No published research has examined the burden of self-neglect on family members.
- A brief psychoeducational intervention on self-neglect could provide support to family members.

CHAPTER 2

SELF-NEGLECT: TOWARD CONCEPTUAL CLARITY

Mary Rose Day

Self-neglect may be described as a person's unwillingness or inability to provide the goods or services necessary to care for his or her own life needs. Self-neglect is increasingly being recognized as an important public health issue with many serious adverse outcomes. It can be accompanied by poor health, malnutrition, hoarding, and squalid home environments on a continuum of severity. Older adults are particularly vulnerable to self-neglect, thus aging populations will increase prevalence risk. Conceptualization of self-neglect has evolved since the 1950s, and a range of conceptual models and frameworks have been proposed. There is no overarching self-neglect theory, thus research is required to clarify further the conceptualizations and measurement of the phenomenon. As there is no standardized universally accepted definition of self-neglect assessment, provision of services and legislative approaches can vary across jurisdictions.

Since the 1950s, a range of conceptual models and frameworks for understanding self-neglect has been proposed. There is, however, no standardized universally accepted definition of self-neglect. Assessment, provision of services, and legislative approaches vary across jurisdictions. In this chapter, definitions of self-neglect and conceptual and theoretical issues are explored.

DEFINITIONS OF SELF-NEGLECT

The concept of self-neglect was first identified in the 1950s, and since then a variety of terms have been used to describe and define self-neglect in the health care and social services literature (Lauder, Roxburg, Harris, & Law, 2009). The terms associated with the concept of self-neglect include *social breakdown syndrome* (McMillan & Shaw, 1966), *senile recluse* (Post, 1982), *senile squalor syndrome* (Clark, Mankikar, & Gray, 1975; Sheikh & Yesavage, 1986), *gross self-neglect* (Cybulska & Rucinski, 1986), *Diogenes syndrome* (Reyes-Ortiz, Burnett, Flores, Halphen, & Dyer, 2014), and *domestic squalor* (Snowdon, Halliday, & Banerjee, 2012).

The term *Diogenes syndrome* was first conceived by Clark et al. (1975) in the United Kingdom and is sometimes used in the diagnosis of self-neglect (Pavlou & Lach, 2006). Diogenes syndrome is defined as extreme self-neglect, domestic squalor, social withdrawal, apathy, a tendency to hoard rubbish (syllogomania), and as lack of shame of living condition (Pavlou & Lach, 2006, p.836).

The symptoms described are distinct behaviors and attributes at the extreme end of the trajectory (such as extreme squalor, unhygienic conditions, chosen isolation, service refusal, and propensity to collect objects) and would not be representative of all self-neglect cases. Self-neglect in older people shares some features of geriatric syndrome, such as multifactorial etiology and associated mortality. However, evidence that self-neglect is a syndrome is limited as it does not take account the broader social and cultural influences involved (Braye, Orr, & Preston-Shoot, 2011; Halliday, Banerjee, Philpot, & MacDonald, 2000; Lauder et al., 2009; Pavlou & Lach, 2006).

The term *domestic squalor* is used to describe extremely neglected living conditions. According to the Department of Health, Australia, "squalid dwelling or living space (as opposed to clothing or appearance) refers to somewhere that is filthy, unclean or foul indicating extreme self-neglect through lack of care, cleanliness or general neglect" (2012, p. 14). The term domestic squalor is included within the definition of *Diogenes syndrome* provided by Pavlou and Lach (2006). Professionals in Australia discriminate between self-neglect and squalor. Self-neglect is described as personal neglect of self and squalor as extreme environmental neglect (McDermott, 2008).

The National Center on Elder Abuse (NCEA; Teaster et al., 2006) defined self-neglect as:

> Adults inability, due to physical or mental impairment or diminished capacity, to perform essential self-care tasks including obtaining essential food, clothing, shelter and medical care obtaining goods and services necessary to maintain physical health, mental health or general safety; and/or managing one's own financial affairs. (p.10)

This definition excludes mentally competent older people, who understand the consequences of their decisions and make a conscious and deliberate decision to engage in acts that threaten their own health or safety as a matter of personal choice. A central issue for addressing self-neglect is the assessment of the person's decision-making capacity and willingness and ability to live safely and independently in the community.

To provide greater clarity for services, the National Association for Adult Protective Services (2008) provided the following definition:

> Self-neglect is the result of an adult's inability, due to physical and/or mental impairments or diminished capacity, to perform essential self-care tasks including: providing essential food, clothing, shelter, and medical care; obtaining goods and services necessary to maintain physical health, mental health, emotional well-being and general safety; and/or managing financial affairs. (National Committee for Prevention of Elder Abuse, 2008, p. 5)

The key concepts within this definition are "individual's competence" and addressing the person's "health and safety needs."

The Department of Job and Family Services, Ohio, provides a statewide policy definition of self-neglect within a definition of neglect. It defines self-neglect as "the failure of an adult to provide for self the goods or services necessary to avoid physical harm, mental anguish, or mental illness or the failure of a caretaker to provide for such goods or services." (2016, p. 1)

The Elder Justice Act (EJA, 2010) defined self-neglect as:

> An adult's inability due to physical or mental impairment, or diminished capacity, to perform essential self-care tasks including (A) obtaining essential

food, clothing, shelter, and medical care; (B) obtaining goods and services necessary to maintain physical health, mental health . . . (C) managing one's own financial affairs. (p. 785)

This definition offers a comprehensive and concise conceptualization of self-neglect. Embracing this definition for research would provide standardization and would make results more comparable (White, 2014).

A collaboration between nurse researchers in the United States and Scotland led to the development of the North American Nursing Diagnosis Association (NANDA) diagnosis and definition of self-neglect as:

The inability (intentional or non-intentional) to maintain socially and cultur-ally accepted standard of self-care with the potential for serious consequences to the health and wellbeing of the self-neglecters and perhaps even to their community. (Gibbons, Lauder, & Ludwick, 2006, p.16)

This definition is holistic and captures the intentional and choice factors as well as the sociocultural influence of the behavior and potential of the negative impact of self-neglect for the individual, his or her family, and the community. Gibbons et al. (2006) differentiated intentional self-neglect (lifestyle, choices, maintaining control, personality type, and fear of institutionalization) from nonintentional self-neglect (cognitive impairment, functional impairment, psychiatric illness, substance abuse, and major life stresses) and developed criteria to support health care providers in identifying self-neglect (p. 15). This definition has been adopted by a number of researchers (Day & McCarthy, 2016; Iris, Ridings, & Conrad, 2010).

Numerous definitions of self-neglect exist. Definitions and conceptualiza-tions of what constitutes self-neglect can vary across disciplines, communities, and cultures. The absence of a widely accepted definition of self-neglect to inform practice and research has created challenges for both research and practice (Dyer, Goodwin, Pickens-Pace, Burnett, & Kelly, 2007; Gibbons et al., 2006). Neglect and self-neglect are often categorized and grouped with elder abuse (NCEA, 2016). Some definitions include abandonment with neglect and self-neglect with neglect (Department of Job & Family Affairs, 2016). Self-neglect has been described as "the orphan in the spectrum of abuse and neglect" (O'Brien, 2014, p.94). The concept of self-neglect, its ideology, and the way it is viewed can have different layers of meaning and interpretation.

CONCEPTUALIZING SELF-NEGLECT

Multiple conceptualizations of self-neglect exist and have evolved over time. Historically, a concept analysis by Reed and Leonard (1989) reviewed the literature on suicidology and noncompliance and identified 20 terms related to self-neglect, which include: *suicide, self-destruction, noncompliance,* and *indirect life-threatening behaviors*. The antecedents identified are self-care regimen prescribed to prevent physical illness; persons possessing knowledge of self-care regimen, and available cognitive, psychomotor, and material resources (p.46). The defining attributes include that the behavior has to be harmful and without any specific purpose, not intended to end one's life immediately, has cumulative effects over time, and repetitive patterns pervading several dimensions of self-care (Reed & Leonard, 1989).

A concept analysis by Day (2016) identified antecedents to self-neglect as multiple comorbidities, mental health issues, and absence of social networks. The presence of one or more comorbidities can increase the risk for executive dysfunction (Dyer et al., 2007). Executive dysfunction can affect the capacity for self-care and protection and can impede decision making and problem solving for a safe independent life (Hildebrand, Taylor, & Bradway, 2013). The defining attributes of self-neglect are described as environmental neglect and cumulative behaviors and deficits (intentional or unintentional). Environmental neglect is a significant factor when defining self-neglect (Day & McCarthy, 2016; Lauder, Scott, & Whyte, 2001). Cumulative behaviors and deficits can consist of malnourishment, poor hygiene, poor grooming, failure to pay bills, noncompliance with medication, poor health and self-care regimens, withdrawal/poor engagement, fear, aggressive behaviors, misplaced trust, and noncooperation or willingness to accept assistance (Dong, Simon, Beck, & Evans, 2010; Dyer et al., 2006; Iris et al., 2010; Turner et al., 2012).

The concept analysis of self-neglect by Reed and Leonard (1989) predominantly focused on theoretical and conceptual literature on suicidology and noncompliance and spanned from 1970 to 1988. Reed and Leonard (1989) suggested that harmful and life-threatening behaviors may not be intentional and result from emotional or organic mental impairment. They concluded that although self-neglect was clinically apparent, sparse literature existed on self-neglect. The concept analysis of self-neglect by Day (2016) was based on a review of empirical and conceptual self-neglect literature spanning 1989 to 2015, and added to the body of knowledge. Day (2016) concluded that self-neglect can manifest both externally and internally and its defining attributes are environmental neglect and cumulative behaviors and deficits that could be intentional or nonintentional. Day (2016) discussed operationalized measures and dimensions of self-neglect and presented a conceptual definition for elder self-neglect that,

> encompasses environmental neglect and cumulative behaviors and deficits, with potential for serious adverse outcomes that impacts on health, safety and well-being of the person themselves and may extend beyond to the community. (p. 9)

This recent concept analysis of self-neglect adds to the body of knowledge and is an important stage in the theory development.

SELF-NEGLECT THEORY AND FRAMEWORKS

There is no one theory that can explain self-neglect (Paveza, Vandeweerd, & Laumann, 2008). According to Lauder et al. (2001), the concept of self-neglect is socially constructed and is the product of a series of social judgments that are influenced by social, cultural, and professional values. Bozinovski (2000) grounded his theory on the seminal study of people who self-neglect and identified two social psychological processes: preserving and protecting identity; the central theme was explained as maintaining continuity (Bozinovski, 2000). Lauder et al. (2009) support a broader conceptualization of self-neglect. Gibbons (2009) concluded that self-neglect theory consists of two main concepts: self-care agency and deliberate action. Thus self-neglect is more related to readiness and ability of individuals to meet complex contextual health and social care factors than the aging process; and a theoretical framework for self-neglect needs to incorporate medical culture (Gibbons, 2009). Some authors suggest that self-care theory explains only some features of self-neglect (Lauder, 2001; Pavlou & Lach, 2006).

A number of conceptual models and frameworks have been proposed to explain and investigate self-neglect (Day & McCarthy, 2016; Dyer et al., 2007; Iris et al., 2010; Pavez et al., 2008). Dyer et al. (2007) explained an etiological model of elder self-neglect based on more than 500 cases and described it as multiple deficits in physical, social, and medical domains as risk factors for elder self-neglect. Cognitive, nutritional, and mental health deficits are viewed as precipitating factors that lead to ED and impairment in the activities of daily living. These, coupled with inadequate social support networks, put older adults at risk and vulnerable to self-neglect.

Paveza et al. (2008) described a risk vulnerability model that focuses on internal and external risk factors as a framework for the study of self-neglect. This model defines elements of risk and vulnerability that could be used to address preventative as well as intervention strategies.

Iris et al. (2010) used concept mapping and experts in the development of a conceptual elder self-neglect model to aid understanding and conceptualization. The findings identified seven hierarchical clusters/dimensions: physical living conditions (inability to care for self), mental health, financial issues, personal living conditions (lifestyle choice), physical health, social network, and personal endangerment. These capture the physical/psychosocial and environmental influences and take into account a wide array of individual and population-level determinants of health (Iris et al., 2010). The physical living conditions and mental health dimensions were the most distinct constructs in the conceptual framework of self-neglect. The conceptual model supports findings that depressive symptoms and cognitive impairment are significant predictors of self-neglect (Gibbons, 2009; Paveza et al., 2008). The elder self-neglect conceptual model (Iris et al., 2010) offers further insight into the determinants and etiology of self-neglect and predisposing influences.

These various conceptualizations have led to different measures of self-neglect. Iris, Conrad, and Ridings (2014) developed a 25-item ESNA (elder self-neglect assessment) and a 62-item ESNA tool. Results from Rasch analysis identified two broad categories: behavioral characteristics and environmental factors. Day and McCarthy (2016) developed a 37-item self-neglect measurement instrument using exploratory factor analysis (EFA). Results from EFA identified a five-factor structure: environment, social networks, mental and behavioral liability, health avoidance, and self-determinism. Burnett et al. (2014) used latent class analysis and identified four subtypes of elder self-neglect as physical and medical neglect, environmental neglect, global neglect, and financial neglect. Greater self-neglect severity is associated with poorer cognition, mental health issues, and substance abuse.

In summary, there is no one all-encompassing explanatory model of elder self-neglect. Self-neglect is a multifaceted entity and is linked to a range of etiologies (Burnett et al., 2014). The frameworks presented include internal and external risk factors (Paveza et al., 2008), dimensions of self-neglect (Iris et al., 2010), behavioral characteristics, and environmental factors (Iris et al., 2014), factor structure (Day & McCarthy, 2016), and subtypes of self-neglect (Burnett et al., 2014). There is a complex interplay among physical, psychosocial, and environmental risk factors. Health and social care professionals need to understand self-neglect in the context of an individual's life experiences and to consider its trajectory in older adults who are self-neglecting (Band-Winterstein, Doron, & Naim, 2012).

CONCLUSION

Self-neglect is a serious and common public health issue that can present unique challenges for health and social care professionals, especially among the elderly. Self-neglect can present along a continuum of severity and includes a complex array of behavioral and environmental issues. Self-neglect is associated with serious adverse health outcomes, including early mortality, signifying the high importance of addressing self-neglect. There is no standardized and universally accepted definition of self-neglect and conceptual clarity remains elusive. This chapter explores definitions of self-neglect, conceptualizations of self-neglect, and self-neglect theory and frameworks. The nature of self-neglect is that it remains largely hidden and unreported.

IMPLICATIONS FOR RESEARCH AND PRACTICE

- The concept of self-neglect was first identified in the early 1950s.
- Definitions vary and lack of conceptual clarity has impacted research and practice.
- Self-neglect and its associated multifactorial etiology and comorbidities, including depression and functional decline, are associated with serious adverse outcomes.
- Several conceptualizations of self-neglect exist, that focus on behavioral characteristics, environmental factors, dimensions and subtypes, risk factors, and vulnerabilities that can assist in clinical practice and research.

REFERENCES

Band-Winterstein, T., Doron, I., & Naim, S. (2012). Elder self-neglect: A geriatric syndrome or a life course story? *Journal of Aging Studies, 26*(2), 109–118.

Bozinovski, S. (2000). Older self-neglecters: Interpersonal problems and the maintenance of self continuity. *Journal of Elder Abuse & Neglect, 12*(1), 37–56.

Braye, S., Orr, D., & Preston-Shoot, M. (2011). *Self-neglect and adult safeguarding: Findings from research* (SCIE Report No. 46). London, UK: Social Care Institute for Excellence.

Burnett, J., Dyer, C. B., Halphen, J. M., Achenbaum, W. A., Green, C. E., Booker, J. G., & Diamond, P. M. (2014). Four subtypes of self-neglect in older adults: Results of a latent class analysis. *Journal of the American Geriatrics Society, 62*(6), 1127–1132. doi:10.1111/jgs.12832

Clark, A. N., Mankikar, G. D., & Gray, I. (1975). Diogenes syndrome. A clinical study of gross neglect in old age. *Lancet, 1*, 366–368.

Cybulska, E., & Rucinski, J. (1986). Gross self-neglect in old age. *British Journal of Hospital Medicine, 36*, 21–25.

Day, M. R. (2016). Elder self-neglect: A concept analysis. In J. J. Fitzpatrick & G. McCarthy (Eds.), *Nursing concept analysis: Applications to research and practice*. New York, NY: Springer Publishing.

Day, M. R., & McCarthy, G. (2016). Self-neglect: Development and evaluation of a self-neglect (SN-37) measurement instrument. *Archives of Psychiatric Nursing, 30*(4), 480–485. doi: 10.1016/j .apnu.2016.02.004

Department of Health. (2012). *Discussion paper on hoarding and squalor.* Melbourne, Victoria, Australia: Ageing and Aged Care Branch, Victorian Government.

Department of Job and Family Services. (2016). Fact sheet Ohio. Retrieved from http://jfs.ohio.gov/ factsheets/APS_FactSheet.pdf

Dong, X., Simon, M., Beck, T., & Evans, D. (2010). A cross-sectional population based study of elder self-neglect and psychological, health, and social factors in a biracial community. *Aging and Mental Health, 14*(1), 74–84.

Dyer, C. B., Goodwin, J. S., Pickens-Pace, S., Burnett, J., & Kelly, P. A. (2007). Self-neglect among the elderly: A model based on more than 500 patients seen by a geriatric medicine team. *American Journal of Public Health, 97,* 1671–1676.

Dyer, C. B., Kelly, P. A., Pavlik, V. N., Lee, J., Doody, R. S., Regev, T., . . . Smith, S. M. (2006). The making of the Self-Neglect Severity Scale. *Journal of Elder Abuse & Neglect, 18*(4), 13–24.

Elder Justice Act. (2010). Patient Protection and Affordable Care Act. Public Law 111-148. Washington, DC: United States Government.

Gibbons, S. (2009). Theory synthesis for self-neglect: A health and social phenomenon. *Nursing Research, 58*(3), 194–200.

Gibbons, S., Lauder, W., & Ludwick, R. (2006). Self-neglect: A proposed new NANDA diagnosis. *International Journal of Nursing Terminologies and Classifications, 17,* 10–18. doi:10.1111/j.1744-618X.2006.00018.x

Halliday, G., Banerjee, S., Philpot, M., & MacDonald, A. (2000). Community study of people who live in squalor. *Lancet, 355,* 882–886.

Iris, M., Conrad, K. J., & Ridings, J. (2014). Observational measure of elder self-neglect, *Journal of Elder Abuse & Neglect, 26*(4), 365–397. doi:10.1080/08946566.2013.801818

Iris, M., Ridings, J. W., & Conrad, K. J. (2010). The development of a conceptual model for understanding elder self-neglect. *The Gerontologist, 50*(3), 303–315.

Lauder, W. (2001). The utility of self-care theory as a theoretical basis for self-neglect. *Journal of Advanced Nursing, 34*(4), 545–551.

Lauder, W., Roxburgh, M., Harris, J., & Law, J. (2009). Developing self-neglect theory: Analysis of related and atypical cases of people identified as self-neglecting. *Journal of Psychiatric and Mental Health Nursing, 16*(5), 447–454.

Lauder, W., Scott, P. A., & Whyte, A. (2001). Nurses' judgments of self-neglect: A factorial survey. *International Journal of Nursing Studies, 38*(5), 601–608. doi:10.1016/S0020-7489(00)00108-5

McMillan, D., & Shaw, P. (1966). Senile breakdown in standards of personal and environmental cleanliness. *British Medical Journal, 2*(5521), 1032–1037.

National Center on Elder Abuse. (2016). Definitions of elder abuse. Retrieved from https://ncea.acl .gov/faq/index.html#faq1 with the title changing to "What is elder abuse?"

O'Brien, J. (2014). Elder abuse and neglect: A role for physicians. In *Elder abuse and its prevention: Workshop Summary.* Washington, DC: National Academy of Sciences.

Paveza, G., Vandeweerd, C., & Laumann, E. (2008). Elder self-neglect: A discussion of a social typology. *Journal of the American Geriatrics Society, 56,* S271–S275. doi:10.1111/j.1532-5415.2008.01980.x

Post, F. (1982). Functional disorders. In R. Levy & F. Post (Eds.). *The psychiatry of late life* (pp. 180–181). Oxford, UK: Blackwell Scientific Publications.

Reed, P. G., & Leonard, V. E. (1989).An analysis of the concept of self-neglect. *Advances in Nursing Science, 12*(1), 39–53.

Reyes-Ortiz, C. A., Burnett, J., Flores, D. V., Halphen, J. M., & Dyer, C. B. (2014). Medical implications of elder abuse: Self-neglect. *Clinics in Geriatric Medicine, 30*(4), 807–823. doi:10.1016/j.cger.2014.08.008

Snowdon, J., Halliday, G., & Banerjee, S. (Eds.). (2012). *Severe domestic squalor.* Cambridge, UK: Cambridge University Press.

Teaster, P. B., Dugar, T., Mendiondo, M., Abner, E. L., Cecil, K. A., & Otto, J. M. (2006). *The 2004 survey of adult protective services: Abuse of adults 60 years of age and older.* Washington, DC: National Center on Elder Abuse. Retrieved from http://www.napsa-now.org/wp-content/uploads/2012/09/2-14-06 -FINAL-60+REPORT.pdf

ISSUES CONCERNING THE SELF-NEGLECTING INDIVIDUAL

CHAPTER 3

MENTAL HEALTH ISSUES AND SELF-NEGLECT

Barbara Cohen

Self-neglect is a concept that can be utilized to describe patterns of behavior across the life span of an individual. Definitions of self-neglect include exhibiting behaviors, such as poor personal hygiene, living in squalor, social withdrawal, hoarding of goods, relapse into serious mental states endangering health and well-being, and/or failing to take actions to avoid loss of housing or services such as electricity or heat. Careful assessment of increasing patterns of self-neglect can prompt caregivers and health care professionals to take steps to protect the well-being of those in need of care and support. Use of community resources and professional organizing services, such as specialists in hoarding and prompt psychiatric assistance, including supportive therapy, nutritional supplements, medication support, and hospitalization as needed, may assist individuals and their families avoid permanent consequences of self-neglect.

Self-neglect is frequently a hallmark of the onset of mental illness in individuals, regardless of the age of onset. This chapter explores the impact of mental illness on self-neglect and the interplay between mental health and the development of self-neglect. Care for those with acute or chronic mental illness so as to avoid the consequences of self-neglect is addressed. Boundary issues involving balancing patient autonomy and clients' safety needs are highlighted. Legal protections available to individuals existing in situations created by self-neglect are discussed. Case studies regarding inconsistencies in judgments (judicial, public, or professional) also are included.

Self-neglect has been defined as the failure of an individual to provide self-care. This failure can arise out of denial or avoidance of expected "normal" social controls and limits on personal behavior (Gunstone, 2003) and can include:

> The development of serious physical disability or illness, as a result of neglect; a relapse into a serious mental state that would endanger general health and well-being, clearly identified as caused by neglect of self and/or treatment; and the development of a serious environmental health problems that may endanger the individual, careers or other visitors. (Morgan, 1998, p. 281)

Day (2010) has defined self-neglect in many older people as the inability or unwillingness to provide themselves goods or services to meet their basic needs. Self-neglect behavior can include a lack of personal hygiene, wearing soiled clothing, and using soiled bedding. The person may live in squalor in a disheveled home environment containing uneaten food, animal excrement, and/or vermin. Individuals may appear apathetic, unconcerned about their living circumstances, and may also exhibit social withdrawal and maintain no personal contacts. Possessions may be hoarded, bringing individuals to the attention of neighbors, the community, or the local authorities. Paranoid or suspicious behaviors can be seen in relation to personal or community welfare (Day, Leahy-Warren, & McCarthy, 2016; Hettiaratchy & Manthorpe, 1989).

Self-neglect can involve the refusal of a person to obtain adequate basic needs required to sustain life such as food, water, clothing, shelter, and medication. Self-neglect may also involve the failure to pay bills, resulting in significant risks to the individual or loss of services such as electricity, heat, or even the loss of a person's residence.

Mental illness can signal its arrival in many ways. One of the consistent hallmarks across the spectrum of mental illness is that of self-neglect. Self-neglecting behaviors, together with the symptoms of mental illness, require urgent referral for care (Deakin & Lennox, 2013; World Health Organization [WHO], 2016). Schizophrenia, dementia, alcohol or substance abuse, or psychosis are frequently diagnosed antecendents to self-neglect, particularly in older clients (Day, Leahy-Warren, & McCarthy, 2013; Reyes-Ortiz, Burnett, Flores, Halphen, & Dyer, 2014). Nurses and other health professionals providing care for individuals who have received a diagnosis of mental illness may view an increase in self-neglect as an urgent sign to increase the support and services in an effort to avoid further decline and ultimate hospitalization. Self-neglect frequently signals the onset or relapse of mental illness. Self-neglect is present in a variety of psychotic disorders. Deakin and Lennox (2013) describe symptoms of self-neglect as possibly heralding the onset or exacerbation of schizophrenia, schizo-affective disorder, drug-induced psychosis, personality disorders, and epilepsy disorders. It is an urgent signal for the cargiver and health care provider, heralding possible declines in mental health and increasing the need for heightened observation and a possible change in the care plan.

Self-neglect has been identified as a cause of Wernicke–Korsakoff syndrome resulting in significant malnutrition (Cocksedge & Flynn, 2014). Self-neglect arising out of mental illness also results in delayed diagnoses of breast and cervical cancer (Aggarwal, Pandurangi, & Smith, 2013) due to clients' failure to participate in preventative health care screening and subsequent treatment.

In caring for those with intermittent or ongoing self-neglect issues in the community, it is necessary for health and social care professionals to be alert to initial warning signs such as sudden weight loss, sleeplessness, and inattention to personal hygiene. As issues of self-neglect become more severe, clients become more endangered by eating spoiled food, failing to pay bills resulting in the termination of heat or electricity, or hoarding and building up clutter leading to unsafe environments. It is suggested that practitioners address smaller consistent declines with the client or, if that is not possible, with the designated caregiver or with the authorized decision maker.

Homelessness or a history of homelessness in combination with mental illness can contribute to self-neglect given the self-care challenges facing those without a permanent residence, address, or method of contact. Formerly homeless individuals may continue to self-neglect even when placed in supportive living environments. Common supportive-living-environment issues for those who self-neglect include hoarding of possessions, such as clothing and food, all of which contribute to squalor and infestations of cockroaches, flies, bedbugs, and other vermin. Additional challenges remain in the areas of self-grooming.

Community health workers and community health nurses are in the unique position of visiting these individuals in their home environment (Anthony, 2015; Day et al., 2016). Situations of self-neglect in communal living environments can create hazards for other residents living in the same or nearby residences. Those working in mental health facilities, supportive environments, naturally occurring retirement communities (NORCs), and assisted living environments may not always have the expertise to manage situations of extreme self-neglect (Bratiotis, 2013; Braye, Orr, & Preston-Shoot, 2013; Johnson, 2015). Appropriate managerial support and supervision are required (Braye, Orr, & Preston-Shoot, 2015), as is additional training (Day & McCarthy, 2015).

RESPONSES TO MENTAL ILLNESS

An issue concerning mental illness associated with self-neglect is whether the person has the capacity to make decisions or is in need of involuntary commitment to a mental health facility (Lauder, Ludwick, Zeller, & Winchell, 2006). Before making a decision, one must consider other services and options in an attempt to avoid involuntary commitment. Nurses may make a referral to a community health nurse or to acute mental health services. In addition, client education, referral for house cleaning services, Meals on Wheels, and medication review and re-evaluation may be solicited (Lauder et al., 2006). Furthermore, a client's competence must be assessed.

The finding of incompetence or reduced capacity often indicates that the client is a danger to herself or himself or others (Involuntary Admission on Medical Certification, 2015). The decision making that flows from the determination of incompetence gives rise to restriction or removal of individual liberty. This is not always in the best interests of the client. An older person with mental health issues may have his or her health care decisions delegated to others. One cannot predict the outcome of current involuntary commitment cases based upon review of prior decisions. Obvious harmful risk factors, such as lack of safe housing, must be weighed against less socially acceptable client behaviors that do not carry direct risk of harm. Evaluation and assessment needs to address life history and story, client's capacity and support networks, occurrence, immanency, frequency of self-neglecting behavior, severity and consequences of behavior, and life history (MacLeod & Stadnyk, 2015). Legal cases addressing involuntary commitment do not guarantee a good outcome for the client.

Legal cases concerning involuntary commitment of homeless individuals who appear disheveled, paranoid, and/or beg for money reveal disputes even among legal authorities as to what constitutes self-neglect (White, 2014, pp. 134–135). Court hearings may subject older individuals to involuntary commitment (resulting in the ultimate reduction in liberty) utilizing the testimony of generalists and family members rather than that of the gerontologists who are in a better position to provide expert opinions with respect to their clients' state of mind and capabilities (Dus, 2016). Civil involuntary commitment leads to significant curtailment of individual liberty. To warrant involuntary commitment requires the highest standard of clear and convincing evidence of potential harm to the self and others, coupled with the presence of mental illness. For example, the United States Supreme Court in *Addington v. Texas* (1979) held that "clear and convincing proof" is required by the Fourteenth Amendment of the U.S. Constitution to involuntarily commit an individual to a mental hospital in a proceeding brought under state law. Chief Justice Burger, writing for the Court in *Addington v. Texas* (*supra*, at 425–428, 431), sets forth, in pertinent part, the reasoning by which that court arrived at the "clear and convincing" standard:

> This Court repeatedly has recognized that civil commitment for any purpose constitutes a significant deprivation of liberty that requires due process

protection. . . . Moreover, it is indisputable that involuntary commitment to a mental hospital after a finding of probable dangerousness to self or others can engender adverse social consequences to the individual. . . . The state has a legitimate interest under its *parens patriae* powers in providing care to its citizens who are unable because of emotional disorders to care for themselves; [and] the state also has authority under its police power to protect the community from the dangerous tendencies of some who are mentally ill. . . . Loss of liberty calls for a showing that the individual suffers from something more serious than is demonstrated by idiosyncratic behavior.

The preceding response illustrated the powers of the state in providing for citizens and the balancing of this against the definition of liberty and the requirement for indisputable evidence. The individual's liberty interest in the outcome of a civil commitment proceeding is of such weight and gravity compared with the state's interests in providing care to its citizens who are unable, because of emotional disorders to care for themselves and in protecting the community from the dangerous tendencies of some who are mentally ill, that due process requires the state to justify confinement by proof more substantial than a mere preponderance of the evidence (*Addington* v. Texas, 1979, p. 441).

From this imperative created by the Supreme Court of the United States, the highest law of the land, it is clear that individuals may be committed only in the presence of clear and convincing evidence. Individuals may not be deprived of life's liberty merely upon presentation of evidence demonstrating self-neglect or harm to self or others.

However, as explained in the following, the judiciary does not always agree on the criteria of what constitutes clear and convincing evidence of the ability of an individual to self-care. This difficulty in effectively and consistently coming to a conclusion about self-neglect in an older adult and the dangers to those living in the community due to individual discretion by an evaluator may inadvertently result in impingement upon an older adult's liberty. Case Study 1, profiling the circumstances of Gregory M (2012), is explanatory.

CASE STUDY 1: MR. GREGORY M

Gregory M, a 51-year-old diagnosed with mild to moderate dementia, had a history of head injuries as a result of alcohol-related accidents. This ultimately resulted in Gregory being committed to a 24-hour supervised residence facility in an effort to control his substance abuse and provide him with custodial care. The formerly homeless Gregory was residing in a motel and was independent with most activities of daily living. He came to the attention of the authorities when attempting to dry tobacco in a microwave, causing a fire. Despite the lack of specific testimony on the part of the state's expert that Gregory was totally incapable of caring for himself, or that he posed an imminent danger to himself and/or others, the court decided to affirm the lower court's decision to place Gregory in a supervised residential facility to minimize alcohol-consumption relapse and avoid possible physical personal injury. Despite the fact that the state's expert had no knowledge of recent alcohol abuse by the patient, the court held that there need not be recent acts or omissions to demonstrate incompetence (In the Matter of the Guardianship and Protective Placement of Gregory M, 2012).

To deprive a person of liberty based on the concern that he or she may, at some time in the future, become a danger to himself or herself or others, when less restrictive means are available, is not in the person's best interests. On the other hand, incompetence proceedings and confinement for supervised treatment and decision making can be most appropriate in certain circumstances, as portrayed in Case Study 2.

CASE STUDY 2: MR. USAMAH AL BANA

Mr. Usamah Al Bana, a homeless, wheelchair-dependent individual with a history of multiple strokes, dysarthria, hypertension, Crohn's disease, hyperlipidemia, asthma, chronic anemia, and psychotic disorder not otherwise specified, was compelled at age 69 to accept a guardian to manage his decision making because of mental impairment resulting from his various physical and mental ailments. He had repeatedly discharged himself against medical advice, threatened health care workers and patients, cursed at other patients, and threatened to break Plexiglas with a fire extinguisher and to make a weapon out of it. The probate court investigator reported that Mr. Al Bana had several indications of self-neglect, he was noncompliant with his medical plans, had no family, and was incapable of attending to his activities of daily living. A social worker testified that Mr. Al Bana had lost his apartment after sharing it with a 21-year-old woman who withdrew all of the funds from his bank account (In the Matter of the Guardianship of Usamah Al Bana, 2014).

Case Studies 1 and 2, Gregory M (2012) and Usamah Al Bana (2014), are reflections of two possible results along the spectrum of judicial decision making with respect to individuals alleged to have issues of self-neglect. In Gregory M's case, the court restricted his liberty despite the absence of any evidence of current impairment or immediate danger, and in the face of expert testimony supporting Gregory's continued living on his own with supportive home services, on the likelihood that he might relapse and injure himself. In the case of Usamah Al Bana (2014), it is more clear-cut that the individual in question warranted the appointment of a guardian to oversee his decision making and facilitate his care. Compelling residential treatment services for individuals who are a danger to themselves or others is a rational solution. Compelling residential treatment services for individuals who are capable of self-maintenance with adequate supportive living services may negatively impact health care and financing of care costs for the society's most vulnerable individuals.

Older adults suffering from dementia, Alzheimer's disease, depression, and other mental illness may have the option of receiving appropriate home-based services, including supervised pharmacology, having issues managed in the least restrictive environment. At times, well-meaning individuals, such as the motel owners of Gregory's motel room for homeless individuals, report perceived instances of self-neglect with the end result of increased governmental surveillance and involvement. In the United States, nurses, as mandated reporters concerned about older adults in the community, report cases of self-neglect to adult protective services (APS). Social workers or other APS professionals generally make unannounced visits to the person's home in response to a report of self-neglect.

The timing of visits by APS is such that the visiting professional may find no evidence of self-neglect. On the other hand, there may be circumstances present, such as a recent illness or loss, in which the older adult may be judged to be lacking in self-care skills. In Case Study 3, an 82-year-old former registered nurse called the police station to report an altercation with a neighbor. She was then visited after police officers reported concerns to APS. The report to APS was made by the police officer without any other independent corroboration of "self-neglect."

CASE STUDY 3: Retired Nurse

An 82-year-old retired nurse lives in a private suburban home with several pets, including a large dog. She has lived in this home for more than 50 years. A dispute developed between the woman and the neighbors concerning property boundaries, snow removal, trash disposal, and barking pets. Disagreements escalated, and adult protective services (APS) was called by the local police. The APS social worker arrived unannounced to find an appropriately dressed woman, a clean house, well-cared-for pets, a full refrigerator, a working car, and a checkbook reflecting appropriate financial acumen. No finding of self-neglect was issued.

Had the social worker come a few weeks later following the protracted illness and sudden death of the retired nurse's beloved dog, the situation would have been different. The woman was in a deep depression, the house neglected, the refrigerator nearly empty, and she was less well groomed. The social worker might have come to an incorrect conclusion of self-neglect rather than a temporary inability to care for oneself as symptomatic of a loss. The initial concern of the police and/or neighbors and the fact-finding by the social worker exemplify the notion that professional judgments may vary depending on the timing and the judgment of the professionals (Lauder, Davidson, Anderson, & Barclay, 2005).

Independent individuals who self-neglect, and who are the most reluctant to accept professional assistance, can find themselves involved with APS. Individuals reported to APS, as well as homeless individuals called to the attention of emergency services, are at increased risk of loss of the right of self-determination, liberty, and autonomy—all under the rubric of beneficence. Consistency in judgment may be difficult to achieve (Lauder, Scott, & Whyte, 2001). In some instances, what appears as self-neglect may be related to the lack of financial means to correct a situation, such as performing home repairs. A lack of adequate food may be associated with lack of adequate public transportation or an inability to maintain a car, car repairs, and payments for gas and car insurance in more suburban or rural areas (MacLeod & Douthit, 2015). Careful consideration of the totality of the circumstances is essential so that appropriate accommodations are made and nurse–patient boundaries are respectfully maintained.

Hoarding as a mental health issue can present additional risks to health, safety, and secure housing. Individuals affected by mental illness living in government-supported housing run a great risk of loss of housing in the face of chronic hoarding, vermin, bedbugs, mice, excessive numbers of pets, or animal waste, all of which are not permitted in general by maintenance rules for public housing. Supportive living environments provide services for clients who come into the housing situation already challenged by homelessness and by one or more manifestations of mental illness. It is common for supportive living environments or NORCs to provide social work services to assist clients in reducing clutter and other hazardous hoarding behaviors. Challenges can range from feces smearing by the mentally ill tenant in his or her room to challenges such as animal hoarding.

Animal hoarding has its own parameters and can ultimately lead to situations of self-neglect. Animal hoarding produces squalor and unsanitary and unsafe conditions for the involved individual (see Chapter 6; Day & McCarthy, 2016). The hoarder may have limited insight into the dire straits of the situation (Frost, Patronek, & Rosenfield, 2011). [The author has served as a community mental health nurse in a team environment providing services to tenants with a history of mental illness living in federally subsidized housing. This experience was the backdrop for Case Study 4, described next.]

The nurse caring for this client had been licensed for 5 years, and was in her first community mental health position. This complex situation was beyond her skill level at that time. In retrospect, a more proactive, earlier team approach involving intra-agency cooperation among hotel management, the local humane society, visits by the team psychiatrist, and regular work with a hoarding specialist might have managed the situation with less trauma to the client (Lauder, Anderson, & Barclay, 2005; Lauder et al.,2005).

One way to manage issues is to represent clients' interests at the government-housing level by involving individuals' families and by organizing support (Koenig, Leiste, Spano, & Chapin, 2013; demonstrated in the case reported by Raeburn, Hungerford, Escott, & Cleary, 2015). In this single case study, the mental health nurse practitioner supported clinical treatment, provided care coordination, and advocated with the client to ensure an improved outcome. The client had long-term problems with mood and behavior that resulted in his move into public housing. As the relationship between the nurse practitioner and the patient continued, she came to the conclusion that as the patient's mood swung, so did his ability to maintain a clean and organized environment. In addition to the arrangement of multiple services such as respite and cleaning services, the mental health nurse practitioner also wrote letters on the tenant's behalf to the local housing authorities explaining the patient's condition and advocating for his rights as a person suffering from a variety of mental health challenges. Active advocacy, clearly explaining the hoarding and other situations that are socially unacceptable in communal living environments, avoided adding homelessness to the patient's other long-standing challenges. Nurses must familiarize themselves with eviction proceedings and evidence required to defend vulnerable clients against a loss of public housing. Mental health nurses must become familiar with rules and regulations governing public housing and behaviors in public housing related to potential evictions. Nurses working in the public sector must have a list of legal aid organizations available to assist clients prior to the finality and urgency of an eviction notice.

CASE STUDY 4: Mrs. Mary H

Mary H, a tenant in a single-room occupancy hotel, collected 20 or so cats and lived with them in a one-room apartment (bathroom down the hallway). She permitted the cats to defecate on the roof space abutting her apartment by opening the window and letting them in and out. The roof was covered in cat feces. The apartment was covered in fleas and other flying insects attracted by the feces on the adjoining roof. The apartment smelled strongly of cat urine. The tenant, a client of the community health psychiatric outreach team, was using her public assistance allowance to feed the cats rather than buying food herself. All efforts to decrease the cat population were to no avail. The tenant became severely anxious and depressed every time suggestions aimed at improving the manageability of the situation were made, even in the face of deadlines to take action imposed by the landlord. She was unable to part with even one cat and stated, "they are my children." Ultimately, in the face of zero progress in remedying the situation, the landlord waited until Mary went out for a few hours, called animal rescue, and all but two of the cats were removed. The roof was cleaned and the tenant threatened with eviction should the situation re-occur.

Public housing placement is not easily achieved for those with mental illness. Although public housing is funded, the supply of available apartments is limited and even increased funding cannot cover the costs of all those eligible to receive public housing or subsidized housing vouchers. Eviction proceedings from public housing fail to meet the mandates of several federal programs such as the Americans with Disabilities Act (1990, amended 2009) and the Fair Housing Amendments Act of 1988 (Carter, 2010). Individuals with severe, persistent mental illness face eviction frequently due to self-neglectful behaviors that constitute the symptomatology of their illness without any regard for the consequences of the loss of housing (Carter, 2010). Those consequences can involve homelessness or institutionalization. Evictions of mentally ill, impoverished individuals destroy the stability needed for successful integration and fail to take into account the great difficulty that exists for those with persistent mental illness in obtaining housing at the outset (Carter, 2010).Eviction leading to loss of federal subsidies for housing can exacerbate an individual's symptomatology while increasing his or her odds of prolonged periods of homelessness (Carter, 2010). These circumstances arise when situations of self-neglect are ignored until they become out of control and affect more than just the one tenant with overwhelming smells, bug infestations, or potential fire hazards. Institutionalization is not always an easy or preferred solution as institutionalization may violate patients' rights to live in the least restrictive environment. Hoarders deserve the protection of the Fair Housing Amendments Act (Jahan, 2015; Ronan, 2011) and it is incumbent upon caregivers to provide a prompt referral to legal assistance to maximize the likelihood of protection of individuals' rights.

CONCLUSION

Mental illnesses, such as schizophrenia, dementia, alcohol, and/or substance abuse or psychosis, can lead to the development or exacerbation of self-neglect behaviors like inadequate attention to nutrition and hygiene, excessive collection of possessions, or hoarding of animals. Evidence of self-neglect provides a window into the mental health or illness status of individuals living in the community. Prompt recognition of the seriousness of this pattern of behavior requires prompt intervention to avoid further deterioration in the client's environment, health, and safety. Although there are many external agencies, such as the APS and the judiciary, for declarations of incompetence and possible hospitalization or commitment, these options also have inherent within them the significant curtailment of clients' liberty and autonomy. Practitioners must incorporate specialists both legal and behavioral to provide clients suffering from self-neglect with the broadest opportunities for management and recovery with an eye toward minimizing restriction of clients' rights to self-determination.

IMPLICATIONS FOR RESEARCH AND PRACTICE

Self-neglect is a hallmark of mental illness. When dealing with individuals suffering from self-neglect:
- Use an objective tool to measure the parameters of the situation.
- Involve experts in the field, especially when making judgments about competence.
- Institutionalization constitutes a significant deprivation of liberty.
- Advocate with appropriate authorities to safeguard clients' subsidized housing.
- Involve legal services organizations to obtain protections offered to those individuals managing life with disabilities.

REFERENCES

Addington v. Texas, 441 U.S. 418 (1979).

Aggarwal, A., Pandurangi, A., & Smith, W. (2013). Disparities in breast and cervical cancer screening in women with mental illness: A systematic literature review. *American Journal of Preventive Medicine*, *44*(4), 392–398.

Anthony, M. (2015). Welcome to home healthcare now! *Home Healthcare Now*, *33*(1), 5–6.

Bratiotis, C. (2013). Community hoarding task forces: A comparative case study of five task forces in the United States. *Health & Social Care in the Community*, *21*(3), 245–253.

Braye, S., Orr, D., & Preston-Shoot, M. (2013). *A scoping study of workforce development for self-neglect work*. Leeds, UK: Skills for Care.

Braye, S., Orr, D., & Preston-Shoot, M. (2015). Learning lessons about self-neglect? An analysis of serious case reviews. *Journal of Adult Protection*, *17*(1), 3–18.

Carter, M. P. (2010). How evictions from subsidized housing routinely violate the rights of persons with mental illness. *Northwestern Journal of Law and Social Policy*, *5*, 118–148.

Cocksedge, K. A., & Flynn, A. (2014). Wernicke–Korsakoff syndrome in a patient with self-neglect associated with severe depression. *Journal of the Royal Society of Medicine Open*, *5*(2), 1–3. doi:10.1177/2042533313518915

Day, M. R. (2010). Self-neglect: A challenge and a dilemma. *Archives of Psychiatric Nursing*, *24*(2), 73–75.

Day, M. R., Leahy-Warren, P., & McCarthy, G. (2013). Perceptions and views of self-neglect: A client-centered perspective. *Journal of Elder Abuse & Neglect*, *25*(1), 76–94.

Day, M. R., Leahy-Warren, P., & McCarthy, G. (2016). Self-neglect: Ethical considerations. *Annual Review of Nursing Research*, *34*(1), 89–107.

Day, M. R., & McCarthy, G. (2015).A national cross-sectional study of community nurses and social workers knowledge of self-neglect. *Age and Ageing*, *44*(4), 717–720. doi:10.1093/ageing/afv025

Day, M. R., & McCarthy, G. (2016). Animal hoarding: A serious public health issue. *Annuals of Nursing and Practice*, *3*(4), 1054. Retrieved from http://www.jscimedcentral.com/Nursing/nursing-3-1054.pdf

Deakin, J., & Lennox, B. (2013). Psychotic symptoms in young people warrant urgent referral. *Practitioner*, *257*(1759), 25–28, 3.

Dus, A. (2016). "But I'm not dangerous Judge, I promise!" Evaluating the implications of involuntary civil commitment criteria and outpatient treatment methods on the elderly. *Elder Law Journal*, *23*, 453.

Frost, R. O., Patronek, G., & Rosenfield, E. (2011).A comparison of object and animal hoarding. *Depression and Anxiety*, *28*(10), 885–891. doi:10.1002/da.20826

Gunstone, S. (2003). Risk assessment and management of patients with self-neglect: A 'grey area' for mental health workers. *Journal of Psychiatric and Mental Health Nursing*, *10*(3), 287–296.

Hettiaratchy, P., & Manthorpe, J. (1989). The 'hidden' nature of self-neglect. *Care of the Elderly*, *1*(1), 14–15.

In the Matter of the Guardianship and Protective Placement of Gregory M.: Outagamie County Department of Health and Human Services, Petitioner-Respondent v. Gregory M., Respondent-Appellant. COURT OF APPEALS OF WISCONSIN, DISTRICT THREE 2012 WI App 27; 339 Wis. 2d 492; 809 N.W.2d 901; 2012Wisc. App. LEXIS 82 January 31, 2012, Decided January 31, 2012, Filed.

In the Matter of the Guardianship of Usamah Al Bana, Court Of Appeals of Ohio, Ninth Appellate District, Summit County 2014-Ohio-5783; 2014 Ohio App. LEXIS 5595 December 31, 2014, Decided.

Involuntary Admission on Medical Certification. (2015). New York Mental Hygiene Law, Chapter 27, Title B, Article 9, §9.27.

Jahan, M. (2015). *A policy to protect hoarders: An analysis of Fair Housing Amendments Act, 1988*. Long Beach: California State University.

Johnson, Y. O. C. (2015). Elder self-neglect: Education is needed. *Home Healthcare Now, 33*(8), 421–424.

Koenig, T. L., Leiste, M. R., Spano, R., & Chapin, R. K. (2013). Multidisciplinary team perspectives on older adult hoarding and mental illness. *Journal of Elder Abuse & Neglect, 25*(1), 56–75.

Lauder, W., Anderson, I., & Barclay, A. (2005). A framework for good practice in interagency interventions with cases of self-neglect. *Journal of Psychiatric and Mental Health Nursing, 12*(2), 192–198.

Lauder, W., Davidson, G., Anderson, I., & Barclay, A. (2005). Self-neglect: The role of judgments and applied ethics. *Nursing Standard, 19*(18), 45–51.

Lauder, W., Ludwick, R., Zeller, R., & Winchell, J. (2006). Factors influencing nurses' judgments about self-neglect cases. *Journal of Psychiatric & Mental Health Nursing, 3*, 279–287.

Lauder, W., Scott, P. A., & Whyte, A. (2001). Nurses' judgments of self-neglect: A factorial survey. *International Journal of Nursing Studies, 38*(5), 601–608.

MacLeod, M. Z. K., & Douthit, K. Z. (2015). Etiology and management of elder self-neglect. *Adultspan Journal, 14*(1), 11–23. doi:10.1002/j.2161-0029.2015.00033.x

Morgan, S. (1998). The assessment and management of risk. In C. Brooker & J. Repper (Eds.), *Serious mental health problems in the community: Policy, practice and research* (pp. 263–290). London, UK: Bailliere Tindall.

Raeburn, T., Hungerford, C., Escott, P., & Cleary, M. (2015). Supporting recovery from hoarding and squalor: Insights from a community case study. *Journal of Psychiatric and Mental Health Nursing, 22*(8), 634–639.

Reyes-Ortiz, C. A., Burnett, J., Flores, D. V., Halphen, J. M., & Dyer, C. B. (2014). Medical implications of elder abuse: Self-neglect. *Clinics in Geriatric Medicine, 30*(4), 807–823.

Ronan, K. P. (2011). Navigating the goat paths: Compulsive hoarding, or Collyer Brothers syndrome, and the legal reality of clutter. *Rutgers Law Review, 64*, 235.

White, W. (2014). elder self-neglect and adult protective services: Ohio needs to do more. *Journal of Law and Health, 27*, 130–163.

World Health Organization. (2016). *Schizophrenia fact sheet*. WHO Media Centre. Retrieved from http://www.who.int/mediacentre/factsheets/fs397/en

CHAPTER 4

DELIRIUM AND SELF-NEGLECT

Graham J. McDougall and Marietta P. Stanton

Self-neglect includes a multifactorial etiology and is independently associated with increased mortality. Cognitive impairment and depression are high risk factors for the development of self-neglect. The diagnosis and treatment of self-neglect must be recognized as a pathological condition, which often manifests as confusion and dehydration. Common behaviors of self-neglect, often labeled as eccentric, include the hoarding of objects, newspapers/magazines, mail/paperwork, and/or animals to the extent that the safety of the individual (and/or other household or community members) is threatened or compromised. Delirium, a syndrome affecting the brain, develops from a variety of causes and often leads to a change in consciousness. Self-neglect and delirium are associated and this combination may lead to deleterious outcomes. This chapter focuses on delirium and self-neglect and its relationship with impaired cognitive function.

Good health, both physical and mental, independence in terms of activities of daily living, living in a safe environment, and good social support are important factors for our older adult population. Self-care, physical function, and the ability to live safely and independently at home can deteriorate rapidly for older adults. Delirium from a variety of causes can produce a change in consciousness that compromises the older adults' health, safety, self-care management, and decision making and may lead to self-neglect. According to Mayo Clinical Staff (2015), delirium produces an acute change in consciousness that produces inattention to important details as well as other cognitive and perceptual changes. A summary of symptoms the *Diagnostic and Statistical Manual of Mental Disorders* (5th ed.; *DSM-5*; American Psychiatric Association, 2013) criteria used to define *delirium* include disturbance in attention cognitive changes that develops over a short interval, evidence that the disturbance is secondary to another medical problem, substance intoxication or withdrawal from drugs or alcohol, reduced awareness of the environment, restlessness, hallucinations, and emotional disturbances.

Since February 1990, when the congressional resolution declaring the 1990s the Decade of the Brain was signed into law, the field of neuroscience has grown exponentially and scientists across multiple disciplines have produced studies linking brain function and behavior (Jones & Mendell, 1999). The orbitofrontal cortex (OFC) plays a crucial role in behavior and is a common site for damage resulting from different types of injuries; for example, closed head injuries, cerebrovascular accidents, tumors, and neurosurgical interventions (Jonker, Jonker, Scheltens, & Scherder, 2015). The OFC is a prefrontal cortex region in the frontal lobes of the brain, which is involved in the cognitive processing of decision making (Cavada & Schultz, 2000). The evidence suggests that the OFC is involved in social adjustment and the control of mood, drive, and responsibility. According to Cavada and Schultz (2000), the OFC has links with widespread brain structures and is critically involved in both complex primate behavior as well as human mental and neurological diseases. A review of the research on the OFC region linked the performance of neuropsychological tests to behavior. The results suggest that in patients with OFC lesions, reversal learning is more associated with behavioral disinhibition, and that impairment in recognition of expressed emotion is more associated with socially inappropriate behavior (Tierney, Snow, Charles, Moineddin, & Kiss, 2007). The aims of this chapter are to (a) describe the signs and symptoms of delirium and self-neglect, (b) synthesize the literature on self-neglect and its relationship to impaired cognitive function, and (c) recommend future studies in self-neglect and its relationship with delirium.

BACKGROUND LITERATURE

Delirium is a pervasive problem in the elderly. The prevalence rate of delirium in older adults with dementia ranges from 22% in the community to 89% in the hospitals (Fick, Agostini, & Inouye, 2002). Delirium in patients with dementia is frequently unrecognized due to overlapping symptoms and lack of knowledge of the older adult's baseline mental status, and the tendency to attribute symptoms of delirium to a worsening of dementia symptoms (Fick & Mion, 2008). About 10% to 31% of patients admitted to the hospital have delirium and 14% to 42% of older adults develop delirium as an inpatient (Miller, Govindan, Watson, Hyzy, & Iwashyna, 2015). The onset of delirium may be precipitated by medications, anesthetics, dehydration, alcohol misuse, pain, sensory impairment, chemical imbalances, vitamin deficiencies, and infections (Inouye, 1999).

Osse et al. (2012) reported the incidence of delirium to be 31.3% for 125 adults greater than 70 years of age following cardiac surgery. In addition, preoperative neopterin levels that are too high, poor cognitive function, as well as high cardiosurgical risks were found to be associated with delirium. Postoperative neopterin and homovanillic acid (HVA) levels were also found to be associated with delirium, together with preoperative cognitive functioning. Neopterin is a pteridine (folic acid) present in body fluids, elevated levels of which result from immune system activation, malignant diseases, allograft rejection, and viral infections, especially AIDS. Plasma neopterin may be a candidate biomarker for delirium after cardiac surgery in these older adults.

As many as 83% of mechanically ventilated patients experience delirium (Ritchie, Torbic, DeGrado, & Reardon, 2017). This delirium doesn't end with a stay in the intensive care unit (ICU). This delirium may persist for months after discharge from the hospital. In addition, delirium is an independent predictor of a higher 6-month three-fold increase in mortality (Baranyi & Rothenhäusler, 2013). In another study, Schandl, Bottai, Hellgren, Sundin, and Sackey (2012) found that after a 4-day stay in the ICU, women who did not receive follow-up care experienced significantly greater psychological problems of depression and posttraumatic stress than men. The authors recommended a follow-up rehabilitation intervention after time in the ICU.

Delirium may produce long-term affective dysfunction. Thus, in a follow-up study, 1 year after discharge, 567 ICU survivors were contacted to determine whether any residual anxiety, depression, or posttraumatic stress disorder (PTSD) was present

(Wolters et al., 2016). ICU participants were classified as having experienced no delirium ($n = 270$; 48%), a single day of delirium ($n = 86$; 15%), or multiple days of delirium ($n = 211$; 37%) during ICU stay. Results indicated that 246 subjects (43%) reported symptoms of anxiety, 254 (45%) symptoms of depression, and 220 had PTSD symptoms. The findings did not specifically report the presence of delirium at follow-up. But previously experienced delirium leads to long-term associations among anxiety, depression, and PTSD. The occurrence of delirium during ICU stay did not increase the risk of these long-term mental health problems.

Intrahospital dementia increased the likelihood of dementia three times for as long as 3 years after hospital discharge. Pandharipande et al. (2013) confirmed the high prevalence of executive impairment among previously critically ill patients 3 and 12 months after discharge. The longer the duration of delirium, the more compromised the global cognition and executive function scores at 3 and 12 months. This cognitive impairment impairs self-care capacity.

Risk factors for delirium fall into four major categories: patient physiologic factors, disease factors, treatment-related risks, and environmental risks. Patient physiologic factors, which precipitate delirium, include age, hypertension, dementia, and coma (Inouye, 2006). Other risk factors for delirium include diseases and treatments such as emergency surgery, mechanical ventilation, organ failure, polytrauma, and metabolic acidosis. Environmental risk factors for delirium, which include physical restraints, indwelling catheters, intravenous infusions, and use of centrally acting medications, can cause and intensify delirium (Wade et al., 2012).

The drug burden index has been associated with at least 20% of the 36 million Americans who are 65 years and older and are being prescribed at least one anticholinergic medication. Studies evaluated and identified deficits with the incident rate of 22% of patients in processing speed, psychomotor performance, concentration/attention, problem solving, recall ability, and language skills (Campbell, Perkins, Hui, Khan, & Boustani, 2011). Delirium was frequently identified by disorientation, altered consciousness, disorganized thinking, and fluctuating alertness (Beyzarov, 2012; Cerejeira, Nogueira, Luís, Vaz-Serra, & Mukaetova-Ladinska, 2012). Anticholinergic drugs caused increases in cognitive impairment and the incidence of delirium in nursing home patients on these drugs increased (Landi et al., 2014; Uusvaara, Pitkala, Kautiainen, Tilvis, & Strandberg, 2011). When cognitive and functional status is examined in patients receiving anticholinergics, a number of elderly patients have diminished scores on scales measuring ability to perform activities of daily living (ADL; Pasina et al., 2013; Salahudeen, Duffull, & Nishtala, 2014). This index may provide a useful method for classifying acute care patients who are at risk of delirium (Lowry, Woodman, Soiza, Hilmer, & Mangoni, 2012). After reviewing studies of anticholinergic use among older patients, the reviewers found the relationship among cognitive function and discontinuation of the medication was poorly understood and recommended that more systematic inquiry be initiated on this complex phenomenon (Mangoni, van Munster, Woodman, & de Rooij, 2013).

There are different types of delirium. Hyperactive delirium is the most readily recognized and may include restlessness such as pacing, agitation, rapid mood changes, or hallucinations. Hypoactive delirium may include inactivity or reduced motor activity and lethargy or abnormal drowsiness. Mixed delirium includes both hyperactive and hypoactive symptoms. Individuals can quickly switch back and forth between the two forms (Mayo Clinic Staff, 2015). In some instances, patients who have dementia may also develop delirium. The major difference, of course, between dementia and delirium is that delirium symptoms can fluctuate significantly and frequently throughout the day. With dementia, an individual's memory and thinking skill don't fluctuate as much as with someone experiencing delirium (Mayo Clinic Staff, 2015).

To illustrate delirium, in general, consider Case Study 1, Mrs. M, aged 67.

CASE STUDY 1: MRS. M

Mrs. M is a fairly healthy senior who works and leads an active social life. She begins to feel ill but goes out to work anyway. Several days ago she awoke with a dry nonproductive cough and has had dyspnea on exertion. Mrs. M goes to her company clinic and is immediately put in an ambulance and sent to the hospital's emergency department (ED). Mrs. M remembers walking into the hospital clinic but nothing else after that until 8 days later. She was delirious upon admission to the ED and shortly thereafter to the ICU. Mrs. M was diagnosed with atypical pneumonia. She had a respiratory arrest sometime during the night and was placed on a ventilator. Thereafter, she was sedated to keep her from fighting the ventilator. She was restrained for the entire time she was on the ventilator. She experienced many adventures (like dreams, which she remembers) while sedated and eventually is taken off the ventilator. The restraints are removed. She believes she is awake and alert but she has auditory and visual hallucinations. She sees people sitting in her room when there is no one there. She even sees some bugs on the walls. Of course, she is on high doses of steroids and other medications. A psychiatrist is brought in to determine whether the hallucinations are new or perhaps part of a mental disorder she had prior to the illness. Eventually, he is convinced that hallucinations are part of a delirium that may be connected to the ICU experience as well as some medications that are being given in high doses. To deal with the hallucinations, the medical staff begin decreasing medications especially the steroids and sedatives. With the reduction in steroids, Mrs. M's delirium was reduced and eventually cleared. After a stay in a long-term acute care facility, Mrs. M was discharged home and eventually returned to work and had resumed normal life 3 months later.

Case Study 1 illustrates the importance of reviewing medications and their impact on elders' mental status. The effect achieved by reducing Mrs. M's medications was so profound that it reminds us how critical removing causes for delirium really is. Obviously, if the delirium is due to an illness or disease process the illness or disease has to be cleared as a way to clear the delirium. If delirium is related to medications it is imperative to reduce or discontinue these medications.

The discussion focused on delirium in the hospital ICU, but delirium can occur at home or in other facilities as shown in Case Study 2.

CASE STUDY 2: MRS. F

Mrs. F is an 85-year-old woman with a history of chronic heart failure. She has a pacemaker and has had mitral valve replacement. She has type 2 diabetes, chronic hypertension, hyperlipidemia, and diminished mobility. Mrs. F lives at home and has a home visit by a nurse and a physical therapist three times a week. She takes a long list of medications, including Lasix, which she takes to decrease lower leg edema. Her daughter reported to the nurse that Mrs. F was recently confused and very emotional. She was suddenly incontinent of urine and fell when trying to get into her chair

One outcome related to the consequence of delirium and other cognitive disorders is self-neglect. Self-neglect usually manifests in the behavior of the individual. Global cases of self-neglect are estimated at over 1 million per year (Day, Warren, & McCarthy, 2016). Executive function, often described as executive failure, is a disturbance of the central nervous system, which includes two constellations of inactivity and affects flatness and behavioral and affective disinhibition. Executive failure is often evaluated in three domains: organizational strategy, cognitive flexibility, and attention. Brain function, specifically aspects of executive function, such as planning, inhibition, and spatial working memory, is impaired in adults with self-neglect (Pickens et al., 2014).

SELF-NEGLECT AMONG OLDER ADULTS

Self-neglect has been described as a geriatric syndrome, similar to falls and incontinence (American Psychological Association, 2016; National Center on Elder Abuse, 2010; Pavlou & Lachs, 2006). After reviewing 54 studies, Pavlou and Lachs (2006) found that self-neglect includes a multifactorial etiology, it has a clear independent association with increased mortality, and two other geriatric syndromes (cognitive impairment and depression) are risk factors for self-neglect.

Pavlou and Lachs's epidemiological study determined the contribution of depressive symptoms and cognitive impairment, which were the independent predictors of self-neglect (Abrams, Lachs, McAvay, Keohane, & Bruce, 2002). Longitudinal data were collected from the participants ($N = 2,161$) enrolled in the New Haven Established Populations for Epidemiological Studies of the Elderly. In the New Haven sample, 92 confirmed cases of self-neglect were identified between the years 1982–1991. Of the adults older than 65 years of age, 15.4% had scores on the Center for Epidemiological Depression (CES-D) greater than 16, indicating depression. On the Short Portable Mental Status Questionnaire (SPMSQ), 7.5% of the adults had four or more errors, indicating clinically significant cognitive impairment. The predictors of self-neglect were being male, living alone, a history of stroke, increased depressive symptoms, and cognitive impairment (Caspi, 2014; Charles et al., 2015).

According to Naik, Lai, Kunik, and Dyer (2008), even though some adults are at risk for self-neglect, the capacity to make some decisions may remain intact. However, other decision-making abilities may be diminished. Identifying self-neglect involves determining whether the individual can both make and implement decisions regarding personal needs, health, and safety related to the capacity for self-care and self-protection. The authors also introduced the notion of having the competence to make decisions as a threshold phenomenon dichotomized as intact or not. Aspects of decision-making capacity cross over into the legal realm. Competence is of interest to clinicians and researchers so that self-care ability may be determined. These competency decisions are related to brain function and one's executive function.

In a study of older adults ($N = 130$) who lived alone, the Dementia Rating Scale (score <131) was used as a screening measure to determine individuals greater than 65 years of age at risk of self-neglect (Tierney et al., 2007). Of those 130 individuals screened, 27 experienced a harmful incident over the next 18 months. An incident was defined as harmful if it occurred as a result of self-neglect or disorientation and resulted in physical injury or property loss or damage and required emergency interventions. The predictors of impaired memory and executive functions were significant risk factors for self-neglect.

Many older adults in situations of self-neglect enter the health care system through the ED (Bartley, O'Neill, Knight, & O'Brien, 2011). One study found no relationship between cognitive function and squalor dwelling ($n = 50$) and nonsqualor dwelling ($n = 150$) (Aamodt, Terracina, & Schillerstrom, 2015). In another inquiry into ED admissions ($N = 224$), 85% of those studied were females living alone who had cognitive impairments and had been victims of incidents of harm involving self-neglect or disorientation, resulting in physical injury, property loss, or damage. Of those adults, 10% experienced harmful outcomes and increased depressive symptoms and worse health were predicted (Charles et al., 2015).

CONCLUSION

Delirium is a clinical syndrome with unpredictable outcomes. Despite its high prevalence and long-term consequences, delirium in the ICU and in other clinical areas often goes undetected and untreated. It is often thought of as a benign problem in the ICU. The neurotransmission system is a promising area for the assessment and recognition of this condition and may be enhanced with the inclusion of biomarkers. When the OFC is damaged, injuries, such as closed head injuries, cerebrovascular accidents, tumors, or neurosurgical interventions, can affect aspects of executive function and purposeful self-neglect behaviors (Cavada & Schultz, 2000). Neuropsychological tests include Trails A and B which are reliable performance measures of executive function (Reitan, 1958).

Delirium is not just a condition that occurs in the hospital, but as illustrated in Case Study 2, can occur at home. Paulson, Monroe, Fick, and McDougall (2015) discuss the importance of making providers, family, and informal caregivers aware of delirium. There is evidence related to the management of delirium in the ICU. However, there are really no medications approved by the Food and Drug Administration to treat delirium. The Society of Critical Care Medicine indicates that the primary treatment of delirium is to determine its cause and early prevention. Early prevention is a complete mental and physical evaluation of preventable causes of delirium.

Assessment of delirium, which may ultimately manifest in self-neglect, might be determined early before it develops if biomarkers are used to determine vulnerability. Plasma neopterin may be a biomarker for delirium after cardiac surgery in older adults. The research on neopterin and HVA levels is related to delirium and other aspects of cognitive functioning. The next levels of concern escalate to the failure to provide adequate food and nutrition for oneself, to take essential medications or refusal to seek medical treatment for serious illness. Independent-living difficulties manifest when an individual leaves a burning stove unattended, for example, and is unable to attend to housekeeping. Other ADL concerns include poor hygiene and not wearing suitable clothing for the weather.

Disturbances in cognitive function are associated with the syndrome of self-neglect. Prevention of delirium with nonpharmacological multicomponent approaches is widely accepted as the most effective strategy to delirium (Inouye, 2006). One such program is the Hospital Elder Life Program (Inouye, Bogardus, Baker, Leo-Summers, & Cooney, 2000), which involves a multicomponent intervention approach initiated by highly trained professionals. Another successful effort was the development of an educational brochure for families (Paulson et al., 2015).

The goal of this chapter is to provide insight into families to understand the difference between delirium and dementia. To identify the signs and symptoms of delirium, its causes, and strategies family members can use to prevent delirium.

IMPLICATIONS FOR RESEARCH AND PRACTICE

- The diagnosis and treatment of self-neglect must first be recognized as a pathological condition that often manifests as confusion and dehydration.
- Disturbances in cognitive function, such as delirium, are associated with the syndrome of self-neglect.
- The prevention of delirium with nonpharmacological multicomponent approaches is widely accepted as the most effective strategy for delirium. One such program is the Hospital Elder Life Program, which involves a multicomponent intervention approach initiated by highly trained professionals.
- The THINK mnemonic is helpful in identifying the causes of delirium in ICU patients.
- Future research might emphasize the OFC, because when damaged from closed head injuries, cerebrovascular accidents, or tumors, neurosurgical interventions can affect aspects of executive function and purposeful behaviors.

REFERENCES

Aamodt, W. W., Terracina, K. A., & Schillerstrom, J. E. (2015). Cognitive profiles of elder adult protective services clients living in squalor. *Journal of Elder Abuse & Neglect, 27*(1), 65–73.

Abrams, R. C., Lachs, M., McAvay, G., Keohane, D. J., & Bruce, M. L. (2002). Predictors of self-neglect in community dwelling elders. *American Journal of Psychiatry, 159*(10), 1724–1730.

American Psychiatric Association. (2013). *Diagnostic and statistical manual of mental disorders* (5th ed.). Arlington, VA: American Psychiatric Publishing.

American Psychological Association. (2016). Elder abuse and neglect: In search of solutions. Retrieved from http://www.apa.org/pi/aging/resources/guides/elder-abuse.aspx

Baranyi, A., & Rothenhäusler, H. B. (2013). The impact of S100b and persistent high levels of neuron-specific enolase on cognitive performance in elderly patients after cardiopulmonary bypass. *Brain Injury, 27*(4), 417–424.

Bartley, M., O'Neill, D., Knight, P. V., & O'Brien, J. G. (2011). Self-neglect and elder abuse: Related phenomena? *Journal of the American Geriatrics Society, 59*(11), 2163–2168.

Beyzarov, E. (2012). The anticholinergic cognitive burden. *Pharmacy Times*. Retrieved from http://www.pharmacytimes.com/publications/issue/2012/april2012/the-anticholinergic-cognitive-burden-

Campbell, N., Perkins, A., Hui, S., Khan, B., & Boustani, M. (2011). Association between prescribing of anticholinergic medications and incident delirium: A cohort study. *Journal of the American Geriatrics Society, 59*(Suppl. 2), S277–S281.

Caspi, E. (2014). Does self-neglect occur among older adults with dementia when unsupervised in assisted living? An exploratory, observational study. *Journal of Elder Abuse & Neglect, 26*(2), 123–149.

Cavada, C., & Schultz, W. (2000). The mysterious orbitofrontal cortex. Foreword. *Cerebral Cortex, 10*(3), 205.

Cerejeira, J., Nogueira, V., Luís, P., Vaz-Serra, A., & Mukaetova-Ladinska, E. B. (2012). The cholinergic system and inflammation: Common pathways in delirium pathophysiology. *Journal of the American Geriatrics Society, 60*(4), 669–675.

Charles, J., Naglie, G., Lee, J., Moineddin, R., Jaglal, S., & Tierney, M. C. (2015). Self-report measures of well-being predict incident harm due to self-neglect in cognitively impaired seniors who live alone. *Journal of Alzheimer's Disease, 44*(2), 425–430.

Day, M. R., Leahy-Warren, P., & McCarthy, G. (2016). Self-neglect: Ethical considerations. *Annual Review of Nursing Research, 34*(1), 89–107.

Fick, D. M., Agostini, J. V., & Inouye, S. K. (2002). Delirium superimposed on dementia: A systematic review. *Journal of the American Geriatrics Society, 50*(10), 1723–1732.

Fick, D. M., & Mion, L. C. (2008). How to try this: Delirium superimposed on dementia. *American Journal of Nursing, 108*(1), 52–60.

Inouye, S. K. (1999). Predisposing and precipitating factors for delirium in hospitalized older patients. *Dementia and Geriatric Cognitive Disorders, 10*(5), 393–400.

Inouye, S. K. (2006). Delirium in older persons. *New England Journal of Medicine, 354*(11), 1157–1165.

Inouye, S. K., Bogardus, S. T., Jr., Baker, D. I ., Leo-Summers, L., & Cooney, L. M., Jr. (2000). The Hospital Elder Life Program: A model of care to prevent cognitive and functional decline in older hospitalized patients. *Journal of the American Geriatrics Society, 48*(12), 1697–1706.

Jones, E. G., & Mendell, L. M. (1999). Assessing the decade of the brain. *Science, 284*(5415), 739.

Jonker, F. A., Jonker, C., Scheltens, P., & Scherder, E. J. A. (2015).The role of the orbitofrontal cortex in cognition and behavior. *Reviews in Neurosciences, 26*(1), 1–11.

Landi, F., Dell'Aquila, G., Collamati, A., Martone, A. M., Zuliani, G., Gasperini, B., & Cherubini, A. (2014). Anticholinergic drug use and negative outcomes among the frail elderly population living in a nursing home. *Journal of the American Medical Directors Association, 5*(11), 825–829.

Lowry, E., Woodman, R. J., Soiza, R. L., Hilmer, S. N., & Mangoni, A. A. (2012). Drug burden index, physical function, and adverse outcomes in older hospitalized patients. *Journal of Clinical Pharmacology, 52*(10), 1584–1591.

Mangoni, A. A., van Munster, B. C., Woodman, R. J., & de Rooij, S. E. (2013). Measures of anticholinergic drug exposure, serum anticholinergic activity, and all-cause post-discharge mortality in older hospitalized patients with hip fractures. *American Journal of Geriatric Psychiatry, 21*(8), 785–793.

Mayo Clinic Staff. (2015). Delirium. Retrieved from http://www.mayoclinic.org/diseases-conditions/delirium/basics/definition/con-20033982?p=1

Miller, M. A., Govindan, S., Watson, S. R., Hyzy, R. C., & Iwashyna, T. J. (2015). ABCDE, but in that order? A cross-sectional survey of Michigan intensive care unit sedation, delirium, and early mobility practices. *Annals of the American Thoracic Society, 12*(7), 1066–1071.

Naik, A. D., Lai, J. M., Kunik, M. E., & Dyer, C. B. (2008). Assessing capacity in suspected cases of self-neglect. *Geriatrics, 63*(2), 24–31.

National Center on Elder Abuse. (2010, March). Factsheet: Why should I care about elder abuse? Retrieved from https://ncea.acl.gov

Osse, R. J., Fekkes, D., Tulen, J. H., Wierdsma, A. I., Bogers, A. J., van der Mast, R. C., & Hengeveld, M. W. (2012). High preoperative plasma neopterin predicts delirium after cardiac surgery in older adults. *Journal of the American Geriatrics Society, 60*(4), 661–668.

Pandharipande, P. P., Girard, T. D., Jackson, J. C., Morandi, A., Thompson, J. L., Pun, B. T., . . . Ely, E. W. (2013). Long-term cognitive impairment after critical illness. *New England Journal of Medicine, 369*(14), 1306–1316.

Pasina, L., Djade, C. D., Lucca, U., Nobili, A., Tettamanti, M., Franchi, C., . . . Marcucci, M. (2013). Association of anticholinergic burden with cognitive and functional status in a cohort of hospitalized elderly: Comparison of the Anticholinergic Cognitive Burden Scale and Anticholinergic Risk Scale: Results from the REPOSI study. *Drugs & Aging, 30*(2), 103–112.

Paulson, C., Monroe, T., Fick, D., & McDougall, G. J. (2015). A family focused delirium educational initiative with practice and research implications. *Gerontology & Geriatrics Education, 11,* 1–18.

Pavlou, M. P., & Lachs, M. C. (2006). Could self-neglect in older adults be a geriatric syndrome? *Journal of the American Geriatrics Society, 54*(5), 831–842.

Pickens, S., Ostwald, S. K., Pace, K. M., Diamond, P., Burnett, J., & Dyer, C. B. (2014). Assessing dimensions of executive function in community-dwelling older adults with self-neglect. *Clinical Nursing Studies, 2*(1), 17–29.

Reitan, R. M. (1958). Validity of the Trail Making Test as an indicator of organic brain damage. *Perceptual and Motor Skills, 8,* 271–276.

Render, M. L., Kim, H. M., Welsh, D. E., Timmons, S., Johnston, J., Hui, S., . . . Hofer, T. P. (2003). Automated intensive care unit risk adjustment: Results from a National Veterans Affairs study. *Critical Care Medicine, 31*(6), 1638–1646.

Ritchie, B. M., Torbic, H., DeGrado, J. R., & Reardon, D. P. (2017). Sedation variability increases incidence of delirium in adult medical intensive care unit patients at a tertiary academic medical center. *American Journal of Therapeutics.* [Epub ahead of print]. PMID: 27340907. doi: 10.1097/MJT.0000000000000455

Salahudeen, M. S., Duffull, S. B., & Nishtala, P. S. (2014). Impact of anticholinergic discontinuation on cognitive outcomes in older people: A systematic review. *Drugs & Aging, 31*(3), 185–192.

Schandl, A., Bottai, M., Hellgren, E., Sundin, Ö., & Sackey, P. (2012). Gender differences in psychological morbidity and treatment in intensive care survivors: A cohort study. *Critical Care, 16*(3), R80. doi:10.1186/cc11338

Tierney, M. C., Snow, W. G., Charles, J., Moineddin, R., & Kiss, A. (2007). Neuropsychological predictors of self-neglect in cognitively impaired older people who live alone. *American Journal of Geriatric Psychiatry, 15*(2), 140–148.

Uusvaara, J., Pitkala, K. H., Kautiainen, H., Tilvis, R. S., & Strandberg, T. E. (2011). Association of anticholinergic drugs with hospitalization and mortality among older cardiovascular patients. *Drugs & Aging, 28*(2), 131–138.

Wade, D. M., Howell, D. C., Weinman, J. A., Hardy, R. J., Mythen, M. G., Brewin, C. R., . . . Raine, R. A. (2012). Investigating risk factors for psychological morbidity three months after intensive care: A prospective cohort study. *Critical Care, 16*(5), R192. doi:10.1186/cc11677

Wolters, A. E., Peelen, L. M., Welling, M. C., Kok, L., de Lange, D. W., Cremer, O. L., . . . Veldhuijzen, D. S. (2016). Long-term mental health problems after delirium in the ICU. *Critical Care Medicine, 44*(10), 1808–1813. doi:10.1097/CCM.0000000000001861

CHAPTER 5

HOARDING: FEATURES, ASSESSMENT, AND INTERVENTION STRATEGIES

May Luu and Sheila R. Woody

Hoarding disorder is characterized by persistent distress when attempting to discard, recycle, or donate items from or out of the home. The inability to discard, often in combination with excessive acquiring, results in the accumulation of large volumes of possessions that prevent residents from using rooms for their intended purposes, such as preparing food, socializing, or sleeping in the bed. This chapter provides a brief overview of the features and complications of hoarding disorder. Assessment is explained, including key features used in evaluation. Finally, we describe evidence-based interventions for hoarding, focusing on cognitive behavioral therapy. Motivation enhancement and harm-reduction strategies, as well as community-based interventions, are also discussed.

Hoarding disorder is a new addition to the fifth edition of the *Diagnostic and Statistical Manual of Mental Disorders* (*DSM-5*; American Psychiatric Association, 2013). Although the official status of this diagnostic category is recent, the behavior has been worthy of clinical attention in the literature for several decades, and media reports of dramatic hoarding cases go back nearly 100 years (Faber, 1947). Hoarding prevalence in the general population has been estimated to range between 2.3% and 5.8% (Iervolino et al., 2009; Timpano et al., 2011).

FEATURES AND COMPLICATIONS OF HOARDING

Personal possessions have historically served to convey status, style, and personality. Possessions can also be a source of great pleasure, from the thrill of obtaining the desired item to discovering forgotten cherished objects. Most people can part fairly easily with or forgo buying nonessential items when living spaces become crowded. For people who suffer from hoarding disorder, however, deciding which possessions to let go of is so painful that the decision gets postponed indefinitely. Living conditions can become extremely cluttered and even objectively dangerous. At that point, this private problem can become a public matter, as housing providers, fire departments, building inspectors, or protective services become involved.

Hoarding disorder is characterized by persistent difficulties throwing away (or recycling, donating, etc.) low-value or seemingly worthless items. This difficulty is the result of a strong emotional urge to save the objects; that is, the accumulation is not passive. Consequently, belongings may fill the home to the point where rooms can no longer be used for typical daily activities such as preparing food or sleeping. Many persons who hoard also excessively acquire items, especially items that are free or represent a "good deal." Thus, although extreme clutter is one of the more obvious features of hoarding, an accumulation of stuff is not enough to qualify for a diagnosis of hoarding disorder. Rather, the clutter accumulation must be related to intentionally acquiring and saving items. Clutter that results strictly from physical, sensory, or cognitive deficits that prevent individuals from taking care of the home would not be considered a hoarding disorder (Maier, 2004).

Compulsive hoarding has been associated with an early onset and lifelong progression. Grisham, Frost, Steketee, Kim, and Hood (2006), for example, reported on a sample of 51 hoarding participants —60% recalled developing mild hoarding symptoms by age 12 and 80% by age 18. Subsequently, moderate symptoms began in their 20s and severe symptoms appeared a decade later. Of these participants, 14% no longer met the criteria for a hoarding disorder at some point after symptom onset. These results were largely replicated in another study (Tolin, Fitch, Frost, & Steketee, 2010). Living and being raised in a hoarded home has broad consequences for functioning and enduring effects on children (see Case Study 1).

CASE STUDY 1: JULIANNE

Julianne engaged in compulsive shopping (often for health and beauty items) but had no space in her home. She would come home and drop her purchases, still in their plastic shopping bag. Her stuff, together with many unopened shopping bags, had come to take over all horizontal spaces, including much of the floor. She was unable to use the kitchen because the counters, sink, and stove were stacked with items, and it was not possible to open the refrigerator without moving a large pile of items on the floor. Julianne's condo needed some minor repairs (e.g., the bathroom sink was leaking, the door to her laundry had come off the tracks), but she was terrified of the consequences of calling for maintenance. Her bed was in poor condition because clutter covered the entire bedroom floor high enough to be level with the bed; as a result, she had not been able to change the linens for several years.

Like many people who have problems with hoarding, Julianne had trouble finding and dealing with important paperwork. In a large Internet-based sample of hoarding participants, 20% had failed to file an income tax return at least once in the past 5 years (Tolin, Frost, Steketee, Gray, & Fitch, 2008). Strong social support may be one factor that could slow down the development or buffer the consequences of living in an extremely cluttered home. Unfortunately, hoarding has been associated with family and occupational difficulties (Frost, Ruby, & Shuer, 2012). Moreover, the safety of the resident and neighbors can be threatened because of elevated risks of fire, for example, from combustible materials (e.g., newspapers or clothing) stored on or near heat sources.

Older adults may experience additional complications of hoarding due to the challenges presented by physical illness and cognitive decline. Dong, Simon, Mosqueda, and Evans (2012) found these factors associated with more severe hoarding symptoms among older adults. Although the typical course of development of hoarding problems has not been well documented, physical and cognitive impairments certainly interfere with the ability to address issues related to clutter and household maintenance in a situation where hoarding has already developed. A further hazard for older adults is the risk of falls or the avalanche of possessions that have been piled high. For these and other reasons, concerns for health and safety are often amplified for older residents of hoarded homes than for other age groups.

ASSESSMENT OF HOARDING

As alluded to earlier, hoarding-related problems may come to the attention of authorities and thus require assessment even in cases where the client is uninterested in or even hostile to assistance. A thorough assessment to allow one to determine whether hoarding disorder is the most appropriate diagnosis will usually involve a home visit, although photographs of the home can be used in situations where it is impractical for the clinician to visit the home. Given the stigma associated with hoarding, obtaining consent for an evaluation can involve a considerable investment of the clinician's time to establish a trusting relationship. For clients who are seeking treatment, we recommend first conducting a thorough interview away from the home and then explaining the importance and value of having a home visit as part of the assessment. For clients who are not seeking help, the entire evaluation generally occurs at home, although initial visits may need to take place outside before the client trusts the clinician enough to permit an inspection.

Key features of hoarding need to be assessed to obtain a correct diagnosis and develop a relevant intervention plan. Obviously, the main *DSM-5* criteria should be assessed: difficulty discarding, extreme accumulation of possessions, and functional impairment or distress. The difficulty discarding should represent the intentional saving of items, rather than passive accumulation that can better be attributed to the lethargy of depression, delusions of psychosis, or other problems. The accumulation of possessions is often obvious, with several rooms that are difficult to move around in. Sometimes, however, other members of the household have placed strong limits on how much the individual can acquire. In such cases, the individual may have turned to storage units; we have seen some clients who spend more on storage units than they do on rent. Due to poor or fluctuating insight, the individual may deny functional impairment, but this will become apparent during a home visit as the clinician observes safety issues or obvious obstacles to the performance of activities of daily living. In addition to these diagnostic criteria, excessive acquisition is a specifier that should be taken into account, as the presence of this problem has implications for the treatment plan. Several self-report or clinician-rated tools are available to assist in the thorough assessment of the symptoms of hoarding disorder.

The Saving Inventory–Revised (SI–R; Frost, Steketee, & Grisham, 2004) is a 23-item self-report questionnaire that assesses problems with excessive acquiring, difficulty discarding, and clutter volume. Obviously, a self-report measure is useful primarily for treatment-seeking clients with good or fair insight. This measure has good reliability and construct validity (Frost et al., 2004). Researchers also regularly use this measure (Frost et al., 2004), so clinicians or other human service professionals can compare client responses to benchmark scores in the literature, which may help with understanding symptoms and treatment planning.

The Clutter Image Rating (CIR) Scale is a widely used tool to measure clutter volume (Frost, Steketee, Tolin, & Renaud, 2008; Tolin et al., 2010). The scale comprises nine photographs that depict a room in various states of clutter, beginning with a room that is as tidy as an empty hotel room (labeled "1"). Each photo shows progressively more clutter, up until the last photo (labeled "9"), which has clutter nearly to the ceiling. There is one set of photos for each of three rooms: bedroom, kitchen, and living room. Anyone who has seen the home—clients, family members, clinicians, or other professionals—can use the scale by selecting the photograph that is most similar to the clutter volume in each room. This measure has demonstrated excellent test–retest reliability and a high level of agreement across assessment contexts and between different raters (e.g., self and observer; Frost et al., 2008; Tolin et al., 2010). In addition, this measure is available for free online.

Another tool, the Activities of Daily Living–Hoarding (ADL–H) Scale, can also be used in self-report format or as an observational rating form (Frost, Hristova, Steketee, & Tolin, 2013). This is a 15-item scale that lists activities that are frequently difficult to do in hoarded homes, such as use a bath/shower, answer the door quickly, or eat at a table. Each activity is rated on a 5-point scale from "can do it easily" to "unable to do." The measure has good reliability and established convergent and discriminant validity. The ADL–H is especially useful in identifying functional impairments that can form the basis for collaboratively established treatment goals.

The HOMES multidisciplinary risk assessment tool is similar to the ADL–H, in that it is a brief checklist intended to be used during initial in-home assessments to identify areas of risk in hoarded homes (Bratiotis, Schmalisch, & Steketee, 2011). The measure was created by a multidisciplinary team of professionals from diverse backgrounds who see hoarding cases in the context of their work. HOMES covers the following issues:

- Health (including many ADL as well as pest infestations, ability to locate medications or medical equipment, and squalor such as spoiled food or presence of feces/urine)
- Obstacles (inability to move freely about the home, tripping or fall hazards, or blocked exits)
- Mental health (poor insight, defensive/angry mental state, or confusion)
- Endangerment (threats to the health or safety of vulnerable members of the household)
- Structure and safety (nonfunctioning utilities, hazardous materials, or structural degradation)

Importantly, HOMES goes beyond ADL–H to include imminent safety threats that should be prioritized first and addressed quickly. To date, this tool has not been evaluated in terms of reliability and validity. The greatest strength of this measure is that professionals from multiple backgrounds can use it to communicate about a coordinated plan to assist the resident.

This brief review has described areas to assess in cases of suspected hoarding as well as tools that can guide the assessment. As with any mental health issue, it is also important to consider differential diagnosis and the possibility of comorbid conditions, especially social anxiety and depression (Frost et al., 2013). Cognitive impairment and attention deficit disorder are also of concern because they can directly interfere with the client's ability to organize belongings, persist with decluttering activities, and make decisions about which items to keep.

INTERVENTIONS TO ADDRESS HOARDING

Due to factors such as poor insight, social stigma about hoarding behavior, or fear of the consequences of bringing attention to their home, many of those who suffer from hoarding are reluctant to seek help or accept offered assistance. Most clients are open to the idea of intervention only after pressure from family or friends or in the context of some threatened external consequence such as eviction. Even those who do accept assistance are typically ambivalent about making changes in their relationship with possessions. Passive resistance, such as missed appointments or failure to complete agreed-upon between-session activities, is common. Poor insight, or failure to appreciate the severity of the problem, can rob clients of their motivation to change their behavior (Tolin et al., 2010). Fluctuating insight levels have also been observed throughout the course of treatment (Hartl & Frost, 1999).

This section provides an overview of cognitive behavioral therapy (CBT) for hoarding, an evidence-based treatment for hoarding disorder. After the overview, we discuss challenges and obstacles commonly encountered during hoarding interventions and potential approaches to address these issues, including motivational interviewing (MI) and harm-reduction strategies.

Cognitive Behavioral Therapy

Although researchers have only begun to publish studies about treatment for hoarding disorder within the past 10 years, early findings from a small number of studies support the efficacy of a specialized form of CBT for hoarding. In a small randomized controlled trial, a large effect size was demonstrated, with clinicians observing overall symptom improvements in hoarding clients who received individual CBT for hoarding (Steketee, Frost, Tolin, Rasmussen, & Brown, 2010). On the other hand, none of the 23 clients on the waitlist received the same rating from the evaluators. In another study, Muroff, Steketee, Bratiotis, and Ross (2012) showed large effect sizes during the course of group CBT for hoarding and significantly smaller effect sizes for those receiving bibliotherapy. More broadly, a recent meta-analysis of 10 treatment studies for CBT for hoarding showed large effect sizes for decreasing problems with discarding, acquisition, and clutter (Tolin, Frost, Steketee, & Muroff, 2015).

Although hoarding does seem to be more prevalent among older adults, only two small studies have been specifically conducted within this age group. In a sample of 12 older adults, only three participants had decreased hoarding symptoms, and at the 6-month follow-up, two had relapsed, exhibiting symptoms similar to those seen prior to therapy (Ayers, Wetherell, Golshan, & Saxena, 2011). In an attempt to strengthen the intervention for older adults, Ayers's group (2014) conducted an open trial to test the effects of prefacing CBT with some sessions focused on organizational skills (e.g., creating to-do lists, calendar use, and categorizing). Eight of the 11 participants were considered to be treatment responders. Unfortunately, no follow-up data were available. These preliminary findings are encouraging for future investigations directed toward improving treatment outcomes for older adults. Interestingly, the meta-analysis by Tolin et al. (2015) examined client age as a potential moderator of treatment effects and found younger age was associated with stronger effect sizes only for the excessive acquiring dimension; improvements in difficulty discarding and clutter volume were not related to client age.

CBT for hoarding aims to reduce three key hoarding symptoms: disorganization, difficulty discarding things, and excessive acquisition (Steketee & Frost, 2014). This model relies on a number of presumptions. One of these is that hoarding symptoms are influenced by several factors, such as basic biological (genetic, biochemical, or neurological factors) and psychological vulnerabilities (mood, personality, or past experiences). In turn, these vulnerabilities influence information processing (decision making, categorizing, or attention), as well as maladaptive beliefs about objects and excessive attachment to possessions. Notably, both negative and positive emotions can become important contributors to hoarding behavior. Anxiety and guilt can motivate avoidance, such as putting off decisions about objects as a way to avoid regret about throwing items away. Pride and joy, on the other hand, can intensify the importance of objects, enhancing the individual's valuation of those items. It is important to recognize both the pleasure in ownership and the problems caused by hoarding behavior in order to understand the ambivalence clients experience about making changes.

CBT for hoarding can be conducted in either individual (Steketee & Frost, 2014) or group format (Muroff, Underwood, & Steketee, 2014). The tested versions of the individual protocol involved 26 sessions of 60 to 90 minutes. Many of these sessions occurred in the client's home. In fact, the meta-analysis by Tolin and colleagues (2015) described previously identified a greater number of home-based sessions as a significant moderator of treatment outcome. Because clients frequently cancel, completing 26 sessions took 9 to 12 months in the treatment trials. Group CBT has ranged from 12 to 20 sessions in published studies, but our experience suggests 20 sessions is more reasonable. Again, periodic home-based sessions are useful.

The protocol developed by Steketee and Frost (2014) initially focuses on building rapport and psychoeducation, identifying contributing factors that maintain hoarding behavior, and skills training to improve decision making, problem solving, and organization. In addition, clients undergo direct or imagined exposure to distressing circumstances (e.g., discarding and acquiring). Clinicians also help clients modify maladaptive beliefs related to hoarding. Toward the end of treatment, clinicians and clients discuss relapse prevention strategies to help clients maintain treatment gains.

Although urgent action may be required at the outset to address imminent health or safety risks in the home (e.g., combustible items stored near a heat source or tripping or falls hazards for frail elderly occupants), starting with relationship building and psychoeducation is recommended. This is even more important in working with hoarding than for most client populations. Most hoarding clients who seek treatment are in midlife (Grisham et al., 2006) and have no prior experience of treatment for hoarding (Ayers, Saxena, Golshan, & Wetherell, 2010). Some may have felt coerced to accept treatment (e.g., because of eviction threats or strong family pressure). Mental health professionals who treat hoarding report that the clients have poorer levels of insight and more therapy-interfering behaviors than nonhoarding clients throughout treatment (Tolin, Frost, & Steketee, 2012). It is not surprising that these professionals also reported more frustration with treating hoarding clients compared to nonhoarding clients. Taken together, it seems that both hoarding clients and clinicians can find the intervention process taxing and difficult. Thus, although efforts to build rapport may sometimes be challenging, the therapeutic alliance is critical.

Providing some background information about hoarding disorder and the general approach of CBT may help the client ease into the treatment process, as well as establish a therapeutic alliance. These initial office-based sessions also set the stage for potential future in-home sessions. For some clients, no one has entered their home for many years. Indeed, the clinician's visits may be the first step toward ending a long period of household isolation. This isolation could have occurred for many reasons, but is often related to the client feeling ashamed and ostracized due to living conditions in the home. These experiences could lead clients to feel defensive and wary when other people, including clinicians, want to talk about the client's living conditions or request access to the client's home. However, the first few sessions are essential to building a strong therapeutic alliance, and psychoeducation may be a nonthreatening way to begin treatment.

After the clinician has a good idea about the client's problem areas that need to be addressed, the next step is to collaboratively establish ground rules and treatment goals (Steketee, 2014; Steketee & Frost, 2014). Some common rules that the clinician and client may agree on include that clinicians will refrain from touching or removing items without explicit consent and that clients have the final decision about what happens with each possession. Bringing these issues up in the beginning will facilitate trust and set boundaries for future interactions. Clients' goals often relate to activities of daily living that have been difficult to accomplish given the hoarding behavior. Some case examples from our practice include:

- Meighen's main goals were to clear the stuff off her bed and the floor of her bedroom so she would be able to use the whole bed for sleeping and could approach the bed without stepping on piles of newspapers and clothing. She also wanted to clear enough space at her desk area to be able to use her computer and to do the recommended rehabilitation exercises for her hand, which she had injured in an accident.
- John had made great improvements in making living space in his home due to strong pressure from his landlord, but he still had a rented storage space that he could not really afford on his limited income. He wanted to clear out the storage space, and he also wanted to clear the stuff from his car, which was so full that he could not drive it.

Skills training is a component of CBT for hoarding that sets it apart from most other CBT interventions. Hoarding is a chronic problem, so clients usually have had many years of living in a hoarded home before agreeing to intervention. Some clients also grew up in a hoarded home, so they never developed the everyday skills and habits that most people use to organize and maintain their living space. Protocols for CBT for hoarding (Steketee & Frost, 2014) provide ideas on how to help clients gain these skills, such as filing systems for paperwork or sorting and storing clothing. This skills-training portion can involve helping clients establish logical resting places for various objects in the home (e.g., pet care supplies, sentimental items) as well as practice strategies for keeping items organized and cleared spaces free for other activities such as relaxing, working, or socializing.

Regular scheduled home visits are recommended to ensure a steady engagement in sorting activities and to help clinicians assess client strengths and weaknesses. Going through the sorting process together can help the client create (and stick to) rules for when to keep or discard objects, and can bring out clients' thoughts and beliefs that promote saving and acquiring. For example, Maggie's couch was so covered in bills, receipts, and other papers that she had barely enough room for one person (herself) to sit on it. As her therapist was helping her sort important from unimportant papers, Maggie expressed a belief that if her papers were organized in drawers or file boxes, she would forget about them, which might make her miss an important deadline or even lose a treasured memory. Being present in the home permitted the clinician to provide social support as Maggie made difficult decisions in evaluating the nature of the papers on the couch (e.g., tax papers vs. outdated discount coupons), to suggest some organizational strategies for Maggie to consider, and to hear Maggie's beliefs about the negative consequences of organizing her papers.

By being present in the home, the therapist was also able to teach Maggie techniques, such as the "only handle it once" (OHIO) rule, to help her make more efficient decisions and follow through with them immediately. The OHIO rule dictates that once clients decide on whether to keep or discard an object, the decision is final and the object cannot be handled again. Making this sort of commitment discourages use of a "not sure" pile, which is likely to turn into piles that clients repeatedly reshuffle without making concrete choices about keeping or discarding. Although initially, decisions about objects can take an inordinate amount of time (and involve much anguish over the possibility of making a decision that one might later regret), over time, clients gain confidence in their decision-making abilities and are able to make faster decisions with less distress.

Behavioral experiments and thought-provoking questions can be used to help clients begin to question their predictions about potential negative consequences of letting go of objects. Behavioral experiments are small exposure exercises set up to test the client's predictions. For example, Maggie's therapist could help her to test the idea that she would forget where she put things if they are in a drawer by identifying a location where a certain category of items will be kept, putting those items in the location, and asking Maggie to recall the location a week or 2 later. Treatment protocols for hoarding offer a range of questions that are helpful in encouraging clients to question their assumptions and thoughts about objects as they are making decisions: Do I already have another object like this one? How many will I use within a reasonable time frame? What are my plans for this object? Have I used this item in the past year? Do I really need it?

If excessive acquisition is a concern, then some sessions can focus on resisting acquiring items in various situations (e.g., from a department store, browsing the Internet, in a dumpster) that often trigger this behavior (Steketee & Frost, 2014). These sessions use an anxiety extinction model, similar to exposure to feared situations. The approach begins with creating a hierarchy of situations the client finds it difficult to enter without acquiring anything. The hierarchy gets ordered from easy to most difficult. Starting with easier situations, the clinician accompanies the client in these situations and assists with management of negative emotions while forgoing opportunities to acquire favored items, things that are a "good deal," and so forth.

Motivation Enhancement

Most hoarding clients struggle with motivation to change. For some, engaging with intervention efforts was not their idea, but rather a family member has reached out and asked for assistance or has pressured the client to do so. We frequently see clients miss sessions or fail to complete between-session activities they had agreed to do. This ambivalence about making changes often requires special efforts to help clients become more aware of and invested in their own reasons for change.

Previous research suggests that including motivation enhancement strategies as a prelude to therapy can improve treatment outcomes. For example, Westra and Dozois (2006) found that a brief MI intervention can increase clients' confidence in being able to control their symptoms and also enhance homework compliance throughout CBT, compared to clients who received CBT only. Because of the ubiquity of ambivalence about change in hoarding, CBT protocols typically incorporate motivation enhancement strategies (Steketee & Frost, 2014). This approach may be especially helpful for clients who fail to recognize consequences of hoarding that are clearly evident to others. For those clients who do recognize their own problematic behaviors, use of an MI approach can help address resistance that commonly emerges during interventions, such as reluctance to commit to making changes or fluctuating motivation over time.

The formal MI approach was developed by Miller and Rollnick (1991) as a way to help prepare clients for changing addictive behavior. An MI stance involves the development of a collaborative partnership between the clinician and the client. The approach is nonconfrontational and nonadversarial, emphasizing empathy and a focus on the clients' strengths, autonomy, and capacity to make their own decisions. The clinician's job is to cultivate the clients' balanced perspective on the problem so that they become empowered to make behavioral choices (e.g., when to save or discard) that are more adaptive and in line with their values and goals. Using an MI stance can reduce defensiveness and mistrust, improve problems with motivation and resistance, and improve clients' confidence in their own ability to make changes.

Genuine empathy is foundational to the MI approach (Miller & Rollnick, 2002) and crucial for any intervention for hoarding. Many clients with hoarding behavior have experienced harsh judgment and even ostracism regarding their living conditions. This kind of stigma can leave the client feeling wary about letting anyone, including clinicians, get too close. Recognizing the client's reasons for saving and specific fears about letting go of objects sets the stage for understanding thoughts and beliefs behind these behaviors. This understanding permits the clinician to help the client recognize discrepancies between the saving or acquiring behavior and the client's personal values and goals. Ultimately, the aim is to support the client to discover and remember his or her own personal reasons to make changes.

Another factor that is relevant to motivation enhancement is self-efficacy. In homes that have severe clutter accumulation, creating living space can seem like an overwhelming prospect, and many clients feel demoralized in the face of this enormous task. Clients who feel they are not capable of making progress are less likely to try or to persist when encountering minor barriers. Helping clients to believe in their own abilities thus becomes a self-fulfilling prophecy as clients follow through with their new goals (Steketee & Frost, 2014). Clinicians can support these beliefs by helping to structure small manageable goals (e.g., work for 15 minutes per day on sorting the materials on top of the dining room table) and by providing encouragement and celebration of goal attainment (e.g., "It's great that you were able to work on this every day this week" or "I'm glad to see you were able to keep the doorway clear over the past month").

Harm-Reduction Approach

Harm reduction is most frequently associated with interventions for substance abuse and dependence. The harm-reduction approach was originally developed to minimize harmful consequences of intravenous drug use without stopping the behavior entirely (e.g., providing sanitary needles). Multiple studies support the effectiveness of harm-reduction approaches for clients with alcohol and substance use problems over a variety of different contexts (Logan & Marlatt, 2010). In essence, harm reduction is a guiding principle for selecting treatment goals in the context of clients who engage in behaviors that are potentially harmful for themselves or others when the clients are not ready to completely stop the behavior (Marlatt & Tapert, 1993). Clinicians are increasingly adopting this stance for different clinical problems, and Tompkins and Hartl (2007) extended this approach to hoarding. Although no clinical trials have examined the effectiveness of harm reduction in hoarding, the approach is commonly used in community-based interventions for hoarding (Bratiotis & Woody, 2013).

Within the hoarding context, a harm-reduction stance prioritizes the health and safety of the client rather than decluttering per se. For clients who are not voluntarily seeking intervention, the treatment goals that arise from a harm-reduction approach can be more acceptable and can help them to consent to intervention. We have often seen this scenario in situations like the one involving David, a 73-year-old man who had been hospitalized for many weeks following a major infection. In preparing for his discharge, the transition team did a home visit and discovered there was no room for him to use mobility aids or for home care staff to assist him with activities such as bathing. David was adamant that he did not want anyone else to make decisions about his belongings, and he was too weak to engage in the process in a timely way. He did agree to intervention goals using a harm-reduction perspective, including having some of his belongings moved within the home to create pathways wide enough for a walker and to clear the bathroom of clothing and other items he had stored there.

Overall, as described by Tompkins and Hartl (2007), a harm-reduction strategy for hoarding involves four components: (a) boosting the willingness of the client and others who are involved in the situation (e.g., family members, housing provider) to engage in the intervention, (b) assessing risky or harmful consequences of hoarding behavior, (c) developing a plan for reducing the risks or potential harm, and (d) executing and monitoring the plan. Ideally, the client would be fully cooperative throughout the implementation of all these steps. If the client is not cooperative, the harm-reduction approach ensures these actions are the least restrictive options necessary to manage the risks.

Tompkins and Hartl (2007) go beyond describing the applicability of harm reduction to establishing intervention goals. They specifically address the interpersonal and family context of hoarding. Often, by the time a hoarding case comes to the attention of clinicians, the client's family and friends have engaged in well-intentioned but unsuccessful efforts to help; such actions often damage the relationship with the client. Family members' feelings of rejection are more likely if the hoarding behavior is severe or if the client has low insight about the consequences of the behavior (Tolin, Frost, Steketee, & Fitch, 2008). Recognizing this, along with the negative consequences of social isolation (which is quite common in hoarding), it can be useful to intervene with the client's loved ones to start repairing the relationship.

Several researchers have begun to develop family interventions to increase seeking treatment and readiness for treatment among those engaged in hoarding behavior as well as to increase the well-being of family members. Sampson, Yeats, and Harris (2012) developed a structured six-session support group that permitted family members to discuss the ambiguous losses they had experienced as a result of living in a hoarded home. Such losses included disrupted relationships with family members who hoard, limited time spent with family, loss of normal family experiences (including mealtimes), and loss of the childhood home. Following the support group, participants reported a softening in their negative feelings toward the hoarding family member as well as a change in their perspective. After participating in the group, members felt less focused on getting the home cleaned up and more hopeful that their relationship with the hoarding family member could be repaired.

Harm-reduction interventions for hoarding often involve a team of people (Tompkins & Hartl, 2007). Members usually include the clinician, client, friends and family, and other stakeholders (e.g., housing providers) or agencies (e.g., older adult protective services). Because it is unlikely that one community agency is equipped to deal with all aspects of hoarding (e.g., fire risk, electrical problems, psychological symptoms, threats to eviction, or medication management), building a team brings relevant expertise together in a collaborative approach so that the client receives one consistent message about changes that need to be made in order to achieve basic standards of health and safety. When professionals do not work as a team, clients can become frustrated with receiving different demands and deadlines from each agency (Bratiotis & Woody, 2013). Coordinating efforts can simplify the intervention process, although commitment to the collaborative approach from the various agencies is required.

Formal mechanisms for multiagency intervention for hoarding is growing in popularity, with at least 80 community-based task forces in the United States and Canada (Bratiotis et al., 2011). With this collaborative approach, specific goals of each member of the team can be incorporated into the intervention plan. For example, the Vancouver Hoarding Action Response Team has members from the Fire Prevention Branch of the Fire Department as well as nurses from the local health authority; other agencies may also be involved on a case-by-case basis. The fire inspectors ensure that fire safety issues are addressed, while the nurses make referrals to needed community and health services. They work together to determine intervention goals, based on a harm-reduction model, and the individual on the team who has the best relationship with the client is the main contact for the client. This approach is closely modeled on case management (Bratiotis, Woody, & Lauster, 2016).

TREATMENT CHALLENGES AND FUTURE DIRECTIONS

Although CBT is the most-researched intervention for hoarding disorder, it can still be improved and is not the most appropriate solution for all situations. Individual CBT for hoarding is time-consuming, costly, and may be more suitable for clients with at least moderate insight into the severity and consequences of the problem. Group CBT for hoarding uses the same basic approach, and some researchers have begun to conduct clinical trials of this variation (Gilliam et al., 2011). Conducting treatment in a group format is obviously more cost-effective, and the group provides social opportunities for group members. In addition, clients are sometimes more open to hearing a different perspective about possessions if it is offered by a fellow client than by a clinician. A structured bibliotherapy conducted in group format has also shown to be both effective and cost-efficient (Frost, Pekereva-Kochergina, &

Maxner, 2011); several communities are starting to coordinate Buried in Treasures support groups, based on the popular book by Tolin, Frost, and Steketee (2014).

As hoarding disorder was only recently recognized as a distinct category in the *DSM-5*, research into the phenomenon and effective interventions has only scratched the surface; much more will be discovered in the next few years. For example, depression commonly co-occurs with hoarding, but research has not yet provided guidance for sequencing interventions. Depression obviously saps motivation and energy, both of which are required to persist through the tedious job of sorting hoarded possessions. The treatment plan has to account for this factor as well as any physical disabilities.

Although coordinated community efforts for hoarding is a good start to decreasing frustration for hoarding clients and streamlining intervention goals, logistical problems still need to be resolved. For example, professionals on the team may have different limitations on information sharing. Professionals in some disciplines are bound by laws and ethical codes regarding confidentiality, whereas others have fewer restrictions. When information cannot be freely shared, record-keeping becomes more complicated; who keeps track of which aspects of the client's progress, and how are different parts of the team kept informed? In addition, most community-based intervention teams are well equipped in relation to some aspects of intervention (e.g., social support, animal welfare, or tenancy preservation), but they also have gaps in the services they are able to offer (e.g., funding for removal of unwanted objects, assistance with decluttering).

One factor that increases the complexity and expense of intervention for hoarding is the need for in-home sessions. Home visits are extremely helpful during the assessment phase, as many clients are unable to accurately report on conditions in the home; seeing the home can help the clinician to prioritize treatment goals related to health and safety. Beyond assessment, as mentioned earlier, greater use of in-home sessions is associated with stronger treatment effects (Tolin et al., 2015). Of course, home visits add expense for the clinician's time and transportation, and access maybe poor because of geographic location or even be unfeasible in certain clinical settings. Development of evidence-based strategies, such as the use of distance technology, may greatly improve the feasibility of home visits.

Residents of hoarded homes face tremendous stigma and often have family conflicts. Setting aside social judgment about the virtue of good housekeeping practices, it is not difficult to empathize with a strong connection with objects. Everyone has cherished possessions that evoke important memories or convey social status, just as almost everyone has objects they have been meaning to get rid of but just have not found the time to remove. The ubiquity of humans' valuing of owned objects may explain in part the public fascination with hoarding. Due to its relatively high prevalence rate, clinicians, especially those who make routine home visits, are likely to encounter hoarding at some point in their careers, so it is useful to know more about this complex disorder. As research interest in this topic accelerates, we anticipate more effective and efficient interventions in the coming years.

CONCLUSION

Hoarding disorder involves the acquisition of large volumes of possessions that impinge on every facet of living, coupled with the inability to discard these possessions. Assessment of hoarding includes the use of self-report and clinician-rated tools and measures for assessing specific aspects of the disorder. Assessment of key features is necessary for a correct diagnosis and development of an intervention plan. A range of interventions is described. Research on hoarding and effective interventions is in its infancy, as hoarding disorder has only recently been recognized in the *DSM-5*.

A strong working alliance is a key to successful outcomes when working with individuals who hoard, yet developing and maintaining such an alliance can be challenging. Parting with possessions is typically necessary to create living space and address health and safety concerns, but discarding (or recycling or donating) generates substantial distress. A strong alliance, based on mutual warmth and respect, can help the client to tolerate and recover from negative emotions and can also help the clinician to maintain a collaborative stance in which the client makes all decisions about his or her own possessions. Such a collaborative approach fosters the setting of feasible and meaningful treatment goals, which in turn enhances the client's investment and motivation for change.

IMPLICATIONS FOR RESEARCH AND PRACTICE

Several self-report and clinician-rated tools are available for assessing aspects of hoarding disorder.
- The SI–R is a self-report measure that assesses the core diagnostic features of hoarding, including difficulty discarding, excessive acquisition, and clutter accumulation, and is most suitable for clients with good or fair insight.
- To measure and communicate with other human service professionals about clutter volume, the CIR tool is recommended. Clients or clinicians select photos to indicate the level of clutter present in the main living areas.
- Both the ADL–H and the HOMES are useful clinician-rated tools that are also appropriate for interdisciplinary consultation. Both tools are helpful in identifying problems with everyday activities due to clutter (e.g., sleeping in bed, cooking in kitchen).
  - In addition, HOMES targets health and safety threats (e.g., vulnerable persons present in the home, blocked exits).
  - Although HOMES was developed with wide consultation from frontline professionals, reliability and validity have not been formally evaluated for this measure.

REFERENCES

American Psychiatric Association. (2013). *Diagnostic and statistical manual of mental disorders* (5th ed.). Arlington, VA: American Psychiatric Press.

Ayers, C. R., Saxena, S., Espejo, E., Twamley, E. W., Granholm, E., & Wetherell, J. L. (2014). Novel treatment for geriatric hoarding disorder: An open trial of cognitive rehabilitation paired with behavior therapy. *American Journal of Geriatric Psychiatry, 22*, 248–252. doi:10.1016/j.jagp.2013.02.010

Ayers, C. R., Saxena, S., Golshan, S., & Wetherell, J. L. (2010). Age at onset and clinical features of late life compulsive hoarding. *International Journal of Geriatric Psychiatry, 25*(2), 142–149. doi:10.1002/gps.2310

Ayers, C. R., Wetherell, J. L., Golshan, S., & Saxena, S. (2011). Cognitive-behavioral therapy for geriatric compulsive hoarding. *Behaviour Research and Therapy, 49*, 689–694. doi:10.1016/j.brat.2011.07.002

Bratiotis, C., Schmalisch, C. S., & Steketee, G. (2011). *The hoarding handbook: A guide for human service professionals*. New York, NY: Oxford University Press.

Bratiotis, C., & Woody, S. (2013). Community interventions for hoarding. In R. O. Frost & G. Steketee (Eds.), *The Oxford handbook of hoarding and acquiring* (pp. 316–330). New York, NY: Oxford University Press.

Bratiotis, C., Woody, S. R., & Lauster, N. (2016). *Case management: An intervention strategy for addressing hoarding*. Manuscript submitted for publication.

Dong, X., Simon, M. A., Mosqueda, L., & Evans, D. A. (2012). The prevalence of elder self-neglect in a community-dwelling population: Hoarding, hygiene, and environmental hazards. *Journal of Aging and Health, 24,*507–524. doi:10.1177/0898264311425597

Faber, H. (1947). Homer Collyer, Harlem recluse, found dead at 70. *New York Times*, 22.

Frost, R. O., Hristova, V., Steketee, G., & Tolin, D. F. (2013). Activities of Daily Living Scale in hoarding disorder. *Journal of Obsessive-Compulsive and Related Disorders, 2,* 85–90. doi:10.1016/j.jocrd.2012.12.004

Frost, R. O., Pekereva-Kochergina, A., & Maxner, S. (2011). The effectiveness of a biblio-based support group for hoarding disorder. *Behaviour Research and Therapy, 49*(10), 628–634. doi:10.1016/j.brat.2011.06.010

Frost, R. O., Ruby, D., & Shuer, L. J. (2012). The Buried in Treasures workshop: Waitlist control trial of facilitated support groups for hoarding. *Behaviour Research and Therapy, 50,* 661–667. doi:10.1016/j.brat.2012.08.004

Frost, R. O., Steketee, G., & Grisham, J. (2004). Measurement of compulsive hoarding: Saving Inventory—Revised. *Behaviour Research and Therapy, 42,* 1163–1182.

Frost, R. O., Steketee, G., Tolin, D. F., & Renaud, S. (2008). Development and validation of the clutter image rating. *Journal of Psychopathology and Behavioral Assessment, 30,* 193–203. doi:10.1007/s10862-007-9068-7

Gilliam, C. M., Norberg, M. M., Villavicencio, A., Morrison, S., Hannan, S. E., & Tolin, D. F. (2011). Group cognitive-behavioral therapy for hoarding disorder: An open trial. *Behaviour Research and Therapy, 49*(11), 802–807. doi:10.1016/j.brat.2011.08.008

Grisham, J. R., Frost, R. O., Steketee, G., Kim, H., & Hood, S. (2006). Age of onset of compulsive hoarding. *Journal of Anxiety Disorders, 20,* 675–686. doi:10.1016/j.janxdis.2005.07.004

Hartl, T. L., & Frost, R. O. (1999). Cognitive-behavioral treatment of compulsive hoarding: A multiple baseline experimental case study. *Behaviour Research and Therapy, 37,* 451–461. doi:10.1016/S0005-7967(98)00130-2

Iervolino, A. C., Perroud, N., Fullana, M. A., Guipponi, M., Cherkas, L., Collier, D. A., & Mataix-Cols, D. (2009). Prevalence and heritability of compulsive hoarding: A twin study. *American Journal of Psychiatry, 166,* 1156–1161. doi:10.1176/appi.ajp.2009.08121789

Logan, D. E., & Marlatt, G. A. (2010). Harm reduction therapy: A practice-friendly review of research. *Journal of Clinical Psychology, 66,* 201–214.

Maier, T. (2004). On phenomenology and classification of hoarding: A review. *Acta Psychiatrica Scandinavica, 110,* 323–337. doi:10.1111/j.1600-0447.2004.00402.x

Marlatt, G. A., & Tapert, S. F. (1993). Harm reduction: Reducing the risks of addictive behaviors. In J. S. Baer, G. A. Marlatt, & R. J. McMahon (Eds.), *Addictive behaviors across the lifespan: Prevention, treatment, and policy issues* (pp.243–273). Thousand Oaks, CA: Sage

Miller, W. R., & Rollnick, S. (1991). *Motivational interviewing: Preparing people to change*. New York, NY: Guilford Press.

Miller, W. R., & Rollnick, S. (2002). *Motivational interviewing: Preparing people to change* (3rd ed.). New York, NY: Guilford Press.

Muroff, J., Steketee, G., Bratiotis, C., & Ross, A. (2012). Group cognitive and behavioral therapy and bibliotherapy for hoarding: A pilot trial. *Depression and Anxiety, 29,* 597–604. doi:10.1002/da.21923

Muroff, J., Underwood, P., & Steketee, G. (2014). *Group treatment for hoarding disorder: Therapist guide*. New York, NY: Oxford University Press.

Sampson, J. M., Yeats, J. R., & Harris, S. M. (2012). An evaluation of an ambiguous loss based psycho-educational support group for family members of persons who hoard: A pilot study. *Contemporary Family Therapy, 34*, 566–581. doi:10.1007/s10591-012-9214-6

Steketee, G. (2014). Individual cognitive and behavioral treatment for hoarding. In R. O. Frost & G. Steketee (Eds.), *The Oxford handbook of hoarding and acquiring* (pp. 260–273). New York, NY: Oxford University Press.

Steketee, G., & Frost, R. O. (2014). *Treatment for hoarding disorder: Therapist guide* (2nd ed.). New York, NY: Oxford University Press.

Steketee, G., Frost, R. O., Tolin, D. F., Rasmussen, J., & Brown, T. A. (2010). Waitlist-controlled trial of cognitive behavior therapy for hoarding disorder. *Depression and Anxiety, 27*, 476–484. doi:10.1002/da.20673

Timpano, K. R., Exner, C., Glaesmer, H., Rief, W., Keshaviah, A., Brahler, E., & Wilhelm, S. (2011). The epidemiology of the proposed *DSM-5* hoarding disorder: Exploration of the acquisition specifier, associated features, and distress. *Journal of Clinical Psychiatry, 72*, 780–786. doi:10.4088/JCP.10m06380

Tolin, D. F., Fitch, K. E., Frost, R. O., & Steketee, G. (2010). Family informants' perceptions of insight in compulsive hoarding. *Cognitive Therapy and Research, 34*(1), 69–81. doi:10.1007/s10608-008-9217-7

Tolin, D. F., Frost, R. O., & Steketee, G. (2012). Working with hoarding vs. non-hoarding clients: A survey of professionals' attitudes and experiences. *Journal of Obsessive-Compulsive and Related Disorders, 1*(1), 48–53. doi:10.1016/j.jocrd.2011.11.004

Tolin, D. F., Frost, R. O., & Steketee, G. (2014). *Buried in treasures: Help for compulsive acquiring, saving, and hoarding* (2nd ed.). New York, NY: Oxford University Press.

Tolin, D. F., Frost, R. O., Steketee, G., & Fitch, K. E. (2008). Family burden of compulsive hoarding: Results of an internet survey. *Behaviour Research and Therapy, 46*, 434–443. doi:10.1016/j.brat.2007.12.008

Tolin, D. F., Frost, R. O., Steketee, G., Gray, K. D., & Fitch, K. E. (2008). The economic and social burden of compulsive hoarding. *Psychiatry Research, 160*, 200–211.

Tolin, D. F., Frost, R. O., Steketee, G., & Muroff, J. (2015). Cognitive behavioral therapy for hoarding disorder: A meta-analysis. *Depression and Anxiety, 32*(3), 158–166. doi:10.1002/da.22327

Tompkins, M. A., & Hartl, T. L. (2007). *Digging out: Helping your loved one manage clutter, hoarding, and compulsive acquiring*. Oakland, CA: New Harbinger Publications.

Westra, H. A., & Dozois, D. J. (2006). Preparing clients for cognitive behavioral therapy: A randomized pilot study of motivational interviewing for anxiety. *Cognitive Therapy and Research, 30*(4), 481–498.

CHAPTER 6

ANIMAL HOARDING

Bronwen Williams

Animal hoarding is under-recognized and poorly understood, but is believed to occur in most communities and cultures. Animal hoarding creates considerable risks to the individuals involved, especially older and vulnerable adults, as well as those trying to support or help them and the wider community. It can cause significant suffering to the animals hoarded. It is often accompanied by considerable self-neglect. Animal hoarding requires a multi-agency approach; however, professionals regularly dismiss situations of animal hoarding as simply being a lifestyle choice. Nurses and other health professionals have a role in identifying possible animal-hoarding situations. This chapter aims to increase the awareness of animal hoarding by providing a brief overview and definition of animal hoarding; epidemiology; characteristics of animal hoarders; risks assessment; types of hoarding, and multidisciplinary interventions.

Around half of all households in the United Kingdom (Reynolds, 2006) and two thirds of all households in the United States own a companion animal. Many of these pets are considered family members (Herzog, 2011). In cases of blindness or cognitive disorders in children such as autism, having an animal in the home is considered therapeutic. Therefore, many older adults, with whom health professionals work, are likely to own animals or live in environments where animals are kept. The companionship and therapeutic value provided by animals on physical and psychological well-being in older adults are acknowledged (Cherniack & Cherniack, 2014; Matchock, 2015; Williams, 2015). However, when animal ownership changes to hoarding the risks to humans, animals, and communities can be high.

Hoarding behavior as a diagnosis is listed in the fifth edition of the *Diagnostic and Statistical Manual of Mental Disorders* (DSM-5; American Psychiatric Association [APA], 2013). The *DSM-5*'s criteria for hoarding include the need to keep belongings, difficulty in discarding or parting with them, experiencing distress when this occurs, the building up of clutter that impairs living areas, and impairments in the individual's functioning. However, it is not yet clear from research or the *DSM-5* whether the hoarding of animals can be included within a hoarding disorder classification, as the types of hoarded objects are not defined (Frost, Patronek, Arluke, & Stekette, 2015). *Animal hoarding* is defined as "the accumulation of a large number of animals and a failure to provide minimal standards of nutrition, sanitation, and veterinary care and to act on the deteriorating conditions of the animals (such as disease, starvation, or death) and the environment (such as severe overcrowding or extremely unsanitary conditions)" (APA, 2013, p. 249). Animals are generally considered to be owned property and therefore can be deemed "property" that is hoarded. Although animal hoarding is mentioned within the description of hoarding (Patronek & Nathanson, 2016), many authors highlight that animal hoarding appears to be different than the hoarding of objects (Frost, Patronek, & Rosenfield, 2011; Patronek & Ayers, 2014; Patronek & Nathanson, 2009; Slyne, Tolin, Stekette, & Frost, 2013).

Animal hoarding can create numerous health and safety risks, with serious, and sometimes fatal, consequences for both humans and animals. Yet animal-hoarding research has not yet received the same recognition and examination as hoarding of objects (Patronek & Nathanson, 2009). Animal hoarding has, for some years, received media attention, which has fuelled a fascination by the public, and the hoarding is often viewed as humorous. This belittles the problem, which inflicts a terrible and often life-threatening existence on those humans and animals living within a hoarded environment. The British Psychological Society (2015) called for the media to address all forms of hoarding in a more appropriate and sensitive manner, but it is not yet evident whether this guidance will be accepted and applied. Some hoarders are prosecuted for animal cruelty and no identification or association is made to animal hoarding. Animal hoarding is poorly understood; prosecution is often an incomplete solution and fails to address the possible physical or mental health components of animal hoarding (Patronek & Ayers, 2014).

Animal hoarding appears to differ from object hoarding in a number of ways. A more significant lack of insight can be apparent in those who hoard animals than those who hoard objects (Patronek & Nathanson, 2016). There tends to be considerably more squalor in animal hoarding, with even basic sanitation unavailable (Frost et al., 2011; Patronek & Nathanson, 2016). Whereas object hoarders tend to keep almost any item, animal hoarders are specific in what they keep, usually only one species of animal; some are known to keep different types of animals as well. Most object hoarders passively acquire items, whereas some types of animal hoarders also acquire passively, many actively seek out more animals. Object hoarding may be more prevalent in men, whereas animals are hoarded more frequently by women. Animal hoarding usually occurs later in life, whereas object hoarding often starts in childhood (Frost et al., 2011).

EPIDEMIOLOGY OF ANIMAL HOARDING

Animal hoarding is believed to occur in most communities (Clavo et al., 2014; Patronek, 1999) and is both under-recognized and under-reported. Its prevalence is unknown as no large-scale epidemiological studies on animal hoarding have been undertaken (Patronek & Ayes, 2014). However, animal hoarding is more prevalent than is often realized; approximately 3,000 new cases of animal hoarding are reported annually in the United States (Arluke & Patronek, 2013; Calvo, Duarte, Bowen, Bulbena, & Fatjó, 2014). Arluke and Patronek (2013) estimate (using current numbers of reported cases) that in the United States there would be a minimum of 5,100 cases for the entire population, which would involve nearly a quarter of a million animals per year. As there is an under-reporting of animal hoarding it is likely that the numbers are higher (Arluke & Patronek, 2013).

Animal hoarding causes "starvation, illness, and death of animals, neglect of self and others and household destruction" (Patronek & Nathanson, 2009, p. 275), with consequences for communities and agencies. The ownership, or the keeping of a number of animals is, in itself, not indicative of animal hoarding (Patronek, 1999), rather it is the manner in which the animals are kept that indicates a problem. In an animal-hoarding situation, animals are kept in an environment that does not meet their individual and species needs, usually through lack of care, inadequate or inappropriate diet, and little or no exercise or veterinary attention (Castrodale et al., 2010). Calvo et al. (2014) found that in most cases no food or water is available for the animals. Animals are generally left undernourished and are unwell. They frequently die and it is not unusual for their bodies to remain in hoarded environments; left to decompose or, quite commonly, stored in freezers (Arluke & Patronek, 2013). Hoarded animals, when removed from a hoarding situation, tend to have poor outcomes (Arluke & Patronek, 2013). Most need to be euthanized because of severe health problems; many that do survive are not suitable for new homes as they are unsocialized and have profound behavioral problems (Patronek & Nathanson, 2009).

Cats tend to be the type of animal most often hoarded, yet in Australia, dogs were the most commonly hoarded species (Joffe, O'Shannessy, Dhand, Westman, & Fawcett, 2014). Other animals hoarded frequently include small mammals, birds, reptiles, and larger animals such as horses, cattle, goats, and sheep (Arluke & Frost, 2002). Often different species are hoarded within the same environment. Native wildlife may also be hoarded (Ockenden, De Groef, & Marston, 2014). Svanberg and Arluke (2016) describe a well-known Swedish case in which a 68-year-old woman was found to be keeping 11 wild swans in a small apartment.

The properties where animal hoarding occurs are usually ordinary, average-sized homes, but vehicles can also be used (Berry, Patronek, & Lockwood, 2005). The average number of hoarded animals is 40, but can be fewer (Calvo et al., 2014), and may be in the hundreds (Frost & Steketee, 2010). Animals can be kept within a property and allowed free access to all areas, or kept in crates or cages that are sometimes stacked on top of each other (Arluke et al., 2002); in some hoarding situations animals are kept outdoors (Calvo et al., 2014). It is worth noting that animal hoarders do not always live at the hoarded property (Calvo et al., 2014). However, professionals should also be aware that there do not need to be unusually large numbers of animals being kept to make it a hoarded situation; rather it is the lack of adequate care for the animals that begins to define an environment as an animal hoard. Professionals and agencies also need to be aware that animal hoarders do not always present as the stereotypical isolated "cat lady."

CHARACTERISTICS OF ANIMAL HOARDERS

The general perception of animal hoarders is that they are female, older and solitary, probably keeping a number of cats, which, to a certain extent, is supported by research (Frost et al., 2015). Evidence shows that animal hoarders are typically middle-aged or older, 75% are female (Arluke & Frost, 2002; Frost & Steketee, 2010), are more likely to live alone, be secretive (Patronek & Hoarding of Animals Research Consortium [HARC], 2001), and to be socially isolated (Patronek & Nathanson, 2009). However, this is not always the case. A Spanish study by Calvo et al. (2014) found that just under half of animal hoarders were men. Steketee and colleagues (2011) identified that just over 50% of animal-hoarding households had other persons living within it, in addition to the identified hoarder. Similarly, Ockenden et al. (2014), who studied 22 animal hoarders in Australia, found that more than half had other people living with them, four (18%) of whom were parents or elderly family members. Therefore, health professionals should bear in mind that older people may be living within an animal-hoarding situation in which a partner or a younger relative is the person with the hoarding behavior. The problem of animal hoarding may also relate to social breakdown and highly complex living situations, a consequence of "personal, familial, neighborhood, or community social problems" (Arluke & Patronek, 2013, p.203). The literature is clear that some form of mental health issue is a consistent theme in those who hoard animals.

Animal Hoarding and Mental Health Issues

Most animal hoarders have coexisting mental health problems; often complex illnesses, which can include significant psychotic disorders, depression, anxiety, and posttraumatic stress disorder (Patronek, Loar, & Nathanson, 2006). A usual and problematical issue that occurs in those who hoard animals is rigid thinking. Individuals present with what might be seen as delusional thinking as they argue that their animals are well and happy when it is very evident that this is not the case (Calvo et al., 2014; Reinisch, 2008; Vaca-Guzman & Arluke, 2005). These rigid belief systems are usually combined with high levels of emotional attachment to the animals (Patronek & Nathanson, 2009). Hoarders often believe that they have a special affinity with their animals, that they are able to understand the animals' needs better than anyone else, and some describe having an almost telepathic or magical connection with their animals (Frost & Steketee, 2010).

Saldarriaga-Cantillo and Rivas (2015) report on a case they term *Noah syndrome,* a variant of Diogenes syndrome. Diogenes syndrome is a behavioral disorder in older people that presents with extreme self-neglect and hoarding tendencies. Noah syndrome is described as the hoarding of animals, combined with an absence of awareness of the impact of the conditions on both the humans and the animals involved (Saldarriaga-Cantillo & Rivas, 2015). The existence of comorbid mental health problems, often complex ones, in those who hoard animals means that skilled and detailed assessments are required.

ASSESSMENT

Animal hoarders, in addition to holding fixed beliefs about their animals and their care, often have rigid beliefs about the world, seeing it as a hostile place and are suspicious of anyone trying to help them. Patronek and Nathanson (2009) have found that animal hoarders tend to be hyper vigilant and have exaggerated threat appraisal. It is suggested that those working with them avoid official paraphernalia (Patronek & HARC, 2001) and not use arguments or persuasion to try to get the individual to change his or her behavior. Workers should be mindful that animal hoarders' primary relationships tend to be with animals rather than humans (Patronek & Nathanson, 2009). The building of trusting and therapeutic relationships is key but is likely to take time and persistence. Health professionals also need to be conscious of any risk of violence from the hoarder. It can be useful to seek someone to assist in engaging with the individual, perhaps a family member, friend, or a veterinary surgeon if appropriate.

The client's physical ability to care for his or her animals should be assessed. This requires those undertaking the assessment to know what types and what numbers of animals are being kept. Older or unwell animals require time for their care, as do those species or breeds with special requirements, such as the grooming of long coats. These issues need to be considered, with animal welfare guidance and advice on care sought, if necessary. The client's mental capacity, his or her ability to understand the animals' requirements, how this affects the care given, and how the client make decisions for the animals in his or her care also needs to be assessed (Patronek & Nathanson, 2016). It does appear that there are different "types" of animal hoarders and each responds differently to assessment and interventions.

TYPES OF ANIMAL HOARDING AND POSSIBLE APPROACHES TO TREATMENT

Three types of animal hoarding have been proposed: overwhelmed caregiving, rescuing, and exploitative hoarding (Frost & Steketee, 2010; Patronek et al., 2006). Often the precipitating factor for the hoarding individual, is a loss of some kind (Frost & Steketee, 2010). A sudden onset of animal hoarding has been linked to a relationship breakdown or significant health crisis. Patronek and Nathanson (2009) suggest that animal hoarding may be associated with complex grief reactions. Health professionals working with older people should be aware of this, as these life events may be common in their client group. No matter what type of animal hoarding is occurring, evidence shows that when animals are removed from a hoarding situation, recidivism occurs in almost all cases (Frost & Steketee, 2010; Patronek et al., 2006; Reinish, 2008) with hoarders acquiring more animals quickly, often within a matter of days.

Overwhelmed Caregiving

The first suggested type of animal hoarding, overwhelmed caregiving (Frost & Steketee, 2010), tends to occur gradually, often when there is a change of circumstances for the individual, such as, bereavement, loss of employment, illness, increasing disability, or reduced income. The number of animals increases, often due to the lack of neutering (Patronek & Nathanson, 2009). The overwhelmed caregiving hoarders have significant emotional attachments with their animals, and although they may recognize some of the issues that exist with the animals, they tend to minimize them. Such an individual can become known in the neighborhood as someone who takes in unwanted animals, and people then tend to bring more animals to them, thus compounding the problem (Patronek & Nathanson, 2009). A recent study (Ramos, da Cruz, Ellis, Hernandez, & Reche-Junior, 2013) examined cat owners in Brazil, where the keeping of larger numbers of animals is an accepted norm. They found that those keeping a number of cats differed from those with just one or two in that they had stronger attachments to their animals and were older. Ramos et al. (2013) hypothesize that more intense and different attachment styles may be precursors to animal hoarding.

Overwhelmed caregiving animal hoarders tend to acquire animals passively; often some are aware of the difficulties faced by their animals, and, consequently, may be persuaded to work with public and private agencies (e.g., adult protective services [APS]; public housing authorities; area agencies on aging [AAA]; mental health professionals; law enforcement officers; fire, public health, and code enforcement departments; animal control agencies; veterinarians; health and social care providers; and community leaders; Frost et al., 2015). Building a trusting and therapeutic rapport is essential in allowing an assessment of the client's mental state, which assists the client in receiving appropriate treatment for any comorbid mental and physical disorders. A helpful therapeutic relationship also allows assessment of the client's mental capacity to make decisions about his or her own welfare and that of the animals. Those working with animal hoarders need to have empathy and understanding for the intense relationships and deep attachment these individuals have with the animals they keep. This may be explained by the important role animals can play for individuals who have histories of trauma and have difficulty finding support and closeness from human relationships (Patronek & Nathanson, 2016). Professionals need to understand who is living in the household, whether there are any children and/or vulnerable adults, and make appropriate safeguarding referrals as necessary.

A multi-agency approach supporting the client to reduce the number of animals and improve the environment is key. It is essential to help the individual access veterinary care and neutering for the animals he or she owns, perhaps enlisting the help of animal charities, which may be able to find new homes for some of the animals, with the agreement of the client. Animal charities also often help with the cost of neutering.

Rescuing

In the second type of animal hoarding, rescuing (Patronek et al., 2006) or mission-driven hoarding (Frost & Steketee, 2010), hoarders actively seek and acquire more animals. They tend to be adamant that no animal should be euthanized. It is likely that this type of hoarder states that he or she is running an animal rescue or shelter and often the individual is supported by a significant network of helpers (Patronek et al., 2006). These hoarder are more reluctant to work with agencies and to reduce animal numbers or to improve their conditions (Patronek et al., 2006). Those running what they purport to be animal "rescue" centers tend to be better socially engaged, with their network of supporters helping and sustaining their behavior (Patronek et al., 2006; Patronek & Nathanson, 2009). These networks, therefore, help meet the animal hoarders' psychological and emotional needs.

Professionals working with these types of animal hoarders are likely to find that they are less amenable to help; therefore, prosecution for animal welfare offenses is more likely. Again, wherever possible, assessment of the hoarder's mental health and mental capacity should be undertaken as well as safeguarding referrals made for children and vulnerable adults, if appropriate. Patronek and Nathanson (2009) describe how individuals who have experienced poor parenting or trauma in childhood become unable to empathize with others and fail to recognize signs of distress in others. This may explain why animal hoarders often seem unable to identify that their animals are sick, suffering, and dying when it is apparent to others.

Exploitative Hoarding

The third type of animal hoarding, exploitative hoarding, is less common. Here, those responsible for the hoarding can appear to be charming and persuasive but are in fact controlling. They have a notable lack of empathy or attachment to animals or humans possibly due to antisocial or borderline personality disorders (Frost et al., 2011). The exploitative hoarder may be less easily identifiable by agencies, due to his or her plausibility, but there are major risks to humans and animals living within this type of situation. Professionals involved with these type of animal hoarders need to be very robust in considering the welfare of any children or vulnerable adults living within or coming into contact with the situation. The lack of empathy in exploitative hoarders probably is not restricted to their animals; it is likely to extend to anyone they have within their households or social groups. Workers need to be alert to the initial plausibility and charisma of these types of hoarders and not be drawn into dysfunctional and damaging dynamics.

In recent years, those working in safeguarding children have identified disguised compliance (Dumbrill, 2006), meaning abusers appear to cooperate with agencies but are "merely going through the motions" (Shemmings, Shemmings, & Cook, 2012, p. 130). Some animal hoarders, who are sociable and plausible in their explanations for the conditions of the animals they keep, are skilled in their ability to keep the agencies at bay. It may be possible that there are some similarities between the behaviors of abusive parents and caregivers of children and those who hoard animals and their use of disguised compliance.

With all types of animal hoarders, professionals need to have the ability to build good and robust therapeutic relationships with individuals as well as excellent working relationships with other agencies. Good assessment skills, clear and accurate recording, especially around a wide range of types of risks and with different types of hoarders, are vital.

RISKS

Animal hoarding creates a number of significant, complex risks to people living in the household, people visiting the property, and the surrounding community. Those doing home visits need to be aware of the possible and likely risks present when visiting an animal-hoarding situation. Professionals may only see individuals in surgeries and clinics and so need to be alert to the possibility that their clients may be living in yet unidentified animal-hoarding situations, either as the hoarder or as a member of the hoarded household.

Environmental Risks

In animal-hoarding environments, animals are often allowed free range of the property and there are usually accumulations of feces and urine, with their associated risks to human health, especially when high levels of ammonia are in the air. It is worth noting that older people have a reduced ability to cope with airborne ammonia (Reinisch, 2008). Although those living in the environment may appear to be tolerating this air pollution, those attending such cases can experience eye irritation and have difficulty breathing (Calvo et al., 2014), and agency personnel may require breathing equipment (Patronek & HARC, 2001). In addition to the effect upon the air quality, the large amounts of urine can cause structural damage to the building by causing floorboards and joists to rot (Castrodale et al., 2010), making them unsafe. In some situations, the damage is such that properties have to be demolished (Patronek & HARC, 2001).

Although hoarding of animals seems to be different than the hoarding of objects, clutter and refuse often accumulate in animal-hoarded environment. This is probably due to the inability of the hoarder to keep up with daily tasks and activities, rather than the deliberate keeping of items (Frost & Steketee, 2010). However, accumulations of items and rubbish increase the risk of vermin infestations and the inability to keep the environment appropriately clean. The smell that emanates from animal-hoarding situations is often why properties are reported. In addition, animal-hoarded households tend to have poor or no sanitation (Patronek & Nathanson, 2016; Reinisch, 2008) generally with no kitchen facilities, so that activities of daily living are compromised or impossible.

Risks to or Caused by the Animals

Animals in hoarding situations are often undernourished (Patronek & HARC, 2001) and typically do not receive routine or emergency veterinary attention (Patronek et al., 2006); therefore, dying and dead animals are not uncommon (Berry et al., 2005) with bodies often remaining on the property. Although zoonosis (the transfer of diseases between animals and people) is generally rare, within animal-hoarded households it is much more likely, and older people are more at risk for transmission (Rienisch, 2008). Hoarded animals are usually unsocialized and unwell, and sometimes different species are kept inappropriately together. Fights between animals are likely, as well as aggression toward humans, who may sustain bites and scratches (Joffe et al., 2014). Health professionals need to be alert to clients who present with injuries from animals. Some clients may even become anemic due to numerous flea bites (Joffe et al., 2014).

Risks to Humans

The number of animals, and the associated clutter and rubbish, significantly increase the risk of trips and falls, a real concern for older people. Some vulnerable adults may live within animal-hoarded environments. Reinsich (2008) found that over half of 71 animal-hoarded properties were residences for someone in addition to the hoarder and 21% of these individuals were older people and adults with disabilities.

When animals are removed from a hoarder, a significant grief reaction is likely and nurses and others may be important in supporting clients. Animal hoarders may lose their animals, homes, and possessions if a property is condemned or cleaned out. Because many animal hoarders have a history of abuse and trauma (Patronek & Nathanson, 2016), professionals need to be mindful of the possibility of this and how interventions by agencies may retraumatize these already damaged and vulnerable people. In addition, when agencies intervene, animal hoarders may also be separated from humans who are significant to them.

INTERVENTIONS

As there are wide-ranging risks associated with animal hoarding that affect individuals, the communities and professionals working with the animal hoarders as well as the related agencies need to consider all that can be done to reduce and manage animal-hoarding situations. However, there are no clear, evidence-based interventions identified for those doing psychological work with animal-hoarding clients (Patronek & Nathanson, 2016). The animal hoarder usually presents with rigid thinking, denial of any problems, and the swift reacquisition of animals when those hoarded are removed; this makes interventions by agencies very difficult. Workers can quickly become frustrated, baffled, and exhausted. Patronek and Nathanson (2009) highlight the importance of understanding an animal hoarder's history, relationships with animals, and how these impact upon identity and self-esteem. Frost et al. (2015) identify that simple, and fast approaches to animal hoarding are unlikely to work and that professionals should avoid challenging the distorted and rigid thinking commonly displayed by animal hoarders.

Medical and Psychological Approaches

Although animal hoarding has received little research attention and is poorly understood, it has been suggested that an addictions framework be considered (Reinisch, 2008) for this population. The thinking processes of those involved in animal hoarding are similar to those who have gambling or substance misuse problems (Frost, 2000). Although there is a dearth of psychological approaches, motivational interviewing, a well-recognized and evidence-based intervention for behavior change, especially addictions, has been proposed as a possibly useful approach in animal hoarding (Patronek et al., 2006). Motivational interviewing could also be used to support behavior change in relatives and caregivers to help improve the situation for an older person who is hoarding.

Saldarriaga-Cantillo and Rivas (2015) recommend that hospitalization of animal hoarders be avoided and that antipsychotic medication or antidepressants like selective serotonin reuptake inhibitors (SSRIs) may be of use, as might cognitive behavioral therapy (CBT). However, Patronek and Nathanson (2009) are clear that although SSRIs and CBTs have been used in object hoarding there is no evidence base, as yet, for interventions and treatment for those who hoard animals. It is unknown whether strategies used for object hoarders would help those who hoard animals (Frost et al., 2011). The level of intervention by services, and its likely success, depends on the type of animal hoarder (Patronek et al., 2006). Overwhelmed caregivers are most open to help to reduce the number of animals and to improve the environment (Patronek et al., 2006). For rescuer/mission-driven hoarders, legal processes are more likely to be required and for exploitative hoarders, the removal of animals and prosecution are probably the only options (Patronek et al., 2006). Koenig, Leiste, Spano, and Chaplin (2013) emphasize the importance of professionals visiting the property of a client who is hoarding and working with the client there. However, the risks involved in doing this should be carefully considered and discussed with senior colleagues and other agencies. Depending on the severity of the situation and the environment, this may not be an option.

A Multi-Agency Approach

Castrodale et al. (2010) recognize that an animal-hoarding situation may become a major incident, and multi-agency involvement and cooperation are essential. However, individual agencies tend to fail in intervening early enough in an emerging hoarding situation, often believing that the behavior is a lifestyle choice (Reinisch, 2008). These situations are complex and require the input of different authorities and state agencies such as animal welfare, veterinary professionals, sanitation, public health, mental health, social care services, emergency services, police, housing, and environmental health (Arluke & Patronek, 2013; Day & McCarthy, 2016). However, a lack of agreed-upon protocols for multi-agency approaches can hinder interventions.

Calvo et al. (2014) found that animal-hoarding situations came to light when concerns about the welfare of the animals were reported, not the welfare of the humans involved. Human health and welfare agencies tended not to have animal hoarding on their radar. This is despite substantial self-neglect common in animal hoarders and the usual neglect of any dependents (Reinisch, 2008). McGuire, Kaercher, Park, and Storch (2013) highlight that agencies lacked protocols for dealing with object hoarders and staff received no training about object hoarding. As animal hoarding is less well recognized, it is likely that this will be the case for these situations as well.

Early detection of animal hoarding is essential (Berry et al., 2005).There is a need for animal welfare organizations and human welfare agencies to cross-report, have appropriate policies (Patronek & Ayers, 2014), and to understand each others' roles. Koenig et al. (2013) describe four hoarding teams operating in Kansas that worked with older people who hoarded objects and/or animals. These teams were either organized or informal, and generally included members from animal welfare, law enforcement, mental health, nurses, other health providers, older persons' agencies, social workers, and public health officials. Although these teams may start to address the problems of delivering services to those who hoard, the authors highlight the time required and the costs involved in these interventions. Ongoing and consistent inputs by specialist providers are required. The importance of mental health practitioners being members of these teams is emphasized, but it is recognized that there is a lack of training and understanding of hoarding by those working in mental health. Koenig and colleagues (2013) also identify how the required team members often come from very different perspectives and professional backgrounds. One of the most difficult problems for these teams concerned the ethical issues surrounding capacity and the right for those who hoard to refuse help and input by agencies. A similar study by Bratiotis (2013), also done in the United States, found that the leadership, purpose, funding, and membership were key issues in the viability of hoarding teams. A significant hindrance in the provision of services to those who hoard animals is the current lack of research and an evidence base to enable professional understanding and interventions.

CONCLUSION

Animal hoarding is common yet under-reported and only the most severe cases tend to come to the attention of professionals and agencies. Animal hoarders are most often middle-aged or older females who live alone. Many animal hoarders have coexisting complex illnesses and believe they have a special affinity with their animals. Three types of animal hoarding have been identified and the assessment of associated risk is vitally important. A multi-agency approach to interventions on animal hoarding is recommended.

IMPLICATIONS FOR RESEARCH AND PRACTICE

- A greater awareness and understanding of animal hoarding has the potential to improve the way professionals and agencies intervene and respond.
- The risks associated with animal hoarding need to be understood.
- Animal hoarding requires multidisciplinary and cross-agency responses to help reduce health and safety risks.
- Future research needs to explore the causes and contributing factors present in all types of hoarding.
- Longitudinal studies on animal hoarders and interviews with their children or siblings can provide further insight on animal hoarding.
- The role of multi-agehcy efforts and how efforts are undertaken, as well as the reporting of good outcomes are an area for exploration.

REFERENCES

American Psychiatric Association. (2013). *The diagnostic and statistical manual of mental disorders* (5th ed.). Arlington, VA: American Psychiatric Publishing.

Arluke, A., & Frost, R. (2002). Health implications of animal hoarding. *Health and Social Work, 27*(2), 125–132.

Arluke, A., Frost, R., Stekette, G., Patronek, G., Luke, C., Messner, E., . . . Papazian, M. (2002). Press reports of animal hoarding. *Society and Animals, 10*, 113–135.

Arluke, A., & Patronek, G. J. (2013). Animal hoarding. In M. Brewster & C. Reyes (Eds.), *Animal cruelty: A multidisciplinary approach to understanding*. Durham, NC: Carolina Academic Press.

Berry, C., Patronek, G., & Lockwood, R. (2005). Long term outcomes in animal hoarding cases. *Animal Law, 11*, 167–194.

Bratiotis, C. (2013). Community hoarding task forces: A comparative case study of five taskforces in the United States. *Health and Social Care in the Community, 21*(3), 245–253.

British Psychological Society. (2015). *A psychological perspective on hoarding: DCP good practice guidelines*. Leicester, UK: Author.

Calvo, P., Duarte, C., Bowen, J., Bulbena, A., & Fatjó, J. (2014). Characteristics of 24 cases of animal hoarding in Spain. *Animal Welfare, 23*, 199–208.

Castrodale, L., Bellay, Y., Brown, C., Cantor, F., Gibbins, J., Headrick, M., . . . Yu, D. (2010). General public health considerations for responding to animal hoarding cases. *Journal of Environmental Health, 72*(7), 14–18.

Cherniack, E. P., & Cherniack, A. R. (2014). The benefit of pets and animal-assisted therapy to the health of older individuals. *Current Gerontology and Geriatrics Research, 2014*, 9. doi:10.1155/2014/623203

Day, M. R., & McCarthy, G. (2016). Animal hoarding: A serious public health issue. *Annuals of Nursing and Practice, 3*(4), 1054. Retrieved from http://www.jscimedcentral.com/Nursing/nursing-3-1054.pdf

Dumbrill, G. (2006). Parental experience of child protection intervention: A qualitative study. *Child Abuse & Neglect, 30*, 27–37.

Frost, R. (2000). People who hoard animals. *Psychiatric Times, 17*(4), 24–29.

Frost, R., Patronek, G., Arluke, A., & Steketee, G. (2015). The hoarding of animals: An update, *32*(4), 47–50. Retrieved from http://www.psychiatrictimes.com/addiction/hoarding-animals-update

Frost, R., Patronek, G., & Rosenfield, E. (2011). Comparison of object and animal hoarding. *Depression and Anxiety, 28*, 885–891.

Frost, R., & Steketee, G. (2010). *Stuff: Compulsive hoarding and the meaning of things*. New York, NY: Houghton Mifflin Harcourt.

Herzog, H. (2011). The impact of pets on human health and psychological well-being: Fact, fiction, or hypothesis? *Current Directions in Psychological Science, 20*(4), 236–239. doi:10.1177/0963721411415220

Joffe, M., O'Shannessy, D., Dhand, N., Westman, M., & Fawcett, A. (2014). Characteristics of persons convicted for offenses relating to animal hoarding in New South Wales. *Australian Veterinary Journal, 92*(10), 369–375.

Koenig, T., Leiste, M., Spano, R., & Chaplin, R. (2013). Multidisciplinary team perspectives on older adult hoarding and mental illness. *Journal of Elder Abuse & Neglect, 25*(1), 56–75.

Matchock, R. L. (2015). Pet ownership and physical health. *Current Opinion in Psychiatry, 28*(5), 386–392. doi:10.1097/yco.0000000000000183

McGuire, J., Kaercher, L., Park, J., & Storch, E. (2013). Hoarding in the community: A code enforcement and social service perspective. *Journal of Social Service Research, 39*, 335–334.

Ockenden, E., De Groef, B., & Marston, L. (2014). Animal hoarding in Victoria, Australia: An exploratory study. *Anthrozoös, 27*(1), 33–48.

Patronek, G. (1999). The hoarding of animals: An under recognized public health problem in a difficult to study population. *Public Health Reports, 114*, 81–90.

Patronek, G., & Ayers, C. (2014). Animal hoarding. In R. Frost & G. Steketee (Eds.), *The Oxford handbook of hoarding and acquiring*. Oxford, UK: Oxford University Press.

Patronek, G., & Hoarding of Animals Research Consortium. (2001). The problem of animal hoarding. *Municipal Lawyer, 19*, 6–9.

Patronek, G., Loar, L., & Nathanson, J. (Eds.). (2006). *Animal hoarding: Structuring interdisciplinary responses to help people, animals and communities at risk*. North Grafton, MA: Hoarding of Animals Research Consortium Retrieved from http://vet.tufts.edu/wp-content/uploads/AngellReport.pdf

Patronek, G., & Nathanson, J. (2009). A theoretical perspective to inform assessment and treatment strategies for animal hoarders. *Clinical Psychology Review, 29*, 274–281.

Patronek, G., & Nathanson, J. (2016). Understanding animal neglect and hoarding. In L. Levitt, G. Patronek, & T. Grisso (Eds.), *Animal maltreatment: Forensic mental health issues and evaluations*. Oxford, UK: Oxford University Press.

Ramos, D., da Cruz, N., Ellis, S., Hernandez, J., & Reche-Junior, A. (2013). Early stage animal hoarders: Are these owners of large numbers of adequately cared-for cats? *Bulletin of Human Animal Interaction, 1*(1), 55–69.

Reinisch, A. (2008). Understanding the human aspects of animal hoarding. *Canadian Veterinary Journal, 49*(12), 1211–1214.

Reynolds, A. (2006). The therapeutic potential of companion animals. *Nursing & Residential Care, 8*(11), 504–507.

Saldarriaga-Cantillo, A., & Rivas, N. (2015). Noah syndrome: A variant of Diogenes syndrome accompanied by animal hoarding practices. *Journal of Elder Abuse & Neglect, 27*(3), 270–275.

Shemmings, D., Shemmings, Y., & Cook, A. (2012). Gaining the trust of 'highly resistant' families: Insights from attachment theory and research. *Child and Family Social Work, 17*, 130–137.

Slyne, K., Tolin, D., Steketee, G., & Frost, R. (2013). Characteristics of animal owners among individuals with object hoarding. *Journal of Obsessive-Compulsive and Related Disorders, 2*(4), 466–471.

Steketee, G., Gibson, A., Frost, R. O., Alabiso, J., Arluke, A., & Patronek, G. (2011). Characteristics and antecedents of people who hoard animals: An exploratory comparative interview study. *Review of General Psychology, 15*(2), 114–124.

Svanberg, I., & Arluke, A. (2016). The Swedish Swan Lady: Reaction to an apparent animal hoarding case. *Society and Animals, 24*, 63–77.

Vaca-Guzman, M., & Arluke, A. (2005). Normalizing passive cruelty: The excuses and justifications of animal hoarders. *Anthrozoös, 18*(4), 338–357.

Williams, B. (2015). Service users and their animals: Considerations for mental health professionals. *Mental Health Practice, 18*(7), 32–37.

CHAPTER 7

FARM ANIMALS AND FARMERS: NEGLECT ISSUES

Catherine Devitt and Alison Hanlon

The bond between animal owners and their animals is important for farm animal welfare and farmers' well-being. Understanding the nuances and complexities of this relationship is central to developing interventions that seek to improve the well-being of both animals and farmers. Farmer willingness and capacity are important factors for maintaining animal welfare standards. Yet, farmers are highly exposed to a range of occupational, environmental, and locational stressors that lead to high stress levels, depression, and anxiety, and erode the variables necessary for positive care of animals. Farmers' age, illness, limited availability of farm help, and more severe issues associated with an accumulation of stress and mental illness point to the potential for self-neglect to occur in farmers. This chapter draws on qualitative research to explore the relationship between human problems and farm animal neglect. The chapter concludes with the guiding principles for determining interventions that may help promote farmer and animal well-being.

An overview on the topic of farm animal welfare and neglect, outlining the historical trajectories and core farm animal welfare legislation, is presented first. What follows is an introduction to farm animal welfare in Ireland and a summary of the contemporary agricultural profile. The authors then proceed to explain the importance of the human–animal bond in explaining farm animal welfare outcomes, including neglect, and draws on relevant research from Ireland and elsewhere. Presented in the conclusion are guiding principles on determining the best way forward in the prevention of both animal neglect and self-neglect among farmers.

EMERGENCE OF FARM ANIMAL WELFARE

The latter half of the 20th century witnessed a shift in the organization and implementation of farming practices in Europe. Underpinning this shift were innovations in technology, increasing demand for food at an affordable price, and the provision of financial supports for farmers. Consequently, farming in Europe became more intensified, industrialized, and specialized. Although increased food production allowed for increased food security, these changes also resulted in bigger farms, increased output, and on-farm mechanization, as well as a decline in the ratio of farmers to animals

TABLE 7.1 An Outline of the Five Freedoms Framework for Animal Welfare Provision

Five Freedoms	Five Provisions
Freedom from hunger, thirst, and malnutrition	Ready access to fresh water and a diet to maintain full health and vigor
Freedom from discomfort	Providing a suitable environment, including shelter, and a comfortable resting area
Freedom from pain, injury, and disease	Prevention or rapid diagnosis and treatment
Freedom from fear and distress	Ensuring conditions to avoid mental suffering
Freedom to express normal behavior	Providing sufficient space, proper facilities, and company of the animal's own kind

(D. Fraser, 2008; Hendrickson & Miele, 2009). Although small family farms remain, the trend is for larger industrial farms.

Changes in food-production processes adversely affect farm animal welfare standards, as documented in Ruth Harrison's (1964) book *Animal Machines*, which exposed the deteriorating welfare conditions of farmed animals. One year later, the publication of the Brambell Report (1965) in the United Kingdom helped shape the emergence of legislation on animal welfare, not only in the United Kingdom, but also in Europe (Broom, 2011; Farm Animal Welfare Council [FAWC], 2009; Veissier, Butterworth, Bock, & Roe, 2008). A compassionate human focus toward animals dates back to 1635 in Ireland when the first animal protection law was introduced. Hanlon and Magalhães-Sant' Ana (2014) described the emergence of zoocentrism and increasing societal concerns toward the treatment of animals, leading to a new social ethic for animals (Rollin, 1999). Increased understanding of the association between animal and human health (referred to as "One Health"), acknowledgement of animals as sentient beings, changes in the governance of farming, increased urbanization, and changing rural/urban dynamics have all contributed to changes in human–animal relationships and societal perceptions of appropriate animal welfare conditions. As a consequence, these changes have pushed animal welfare as a topic into mainstream public and political conversations, resulting in regulatory frameworks (Broom, 2016; Buller & Morris, 2003; D. Fraser, 2014). The Five Freedoms and Provisions (FAWC, 1993) is an established framework providing guidance on animal welfare (Table 7.1). The Freedoms identify responsibilities of those who care for animals and the potential for animal neglect.

DEFINING FARM ANIMAL NEGLECT

Animal neglect is a poorly defined concept. In the legal context, it is synonymous with animal cruelty. However, cruelty implies intent, in contrast to neglect, which is associated with an act of omission. Infringements to the Five Freedoms, which are severe and chronic in nature, where no remedial action has been taken (such as appropriate veterinary care), characterize farm animal neglect. Another defining feature is that, in practice, the focus tends to be at an individual farm level. Often reported at individual farmer level are examples of farm animal neglect (Kelly et al.,

2013), which include cases of chronic underfeeding of animals, lack of appropriate veterinary care, or unhygienic housing associated with morbidity and mortality.

FARM ANIMAL WELFARE IN IRELAND—FROM ACTS OF COMMISSION TO ACTS OF OMISSION

The regulatory approach to farm animal welfare in Ireland in the 20th century has witnessed major changes. Until 1980, the principle legislation focused on animal protection and acts of commission, providing grounds for prosecution for animal cruelty. The animals had to have suffered before legal action could be taken. In 1984, the Protection of Animals Kept for Farming Purposes Act (Statutory Instrument Ireland, s13) introduced legal concepts of animal welfare. This represented a conceptual transition from protection and cruelty to safeguarding animal welfare. However, it took a further 16 years to employ legal provisions to support this conceptual change.

In 2000, the European Communities Protection of Animals Kept for Farming Purposes Regulations (Statutory Instrument 127 of 2000) authorized government veterinary inspectors to issue welfare notices—a legal provision to instruct farmers to improve farm animal welfare. The notices were issued when farm animal welfare was compromised by the farmers because of suboptimal housing or management, thus addressing acts of omission. This approach has continued, with one significant change introduced by the Animal Health and Welfare Act in 2013, which contains a new provision regarding the physical and mental competence of the animal owner: Person incapable of taking care of animals (s15, Section 61).

THE HUMAN–ANIMAL BOND AND ITS IMPLICATIONS FOR FARM ANIMAL NEGLECT

A considerable body of literature now exists defining the association between the human–animal relationship, or bond, and animal welfare (Breuer, Hemsworth, Barnett, Matthews, & Coleman, 2000; Fukasawa, Kawahata, Higashiyama, & Komatsu, 2016; Hemsworth & Coleman, 2010; Jääskeläinen, Kauppinen, Vesala, & Valros, 2014; Kauppinen, Vesala, & Valros, 2012; Waiblinger et al., 2006). Aside from good regulation as being important for animal welfare, the bond between animal owners and their animals is fundamental to animal welfare standards, and understanding the nuances and complexities of this relationship is central to developing interventions that seek to improve the welfare and well-being of both animals and their owners (Waiblinger et al., 2006).

In the case of farm animal welfare, both animal and farmer welfare depend on there being a positive bond in place. In opposition, negative or harmful relationships can contribute to animal stress, and reduce animals' ability to produce (Hemsworth & Coleman, 2010; Kauppinen et al., 2012). Individual farmer variables can influence this bond, as well as the desire to improve welfare standards. These variables include how motivated farmers are and whether or not they feel that they have the available time and finances to carry out a particular welfare-oriented action (Kauppinen et al., 2012; Waiblinger et al., 2006). Furthermore, farmer personality, feelings of empathy toward the animals, how satisfied and confident the farmer feels in his or her work, and the extent to which the farmer has the knowledge and skills needed to carry out a particular welfare-oriented action are also important variables in influencing how farm animal welfare outcomes are affected. If farmers feel positive about their work, they are more likely to exhibit positive farmer welfare-related perceptions and behavior, which will transfer to a positive outcome for farm animal welfare. The converse may also occur. Overall, farm animal welfare outcomes are related to farmer attitudes and behavior, and welfare outcomes, whether good or bad, reinforce this relationship. Therefore, a positive human–animal bond can reduce the stress of farming, while improving and maintaining job-satisfaction levels (Hemsworth, 2003; Kolstrup & Hultgren, 2011). A number of sociologists, such as Tovey (2003), argue that for farmers, caring for their animals provides an important element of farmer identity and what it means to be a good farmer (Van Huik & Bock, 2007).

Farmers at Risk

Farmers are particularly at risk of experiencing a range of stressors that may amplify the risk of human self-neglect and erode the relationship between them and their animals. As a profession, farming is vulnerable to high levels of stress, depression, and mental health problems (Firth, Williams, Herbison, & McGee, 2007; C. E. Fraser et al., 2005; Parry, Barnes, Lindsey, & Taylor, 2005), and relative to other professions, farmers experience high suicide rates (Andersen, Hawgood, Klieve, Kõlves, & De Leo, 2010; Cleary, Feeney, & Macken-Walsh, 2012; C. E. Fraser et al., 2005; Lobley, 2005). Social and psychosocial risk factors, which can extend to include not only farmers, but also farm workers and members of the farming family (Kolstrup et al., 2013), can be grouped according to occupational stressors, environmental stressors, and locational stressors (Lizer & Petera, 2007).

In comparison to other types of farming activities, smallholder farmers, rurally isolated farmers, livestock farmers, as well as farmers engaged in manual work at a later stage in life may be more vulnerable to occupational and environmental stress (Cleary et al., 2012; Kolstrup et al., 2013; Parry et al., 2005; Sanne, Mykletun, Moen, Dahl, & Tell, 2004). In addition, a relationship breakdown or death of a partner or family member, age, and an illness can also increase vulnerability to stressors (Fennell, Jarrett, Kettler, Dollman, & Turnball, 2016; Firth et al., 2007), and may activate an on-farm welfare crisis for farmer and farm animal neglect. A farm crisis—such as an animal disease outbreak—can further amplify farmer stress and the potential for a stress disorder (Olff, Koeter, Van Haaften, Kersten, & Gersons, 2005). Although farmers engaged in smallholdings may be more at risk, agricultural intensification can also increase risk exposure to occupational stressors and negatively affect human–animal interactions as animals become dehumanized under intensive systems of production, and farmer empathy may potentially become eroded (Bock, Van Huik, Prutzer, Kling Eveillard, & Dockes, 2007; Porcher, 2006). Experiences of stress, depression, and anxiety are associated with impaired functioning and performance on the farm, as well as compromised farm safety (Haslam, Loughnan, Reynold, & Wilson, 2005; Stallones, Marx, Garrity, & Johnson, 2004). Evidence suggests that some farmers may choose not to ask for help or seek support because of denial, a strong sense of self-reliance and stoicism, and/or a fear of stigma (Devitt, Kelly, Blake, Hanlon, & More, 2015; Hossain, Eley, Coutts, & Gorman, 2008; Morrissey, Clarke, Hynes, & O'Donoghue, 2009; Morrissey, Daly, Clarke, Ballas, & O'Donoghue, 2009). Yet, poor access to appropriate health and psychiatric services because of the rural location and isolation of farms may also help explain the failure of farmers to avail themselves of the necessary social, health, and psychiatric support services.

Focusing on Ireland, in recent times, rural Irish society has witnessed a process of change, underpinned particularly by economic decline and rural restructuring (Furey, O'Hora, McNamara, Kinsella, & Noone,2016).The impact of a changing agricultural and rural context on Irish farmers is evident in Cleary et al.'s (2012) study on pain and distress in rural Ireland. In their qualitative study, the authors attributed stress and disillusionment among Irish farmers to economic vulnerability; changing farm systems; and difficulties related to keeping up with social, cultural, and technological adaptation. Farmers spoke about trying to cope with financial difficulties often associated with small farms, regulations, and the rate of rural change. Older farmers reported feeling marginalized in terms of emerging, modern rural norms (Clearly et al., 2012). According to Macken-Walsh (2011), stories of rural life in Ireland are often based upon narratives of unhappiness and desperation.

Irish farmers have the highest all-cause mortality rate in comparison to other occupational cohorts (Smyth, Evans, Kelly, Cullen, & O'Donovan, 2013). A high proportion of psychiatric inpatient admissions in rural areas (Morrissey, Clarke, et al., 2009; Morrissey, Daly, et al., 2009) are more at risk of suicide and are often directly exposed to suicide (Ní Laoire, 2001). Findings from a 2012 survey on mental health in Ireland observed that 15% of farmers experience mental health problems; however, the majority (72%) would not want others to know about their mental health problem. Furthermore, over 30% would delay seeking treatment and hide their mental health problem (see Change, 2012).

Implications of At-Risk Farmers on Farm Animal Welfare and Neglect

Kelly, More, Blake, and Hanon (2011) and Kelly et al. (2013) researched the identification of key performance indicators for farm animal welfare incidents in Ireland and determined, four indicators of neglect on the farms studied (where an incident of neglect had occurred) using two national databases operated by the Department of Agriculture, Food and Fisheries. The indicators of welfare problems on the case farms included high rates of animal mortality and unburied carcasses, a history of animal welfare problems, issues with animal registering, and poor farm management skills (Kelly et al., 2011). Notably, the researchers observed health issues among farmers, such as alcohol addiction, depression, and problems following the death of a parent, and stress from increased paperwork, which contributed to and underpinned the neglect incident (Kelly et al., 2011). Kelly et al. (2011, 2013) raised important questions about the relationship between problematic human experiences and farm animal welfare in Ireland.

Although farmers recognize the importance of the human–animal bond, they also recognize that ensuring their own sense of well-being and welfare can be difficult (Kauppinen et al., 2012). In the context of human self-neglect, an important defining characteristic associated with farm animal neglect is the psychological state of the farmer (Andrade & Anneberg, 2014; Devitt et al., 2015; Kelly et al., 2011). Furthermore, the affective mental state and intention of the farmer may be a key differential factor between farm animal neglect and animal cruelty. Social, personal and financial problems can combine to disrupt everyday farming patterns, resulting in an inability to manage everyday farming activities, increasing the risks to farm animal welfare standards and the potential for farm animal neglect and self-neglect among farmers (Andrade & Anneberg, 2014; Day, Leahy-Warren, & McCarthy, 2013; Devitt et al., 2015). Andrade and Anneberg (2014) identify "narratives of disruption"—an accumulation of crises in the farmer's life, which can then have consequences for the normal functioning of the human–animal bond (Andrade & Anneberg, 2014).

Research conducted by Devitt et al. (2015) found that age-related (physical) difficulties and a limited availability of farm help affected farmers' ability to carry out everyday farming activities, resulting in incidents of farm animal neglect. Older farmers recalled these difficulties within the wider context of the rural community decline in Ireland, experiences of emigration, changes in farming structure (such as the reduction in the number of smaller farmers), and the reluctance to ask for farm help and to reduce livestock numbers (Devitt et al., 2015). These experiences and situations were associated with less severe animal neglect cases. Drawing on what we know regarding the human–animal bond and its relationship with animal welfare, the range of stressors recalled in the Devitt et al. (2015) study undoubtedly affects farmers' satisfaction, motivation, and work performance (farmer willingness and capacity), and, in turn, potentially undermines the reciprocal relationship between both farmer and animal welfare. In particular, this explains the potential for farm animal neglect among farmers experiencing severe mental health problems.

Devitt et al. (2016) reported poor uptake of engagement with support services among their farmer participants, attributed to "a reluctance to seek on-farm help, a strong sense of self-reliance and farmers' inability to talk openly about their problems, even with family members, leading to problems on the farm" (p.12). Farmers failure to seek support was also reported by veterinarians working with farmers (Devitt, Kelly, Blake, Hanlon, & More, 2013, 2014), and has been attributed to a male narrative that is based upon a feeling of being able to take care of one's own problems (Andrade & Anneberg, 2014; Gullifer & Thompson, 2006).

LINK BETWEEN SELF-NEGLECT AND ANIMAL NEGLECT

Self-neglect is associated with depression, dementia, old age, isolation, poor social networks, economic decline, poor coping, and alcohol and substance abuse (Gibbons, 2009; Pickens et al., 2013). Farmer demographics (older population) and the risk factors they are exposed to—the occupational, environmental, and locational stressors previously outlined—also place them at risk of self-neglect, in particular, variables related to age, poor or reduced social networks, and poor economic circumstances. Recent narratives of self-neglecting younger adults portrayed a history of substantial financial instability, distrust, and substance abuse (Lien et al., 2016). Evidence from Devitt et al. (2015) and Andrade and Anneberg (2014) suggest that a trigger or an incident such as the death of a family member, may propel a farm situation into decline. This is in line with evidence on the variables associated with self-neglect, whereby a traumatic life event, circumstance, or life history often presents as a risk factor (see Day, Leahy-Warren, & McCarthy, 2016). Despite the risk of vulnerabilities for self-neglect increasing as the population ages (Day et al., 2016), there is no data or more qualitative observations on the prevalence of self-neglect among the farming population in Ireland. This is also despite a considerable proportion of that population belonging to an older population cohort already at risk of a range of social and psychological stressors inherent to the farming profession.

CONCLUSION

Strategies aimed at preventing self-neglect among farmers need to be underpinned and informed by an understanding of the range of occupational, locational, and environmental stressors that farmers are exposed to and that are inherent to the farming profession. Although some of these stressors can be controlled or reduced in the form of assistance, such as help with paperwork and on-farm workload, other stressors, such as those related to regulations, hazards of the physical environment, and the rural and at-times isolated nature of farming, will persist. It is recognized that securing farmer well-being is the most important strategy for improving animal welfare once welfare has been compromised (Kauppinen, Vainio, Valros, Rita, & Vesala, 2010).

Key ethical questions arise when we consider how best professionals can or should respond to farm animal neglect where there is a problematic human dimension. The answers to these questions will not be dealt with in this chapter yet their inclusion here should provoke important reflections on the challenges involved: Should the welfare of the farmer be prioritized ahead of the welfare of the animals? Can this occur in tandem? Should the animals be removed from the farm even if this action causes a further decline in farmer well-being? Regardless of the answers, there is a growing recognition that it is difficult to standardize practice when responding to farm animal welfare incidents (Anneberg, Vaarst, & Sandøe, 2013; Devitt et al., 2013, 2014).

Undeniably, the problem requires a comprehensive assessment by veterinarians and/or other professional groups of farmers' competency to care (Andrade & Anneberg, 2014; Devitt et al., 2013). Others recommend a family-centered educational approach that aims to work in partnership with the animal owner to improve human and animal well-being (FAWC, 2007; Williams & Jewell, 2012). This is very much in line with the observations from Devitt et al. (2013) regarding the potential role of family members, neighbors, and local support groups in highlighting concerns about farmer well-being and in assisting officials in achieving a solution for both farmer and the farm animals. Indeed, informal networks within the home and community have traditionally served as important sources of social and physical support for farmers, buffering the effects of stress and mental illness (Kutek, Turnball, & Fairweather-Schmidt, 2011; McLaren & Challis, 2009).

In Ireland, an Early Warning System established in 2004 represents a joint collaborative approach between a number of relevant stakeholders and agencies, including the Irish Farmers Association; the Department of Agriculture, Food and the Marine; the Irish Society for the Prevention of Cruelty to Animals; and, in some regions, the Health Service Executive. The aim of the system is to mitigate the potential for farm animal neglect by identifying and resolving welfare problems before they become critical. Clearly, any way forward needs to start with an understanding among policymakers and implementers, health and veterinarian practitioners on farmers at risk for self and animal neglect, the complexities of the human–animal bond, and the implications for farm animal welfare. Practitioners need to be able to recognize at-risk cases, the signs of self-neglect (such as hoarding, animal hoarding, squalor, reclusivity, or cognitive/functional impairment) and the signs of animal neglect (such as high prevalence of mortality and morbidity of livestock), and know what procedures must be followed in order to bring about a resolution. There can be instances in which cases of animal neglect that may not be animal hoarding or willful neglect of animals but may be incidental and associated with impairment or disability of the person, which impacts the farmers' ability to appropriately care for their animals (Ayers, Dozier, & Bratiotis, 2016). Thus, it is important to identify the underlying factors and causes associated with individuals' behaviors. Assessment of individuals' competency to care for their animals is important. Hence, ensuring that adequate and coordinated cross-reporting structures are in place, which allows the relevant professionals—veterinary, social, and health—to work together to help bring about a solution for all those involved, including the farm animals, is fundamental. This coordinated approach requires tailored information and guidelines for all professionals involved, professional confidence, and a comprehensive yet flexible multiagency structure and protocol that allows for relationship building, learning, and confidential cross-reporting among the relevant agencies (Devitt et al., 2013, 2014).

IMPLICATIONS FOR RESEARCH AND PRACTICE

- Understanding the nuances and complexities of the bond between farmers and their animals is important for developing interventions that seek to improve the welfare and well-being of both farmers and farm animals.
- Addressing self-neglect among farmers requires a multidisciplinary approach between health and social care professionals and veterinarians.
- Research into the impact of farmer mental health and empathy for animal neglect and, more broadly, better insight into early indicators of self and animal neglect in farmers is required.

REFERENCES

Andersen, K., Hawgood, J., Klieve, H., Kõlves, K., & De Leo, D. (2010). Suicide in selected occupations in Queensland: Evidence from the state suicide register. *Australian and New Zealand Journal of Psychiatry, 44,* 243–249.

Andrade, S., & Anneberg, I. (2014). Farmers under pressure. Analysis of the social conditions of cases of animal neglect. *Journal of Agricultural Environmental Ethics, 27,* 103–126.

Animal Health and Welfare Act, Ireland Statutes s15. (2013). Retrieved from https://www.agriculture .gov.ie/media/migration/animalhealthwelfare/legislation/AnimalHealthandWelfareAct060314.pdf

Anneberg, I., Vaarst, M., & Sandøe, P. (2013).To inspect, to motivate—or to do both? A dilemma for on-farm inspection of animal welfare. *Animal Welfare, 22,* 185–194.

Ayers, C. R., Dozier, M. E., & Bratiotis, C. (2016). Social responses to animal maltreatment offenders: Neglect & hoarding. In L. Levitt, T. Grisso, & G. Patronek (Eds.), *Animal maltreatment: Forensic mental health issues and evaluations* (pp. 234–250). London, UK: Oxford University Press.

Bock, B. B., Van Huik, M. M., Prutzer, M., Kling Eveillard, F., & Dockes, A. (2007). Farmers' relationship with different animals: The importance of getting close to the animals. Case studies of French, Swedish and Dutch cattle, pig and poultry farmers. *International Journal of Sociology of Food and Agriculture, 15,* 108–125.

Brambell, R. (1965). *Report of the Technical Committee to Enquire Into the Welfare of Animals Kept Under Intensive Livestock Husbandry Systems,* Cmd. (Great Britain. Parliament, pp. 1–84.), HMSO.

Breuer, K., Hemsworth, P. H., Barnett, J. L., Matthews, L. R., & Coleman, G. J. (2000). Behavioural response to humans and the productivity of commercial dairy cows. *Applied Animal Behavioural Science, 66,* 273–288.

Broom, D. (2011). A history of animal welfare science. *Acta Biotheoretica, 59,* 121–137.

Broom, D. (2016). Sentience and animal welfare: New thoughts and controversies. *Animal Sentience: An Interdisciplinary Journal on Animal Feeling, 1*(5), 11.

Buller, H., & Morris, C. (2003). Farm animal welfare: A new repertoire of nature–society relations or modernism re-embedded? *Sociologia Ruralis, 43*, 216–237.

Cleary, A., Feeney, M., & Macken-Walsh, A. (2012). *Pain and distress in rural Ireland; a qualitative study of suicidal behavior among men in rural areas.* Dublin, Ireland: University College Dublin and Teagasc. Retrieved from www.teagasc.ie/publications/2012/1333/Pain_and_Distress_in_Rural_Ireland_Report.pdf

Day, M. R., Leahy-Warren, P., & McCarthy, G. (2013). Perceptions and views of self-neglect: A client-centred perspective. *Journal of Elder Abuse & Neglect, 33*(2), 145–156.

Day, M. R., Leahy-Warren, P., & McCarthy, G. (2016). Self-neglect, ethical considerations. *Annual Review of Nursing Research, 34*(1), 89–107.

Devitt, C., Boyle, L., Teixeira, D. L., O'Connell, N. E., Hawe, M., & Hanlon, A. (2016). Pig producer perspectives on the use of meat inspection as an animal health and welfare diagnostic tool in the Republic of Ireland and Northern Ireland. *Irish Veterinary Journal, 69*, 2–11.

Devitt, C., Kelly, P., Blake, M., Hanlon, A., & More, S. J. (2013). Veterinarian challenges to providing a multi-agency response to farm animal welfare problems in Ireland: Responding to the human factor. *Revue scientifique et technique (International Office of Epizootics), 32*, 657–666.

Devitt, C., Kelly, P., Blake, M., Hanlon, A., & More, S. J. (2014). Dilemmas experienced by government veterinarians when responding professionally to farm animal welfare incidents in Ireland. *Veterinary Record Open, 1*, e000003.

Devitt, C., Kelly, P., Blake, M., Hanlon, A., & More, S. J. (2015). An investigation into the human element of on-farm animal welfare incidents in Ireland. *Sociologia Ruralis, 55*, 400–416.

European Communities. (2000). Protection of Animals Kept for Farming Purposes Regulations, 2000. Statutory Instrument No. 127/2000.

Farm Animal Welfare Council. (1993). *Second report on priorities for research and development in farm animal welfare.* London, UK: DEFRA Publications.

Farm Animal Welfare Council. (2007). *Report on stockmanship and farm animal welfare.* Retrieved from www.fawc.org.uk/pdf/stockmanship-report0607.pdf

Farm Animal Welfare Council. (2009). *Farm animal welfare in Great Britain: Past, present and future.* Retrieved from www.fawc.org.uk/pdf/ppf-report091012.pdf

Fennell, K., Jarrett, C., Kettler, L., Dollman, J., & Turnball, D. (2016). "Watching the bank balance build up then blow away and the rain clouds do the same": A thematic analysis of South Australian farmers' sources of stress during drought. *Journal of Rural Studies, 46*, 106–110.

Firth, H. M., Williams, S. M., Herbison, G. P., & McGee, R. O. (2007). Stress in New Zealand farmers. *Stress and Health, 23*, 51–58.

Fraser, C. E., Smith, K. B., Judd, F., Humphreys, J. S., Fragar, L. J., & Henderson, A. (2005). Farming and mental health problems and mental illness. *International Journal of Social Psychiatry, 51*, 340–349.

Fraser, D. (2008). *Understanding animal welfare: The science in its cultural context.* Chichester, UK: Wiley-Blackwell.

Fraser, D. (2014). The globalization of farm animal welfare. *Revue scientifique et technique (International Office of Epizootics), 33*, 33–38.

Fukasawa, M., Kawahata, M., Higashiyama, Y., & Komatsu, T. (2016). Relationship between the stockperson's attitudes and dairy productivity in Japan. *Animal Science Journal, 88*(2), 394–400. doi:10.1111/asj.12652

Furey, E., O'Hora, D., McNamara, J., Kinsella, S., & Noone, C. (2016). The roles of financial threat, social support work stress, and mental distress in dairy farmers' expectations of injury. *Frontiers in Public Health, 4*, 126–137.

Gibbons, S. W. (2009). Theory synthesis for self-neglect: A health and social phenomenon. *Nursing Research, 58,* 194–200.

Gullifer, J., & Thompson, A. (2006). Subjective realities of older male farmers: Self-perceptions of ageing and work. *Rural Society, 16,* 80–97.

Hanlon, A. J., & Magalhães-Sant'Ana, M. (2014). Zoocentrism. In H. ten Have (Ed.), *Encyclopedia of global bioethics.* Cham, Switzerland: Springer International. doi:10.1007/978-3-319-05544-2_450-1

Harrison, R. (1964). *Animal machines: The new factory farming industry.* London, UK: Vincent Stuart Publishers.

Haslam, N., Loughnan, S., Reynold, C., & Wilson, S. (2005). Dehumanization: A new perspective. *Social and Personality Psychology Compass, 1*(1), 409–422. doi:10.1111/j.1751-9004.2007.00030.x

Hemsworth, P. H. (2003). Human–animal interactions in livestock production. *Applied Animal Behavioral Science, 81,* 185–198.

Hemsworth, P. H., & Coleman, G.J. (2010). *Human–livestock interactions: The stockperson and the productivity and welfare of intensively farmed animals* (2nd ed.). Oxford, UK: CAB International.

Hendrickson, M., Miele, M., & Morgan, S. L. (2009). Changes in agriculture and food production in NAE since 1945. In B. D. McIntyre, H. R. Herren, J. Wakhungu, & R. T. Watson (Eds.), *International assessment of agricultural knowledge, science and technology for development: North America and Europe (NAE) report, agriculture at a crossroads* (Vol. 4, pp. 20–78). Washington, DC: Island Press.

Hossain, D., Eley, R., Coutts, J., & Gorman, D. (2008). Mental health of farmers in Southern Queensland: Issues and support. *Australian Journal of Rural Health, 16,* 343–348.

Jääskeläinen, T., Kauppinen, T., Vesala, K. M., & Valros, A. (2014). Relationships between pig welfare, productivity and farmer disposition. *Animal Welfare, 23,* 435–443.

Kauppinen, T., Vainio, A., Valros, A., Rita, H., & Vesala, K. M. (2010). Improving animal welfare: Qualitative and quantitative methodology in the study of farmers' attitudes. *Animal Welfare, 19,* 523–536.

Kauppinen, T., Vesala, K. M., & Valros, A. (2012). Farmer attitude toward improvement of animal welfare is correlated with piglet production parameters. *Livestock Science, 143,* 142–150.

Kelly, P. C., More, S. J., Blake, M., & Hanlon, A. (2011). Identification of key performance indicators for on-farm animal welfare incidents: Possible tools for early warning and prevention. *Irish Veterinary Journal, 64,* 13–22.

Kelly, P. C., More, S. J., Blake, M., Higgins, I., Clegg, T. A., & Hanlon, A. J. (2013). Validation of key indicators on cattle farms at high risk of animal welfare problems: A qualitative case-control study. *Veterinary Record, 172,* 314.

Kolstrup, C. L., & Hultgren, J. (2011). Perceived physical and psychosocial exposure and health symptoms of dairy farm staff and possible associations with dairy cow health. *Journal of Agricultural Safety and Health, 17*(2), 111–125.

Kolstrup, C. L., Kallioniemi, M., Lundqvist, P., Kymäläinen, H. R., Stallones, L., & Brumby, S. (2013). International perspectives on psychosocial working conditions, mental health, and stress of dairy farm operators. *Journal of Agromedicine, 18*(3), 244–255. doi:10.1080/1059924X.2013.796903

Kutek, S. M., Turnball, D., & Fairweather-Schmidt, A. K. (2011). Rural men's subjective well-being and the role of social support and sense of community: Evidence for the potential benefit of enhancing informal networks. *Australian Journal of Rural Health, 19,* 20–26.

Lizer, S. K., & Petrea, R. E. (2007). Health and safety needs of older farmers: Part 1. Work habits and health status. *Workplace Health and Safety, 55,* 485–491.

Lobley, M. (2005). Exploring the dark side: Stress in rural Britain. *Journal of the Royal Agricultural Society of England, 166,* 1–8.

Macken-Walsh, A. (2011). Partnership and subsidiarity? Exploring the socio-cultural context of Irish farmers' non-participation in contemporary rural development. *Rural Society Journal, 2,* 1037–1656.

McLaren, S., & Challis, C. (2009). Resilience among men farmers: The protective roles of social support and sense of belonging in the depression suicidal ideation relation. *Death Studies, 33,* 262–276.

Morrissey, K., Clarke, G., Hynes, S., & O'Donoghue, C. (2009). *Examining access to acute and community care psychiatric services for depression suffers in Ireland* (Teagasc REDP Working Paper Series 09-WP-RE-08). Retrieved from www.agresearch.teagasc.ie/rerc/downloads/workingpapers/09wpre08.pdf

Morrissey, K., Daly, A., Clarke, G., Ballas, D., & O'Donoghue, C. (2009). *An examination of psychiatric inpatient admissions in rural Ireland* (Teagasc REDP Working Paper Series 09-WP-RE-10). Retrieved from www.agresearch.teagasc.ie/rerc/downloads/workingpapers/09WP10.pdf

Ní Laoire, C. (2001). A matter of life or death? Men, masculinities, and staying "behind" in rural Ireland. *Sociologia Ruralis, 41,* 220–236.

Olff, M., Koeter, M., Van Haaften, H.,Kersten, P., & Gersons, B. (2005). Impact of a food and mouth disease crisis on post-traumatic stress symptoms in farmers. *British Journal of Psychiatry, 186,* 165–166.

Parry, J., Barnes, H., Lindsey, R., & Taylor, R. (2005). *Farmers, farm workers and work-related stress.* London, UK: Her Majesty's Stationery Office/Health and Safety Executive.

Pickens, S., Ostwald, S. K., Pace, K. M., Diamond, P., Burnett, J., & Dyer, C. B. (2013). Assessing dimensions of executive function in community-dwelling older adults with self-neglect. *Clinical Nursing Studies, 2,* 17–29.

Porcher, J. (2006). Well-being and suffering in livestock farming: Living conditions at work for people and animals. *Sociologie du Travail, 48,* e56–e70.

Protection of Animals Kept for Farming Purposes Act, Ireland Statutes s13. (1984). Retrieved from http://www.irishstatutebook.ie/eli/1984/act/13/enacted/en/html

Rollin, B. E. (1999). *Veterinary medical ethics: Theory and cases.* Amexs: Iowa State University Press.

Sanne, B., Mykletun, A., Moen, B. E., Dahl, A., & Tell, G. S. (2004). Farmers are at risk for anxiety and depression: The Hordal and Health Study. *Occupational Medicine, 54,* 92–100.

Shaw, J., Barley, G., Hill, A., Larson, S., & Roter, D. L. (2010). Communication skills education onsite in a veterinary practice. *Patient Education and Counseling, 80,* 337–344.

Smyth, B., Evans, D., Kelly, A., Cullen, L., & O'Donovan, D. (2013). The farming population in Ireland: Mortality trends during the 'Celtic Tiger' years. *European Journal of Public Health, 23,* 50–55.

Stallones, L., Marx, M.B., Garrity, T.F., & Johnson, T.P. (2004). Attachment to companion animals among older pet owners. *Anthrozoös, 2*(2), 118–124. doi:10.2752/089279389787058127

Tovey, H. (2003). Theorizing nature and society in sociology: The invisibility of animals. *Sociologia Ruralis, 43,* 196–213.

Van Huik, M. M., & Bock, B. B. (2007). Attitudes of Dutch pig farmers towards animal welfare. *British Food Journal, 109,* 879–890.

Veissier, I., Butterworth, A., Bock, B., & Roe, E. (2008). European approaches to ensure good animal welfare. *Applied Animal Behavior Science, 113,* 279–297.

Waiblinger, S., Boivin, X., Pedersen, V., Tosi, M.-V., Janczak, A. M., Visser, E. K., & Jones, R. B. (2006). Assessing the human–animal relationship in farmed species: A critical review. *Applied Animal Behavior Science, 101,* 185–242.

Williams, D., & Jewell, J. (2012). Family-centred veterinary medicine: Learning from human paediatric care. *Veterinary Record, 170*(3), 79–80.

CHAPTER 8

ENVIRONMENTAL NEGLECT

John Snowdon and Graeme Halliday

Environmental neglect can be defined as the failure to care for and protect one's surroundings. It is a behavior that some authors have described as one of the domains of self-neglect, alongside other behaviors that result in diminished self-care. Definitions and concepts of self-neglect are varied, so data on its epidemiology are difficult to establish. Some scales, designed to measure the degree of self-neglect, focus on the neglect of domestic hygiene as a principal feature of self-neglect, whereas others suggest that filth and domestic uncleanliness feature only in the most severe cases of self-neglect. There is a good reason to rate domestic neglect separately from neglect of self-care, and to recognize that the interplay of factors leading to domestic neglect may differ from those that result in a person neglecting to obtain goods and services essential for safety and physical health. Severe domestic squalor is a description of living conditions, not of behavior. Most people who live in very unclean homes have a mental disorder and many lack the capacity to appropriately look after themselves and their dwellings. Some hoard possessions; a larger proportion of them accumulate waste and material that should be discarded. This chapter discusses how best to assess and intervene in such cases, with the ongoing attention to the rights of individuals and to their capacity to attend to their own welfare and the rights of others.

The noun *neglect* means disregard, negligence, or the act or fact of neglecting (*Macquarie Concise Dictionary*, 2009, p. 839). Other sources have cited *carelessness, laxity,* and *dereliction* as synonyms. *Neglecting* means failing to take proper care of, paying little or no attention to, or omitting through indifference or *carelessness*. In this chapter, *environmental neglect* is deemed to mean failure to care for and protect one's surroundings. Rather than discuss varying behaviors and attitudes in relation to the environment in general beyond people's homes, the focus here is on the ways in which individuals may be lax (negligent, careless, or indifferent) in looking after their homes (such as their domestic surroundings).

The first notable mention in the health-related literature concerning research on neglecting the domestic environment was by Shaw (1957). In studying reports by health visitors concerning people in England older than 60 years, 139 reports showed evidence of what Shaw called "social breakdown" (p. 823). Summarizing the data about observations concerning their dwellings, she wrote that "the room in such cases is the epitome of neglect. Dust lies thick everywhere, and cobwebs abound. The windows are barely translucent and the curtains are in shreds. Rubbish, odds and ends and remains of food are found everywhere. The bed is often broken and the sheets, if there are any, are dark grey" (p. 825). In an article in the same journal, Macmillan (1957) described the psychiatric aspects of social breakdown in the elderly.

Nine years later, Macmillan and Shaw (1966) elaborated on their original research in an article titled "Senile Breakdown in Standards of Personal and Environmental Cleanliness." They rated 72 cases on 10 environmental features (floor, walls, ceiling, windows, bed, table, cooker, coal, dirt, and smell) and five personal ones (skin, hair, hands, clothes, and disposal of excreta). They reported that the mental state of the individuals in 34 of the cases was normal (apart from mild reactive depression in 11), but labeled the other 38 people as psychotic: Of these, 24 had dementia, eight had schizophrenia or paranoid psychosis, three were manic depressive, and three were alcoholic. They commented that a particular pattern of personality was seen in many of the 72 cases: that of a domineering, quarrelsome, and independent individual who had rejected the community and abandoned the accepted standards of behavior of the neighborhood.

Clark, Mankikar, and Gray (1975) published personal details of 30 inpatients aged 66 to 92 years, all acutely physically ill when admitted to their geriatric medicine unit. All were known to the social services department and all had been living "in a desperate state of domestic disorder, squalor, and self-neglect" (p. 366). Fourteen died. They titled their paper "Diogenes Syndrome," but provided scant evidence (other than lack of shame and contempt for social organization) for why Diogenes's name should be used as an eponym. There has been confusion about whether the term *Diogenes syndrome* is inclusive or exclusive of those with underlying mental illness or dementia, and most of those working in the field would now agree that the term is a misnomer and should be dropped. Reifler (1996) preferred the term *syndrome of extreme self-neglect* (p. 1411). Lenders, Kuster, and Bispinck (2015) used the term *domestic neglect* when referring to 186 cases of hoarding and squalor in Germany, where the dwellings were described as "uninhabitable."

DEFINITIONS

Which term best describes people living in very unclean conditions? Which term is most appropriate when alluding to the characteristics reported by Macmillan and Shaw (1966), Clark and colleagues (1975), and Halliday, Banerjee, Philpot, and Macdonald (2000) in England, and the cases and series reported by Wrigley and Cooney (1992, Ireland), Wustmann and Brieger (2005, Germany), Chan and colleagues (2007, Hong Kong) and authors from diverse countries around the world? People who do not clean up waste in their homes can be described as neglectful of their domestic environment. A term now commonly used to describe very unclean living conditions resulting from environmental neglect (without referring to whether the occupants are at fault or are themselves unclean) is *severe domestic squalor.* Failure to maintain acceptable standards of personal hygiene and self-care has been referred to as *self-neglecting behavior;* the resulting poor state of self-care could be described as a manifestation of self-neglect.

Squalor

There are basically two types of severe domestic squalor: (a) wet squalor cases, in which people (mainly with frontal lobe pathology and mental illnesses) accumulate waste by not troubling to throw it out (and sometimes actively resist discarding it), and (b) dry squalor cases, in which people hoard and resist discarding so much that their dwelling cannot be kept properly clean. Clinicians who use the term *squalor* as a descriptor for very unclean living conditions have been criticized by community members who regard the word as pejorative. However, it should be emphasized that the term describes an environment and not the people who live there. Alternative words such as *mess* do not adequately convey the extent of the uncleanliness. People may be happy to live and play in messy surroundings but would balk at the idea of living in squalor. It implies a public health risk and emphasizes that the state of the living conditions must not be ignored. The word conveys a requirement for urgent attention and action. It is confronting and shocking. Administering bodies, such as municipal councils and parliaments who are told that squalor has developed in a location for which they are responsible, will recognize a need to deal with the situation effectively, whereas mess can be tolerated. The conditions in cases of severe domestic squalor commonly provoke disgust. This is a fact, whether it sounds pejorative or not.

Domestic squalor lies on a continuum that extends from disorganized living that would benefit from a cleanup to severe domestic squalor that poses significant health risks and requires immediate cleanup (Norberg & Snowdon, 2014). "The term 'severe domestic squalor' is applied when a person's home is so unclean, messy and unhygienic that people of similar culture and background would consider extensive clearing and cleaning to be essential. Accumulations of dirt, grime, and waste material extend throughout living areas of the dwelling, along with presence or evidence of insects and other vermin. Rotting food, excrement and/or odors are likely to cause feelings of revulsion among visitors. As well as accumulation of waste, there may have been purposeful collection and/or retention of items to such a degree that it interferes with occupants' ability to adequately clean up the dwelling" (Snowdon, Halliday, & Banerjee, 2012, p. 11).

Self-Neglect

In contrast to domestic squalor, self-neglect is a much broader, less specific descriptor. Definitions have varied, and Gibbons, Lauder, and Ludwick (2006) decried a lack of national and international agreement about what the term means. They proposed "diagnostic test criteria for identification of self-neglect by health care provider" (p. 15) to assist nurses when planning care and interventions; they aimed to encourage consistency in practice and research. The only essential criterion to be used by health care providers in identifying self-neglect is the lack of personal and/or environmental hygiene. The other five criteria (at least two of which needed to be fulfilled to support the diagnosis) are all related to the provision or acceptance of medical services. Self-neglect was defined by neglect of personal and/or environmental hygiene combined with neglected attention to medical needs. Thus, if a person's hygiene was considered adequate, the criteria for self-neglect were not met even if the person intentionally or unintentionally was neglecting to eat, failing to look after his or her own safety and well-being, and/or ignoring other aspects that contribute to quality of life. The focus of this definition on hygiene and medical services (without including neglect of other aspects of self-care) demands for its expansion.

In 2007, the National Committee for Prevention of Elder Abuse asserted that self-neglect is an adult's inability, due to physical or mental impairment or diminished capacity, to perform essential self-care tasks including (a) obtaining essential food, clothing, shelter and medical care; (b) obtaining goods and services necessary to maintain physical health, mental health or general safety; and/or (c) managing one's own financial affairs" (Reyes-Ortiz, Burnett, Flores, Halphen, & Dyer, 2014, p. 809). It should be noted that hygiene and caring for the domestic environment were not mentioned specifically in this definition and that it purports to state what the neglect is due to, that is, physical or mental impairment or incapacity.

Reyes-Ortiz et al. (2014) also quoted Pavlou and Lachs (2008), who (contrastingly) had described a self-neglecting elder as "a person who exhibits at least one of the following: (1) persistent inattention to personal hygiene and/or environment; (2) repeated refusal of some/all indicated services that can reasonably be expected to improve quality of life; (3) self-endangerment through the manifestation of unsafe behaviors (e.g., persistent refusal to care for a disease)" (p.1842). Pavlou and Lachs (2008) suggested that the inconsistency among definitions was partly because of lack of empirical research, but also because of enormous societal latitude, cultural differences, and individual variability on what constitutes proper attention to health and hygiene. They contrasted the views of those who regarded self-neglect as a medical entity with those who supported a view that self-neglect is a societal problem, and went on to say that medical and psychiatric conditions probably underlie most cases.

DIFFERENTIATING ENVIRONMENTAL NEGLECT FROM NEGLECT OF SELF-CARE

Should inattention to domestic hygiene be mentioned in definitions of self-neglect? It is true that if a person does not adequately care for his or her domestic environment, harm can result to that person? Environmental neglect contributes to diminished self-care. It may have the potential for causing health or injury problems, or (in cases of hoarding) fire damage—but not necessarily. Persons can live in very unclean conditions but still look after themselves well—and even go to work looking so smart that no one would suspect their dwelling is very unclean: the home is neglected, but not the self.

Persistently neglecting to get rid of accumulating waste products and dirt, or to clear away excessive clutter from a dwelling, may pose risks to the occupant(s). Vermin, attracted by readily accessible garbage, can spread disease. Mold, pathogens, and toxins can build up in an unclean environment and may result in physical symptoms. Mounds of accumulated waste and structural damage due to damp or other consequences of long-term neglect may increase the likelihood of accidents and falls and may block egress from a dwelling. The latter may put lives at risk, especially if accumulated inflammable material catches fire. Neglect (inadequate attention) regarding risks to one's own person could be viewed as self-neglect, though it has been found that in many cases where occupants have, for years, neglected to do anything about potentially unhealthy and dangerous domestic environments, they somehow evade illness and physical harm. Thus, long-lasting environmental neglect may result (but not universally) in harm to the self. Harm is a potential, but not a necessary consequence.

However, there is undoubtedly a statistical association between environmental (domestic) neglect and neglect of personal hygiene and cleanliness. Evidence and case studies tell us they commonly occur together. Environmental neglect may also be associated with other forms of neglected self-care in cases where individuals fail to provide themselves with adequate food, water, clothing, or prescribed medication, and/or when they fail to seek medical attention that is clearly indicated (Dong et al., 2010). It could be hypothesized that when environmental neglect and self-neglect coexist, it is usually because of abnormalities or changes in the same region of the brain (e.g., the frontal lobe). Various researchers have asserted that older adults who self-neglect often live in squalor (Burnett et al., 2014; Kelly, Dyer, Pavlik, Doody, & Jogerst, 2008; Poythress, Burnett, Naik, Pickens, & Dyer, 2006), whereas Reyes-Ortiz et al. (2014) stated that self-neglect is characterized by squalor and unsafe living circumstances; they affirmed that it is a result of medical, neurologic, or psychiatric disorders, coupled with lack of capacity for self-care and self-protection. Dyer, Goodwin, Pickens-Pace, Burnett, and Kelly (2007) declared that self-neglect is the inability to provide for oneself the goods or services to meet basic needs, and that "individuals who neglect themselves are typically older persons with multiple deficits in social, functional, and physical domains who, in extreme instances, live in squalor" (p. 1671).

DIFFERING VIEWS CONCERNING DOMAINS OF SELF-NEGLECT

McDermott (2008) noted that self-neglect emerged as an issue in the United States in the late 1970s, when elder abuse was recognized as a social problem. Although there has been considerable variation between the states in their respective definitions of self-neglect (Roby & Sullivan, 2000), the American Bar Association Commission on Law and Aging stated in 2005 that the majority of the states used the term to refer to people who "neglect their needs for nutrition, financial solvency, medical care or adequate shelter" (cited by McDermott, 2008, p. 232). McDermott (2008) declared that in the United States the term self-neglect is used in an all-encompassing manner to describe a person's failure to carry out essential self-care tasks. In contrast, she found that professionals concerned about environmental care and self-care in Australia (community and health services, housing and council staff) draw clear distinctions among behaviors that involve neglect of self-care (self-neglect), extreme neglect of the environment (squalor), and the inability to throw objects away (hoarding). Squalor was perceived as including three elements: vermin, garbage/waste, and resultant odors. In relation to the latter, McDermott noted that the professionals she interviewed used strong adjectives to convey the potency of the smells as well as the overwhelming nature of the environmental circumstances: "filthy, disgusting, horrible, revolting, putrid and oozing." It seems likely that the distinction was partly based on perceptions of unacceptability. Self-neglect and hoarding did not have to be seen as extreme, whereas squalor was viewed as intolerable. Most participants made a clear distinction between hoarding and squalor, the former involving a degree of purposeful organization, whereas squalor was characterized by unorganized accumulations of waste, decomposition, strong odors, and an excess of animals and vermin. Nevertheless, descriptions by participants made it clear that self-neglect, hoarding, and squalor co-existed in a number of their cases; distinctions were not necessarily clear-cut.

Burnett and colleagues (2014) examined the data gathered by adult protective services (APS) caseworkers in Texas in 2004 to 2008 in relation to 5,686 cases of elder self-neglect (defined as the inability, due to physical or mental impairments or reduced capacity, to provide oneself with the necessary resources to maintain physical health, mental health, and overall well-being). Latent class analysis identified four unique subtypes of elder self-neglect, with some 49% manifesting physical or medical self-neglect problems (with a relatively low probability of coexisting mental health neglect), 22% environmental neglect (but with a moderate probability of co-existing physical and medical self-neglect), 21% global neglect, and 9% financial neglect. Global neglect was characterized by high probabilities of physical and medical neglect, mental health neglect, and environmental neglect, and a .42 probability of having social problems. The authors posited that their data provided evidence of differences between subtypes regarding potential targets for intervention and prevention.

Reyes-Ortiz et al. (2014) stated that three domains of self-neglect have been identified: (a) personal hygiene, (b) impaired function (e.g., decline in cognitive function and activities of daily living), and (c) environmental neglect. In their description of Mrs. LJ's circumstances, they demonstrated all three domains being affected, and they referred to this as a case of self-neglect.

Mrs. LJ's case (see Case Study 1) would have fitted well into Macmillan and Shaw's (1966) case series. But various other examples of impaired self-care (i.e., self-neglect) would not have fitted so well, and in those cases, standards of cleanliness would have been of little or no relevance to the interventions that might restore the quality of life. Many such cases would have been rated as showing mild self-neglect. Typically, these would have shown impairment in only one aspect of self-care. Mrs. LJ's case was extreme, in that she had a severely impaired ability to look after her own bodily needs and hygiene or to function well in her environment. Many aspects of self-care were affected. She lived in severe domestic squalor and was markedly self-neglectful.

It appears that some experts and authors regard self-neglect as meaning that an individual is deficient in self-care, whereas others put more emphasis on difficulties in functioning within an environment—particularly in relation to hygiene. Authors discussing how the concept of self-neglect rose to prominence commonly refer to reports of social breakdown in standards of personal and environmental cleanliness as providing the first reports of cases of self-neglect. Ratings of degree of self-neglect may vary from mild to severe, as do ratings of domestic squalor. In cases where moderate or severe domestic squalor coexists with self-neglect (however defined), it would seem sensible and appropriate to rate both self-neglect and squalor, and to specifically record comments about the person's living conditions. Lee and LoGiudice (2012) commented on the diversity and complexity of such cases and recommended a classification based on the symptoms of self-neglect, hoarding, and domestic squalor, and combinations thereof. Dong, Simon, and Evans (2012) identified five domains of self-neglect: hoarding, poor basic personal hygiene, house in need of repair, unsanitary conditions, and inadequate utilities. They reported the prevalence

---

CASE STUDY 1: MRS. L J

Mrs. L J is a 79-year-old widow who has resided in her dwelling (now dilapidated) for 30 years. She has little contact with other people. Mrs. L J has hypothyroidism, hypertension, arthritis, and cataracts; she has not visited her doctor for a year. She does not drink alcohol. The APS have referred her for evaluation. She recently went to jail for multiple unpaid fines for refusing to clean up piles of trash in her backyard. Most of the interior of the house is inaccessible because of clutter. The home is infested with cockroaches and smells of trash and urine. Multiple animals live in the house, including a wild pregnant possum. The kitchen is filthy and there is moldy food in the refrigerator. The bathroom is unusable; she uses a bucket for her excretions. She has extensive dental caries and poor personal hygiene. She has difficulty rising to a standing position, but her physical examination is otherwise normal. She is oriented but her thoughts often appear tangential. She does not cooperate in testing for depression and appears suspicious of the interviewers. Her St. Louis University Mental Status score is 23 out of 30 (normal range 27–30) and she is assessed as having severe executive control dysfunction. The cognitive deficits point to a diagnosis of Alzheimer's disease, and she is assessed as lacking the capacity to remain living independently: She refuses assistance in rectifying her situation and fails to recognize various dangers in her home (Reyes-Ortiz et al., 2014).

of each of these behaviors in an elderly Chicago population. Stating that the person has or had been self-neglecting, without specifying which aspects of care were being neglected, does not clarify whether the person was living in an unclean dwelling, and, if so, whether there was an over-accumulation of waste products (including animal excrement) or clutter or not.

Similarly, of course, it is appropriate for those assessing squalor or hoarding situations to also rate aspects of the occupant's self-care. Dealing with environmental neglect often does not have to be immediate but the personal needs of the occupant may need urgent attention.

TAKING CARE OF ONE'S HOME

Most people have homes. A majority reside long term in dwellings that they own, rent, or pay money to live in. Some live in staffed residential facilities. Others may be homeless. Occupants of houses and apartments acknowledge a responsibility to maintain the cleanliness of their dwellings. Some of us are untidy and somewhat disorganized, but most homes are kept reasonably clean, with ready access to amenities and living areas.

Hoarding is not necessarily abnormal. Hoarding is "storing for future use" and can be acceptable and potentially beneficial, providing the hoarded material does not interfere with daily living activities and the social lives of occupants of the dwelling. When stored material overflows into living areas and blocks access within the dwelling so that usual activities (food preparation, washing, toileting, or socializing) are constrained, the acquiring behavior leads to functional impairment. The person who hoards has an irresistible urge to retain acquired items even when there seem to be overwhelming reasons for discarding at least some. If, in addition, the hoarding causes clinically significant distress or impairment in social, occupational, or other important areas of functioning (including maintaining a safe environment for self or others), and if other criteria stipulated in the fifth edition of the *Diagnostic and Statistical Manual of Mental Disorders* (*DSM-5*; American Psychiatric Association, 2013) are fulfilled, that person can be said to have a hoarding disorder.

Purposeful but excessive hoarding can be viewed as neglectful, in that persons who hoard appear to have neglected to think of the effects on others, let alone the risks and consequences affecting themselves. One potential consequence is that the accumulation of items will result in reduced ability to clean areas that cannot be accessed. The more disorganized the hoarded material is, the more difficult it will be to clear away the cobwebs, dust, insects, and vermin. Pet owners may see their animals climb among the items and leave excrement there. Hoarding may lead to a squalor situation—though "the great majority of subjects with pathological hoarding behavior" are said not to exhibit squalor and self-neglect (Pertusa & Fonseca, 2014, p. 67). Studies of the prevalence of domestic squalor in series of cases of hoarding disorder have yet to be published.

Hoarding needs to be distinguished from nonpurposeful accumulation and retention of items and material (Snowdon, 2015). Some people appear not to care about buildup of dirt and waste in their dwellings. This may be related to personality issues, but there may also be a cultural element: Some groups of people appear not to mind or notice that their domestic surroundings are unclean. Quentin Crisp famously stated that: "About cleaning the rest of the room I did nothing at all ... there was no need to do any housework. After the first four years the dirt doesn't get any worse" (Crisp, 1997, p. 102), but whether he was rebelling against social norms or just advertising personal indolence is debatable. Apathy and unawareness of reasons for maintaining a degree of order and cleanliness in a home may result in accumulation of useless and unneeded material. Clark et al. (1975, p. 366) reported that several of their 30 inpatients with Diogenes syndrome "hoarded useless rubbish (syllogomania)—newspapers, tins, bottles and rags, often in bundles and sacks." Snowdon (1987), referring to 83 people who lived in very unclean conditions, stated that, "marked hoarding was a feature of most cases," with items "piled high" in 36 cases. With hindsight, the word *accumulation* should have replaced *hoarding*: The items had piled high because of the inability or lack of motivation to discard, rather than the resistance to discarding. Halliday et al. (2000) reported that half of the 81 participants in their study of squalor in London had accumulated or hoarded items such as newspapers, bottles, and plastic bags to a major degree. Various case reports have described emptied containers being left lying around in homes, together with wrappings, apple cores, and other items that would generally be viewed as garbage. Stuff accumulates (see Frost & Steketee, 2010) not with an intention of keeping it but because the person has not got around to throwing it into a trash can. Sometimes the person resists attempts to remove the waste items, though commonly this seems to be impulsive opposition and grasping on to their possessions, rather than purposeful retention of specific objects of their choice. In other cases, the person makes little objection to the accumulated garbage being taken away.

Maier (2004) referred to stereotypic and ritualistic behaviors in cases of dementia and chronic schizophrenia, in which acquisition is "just motor activity without clear intention or aim," he favored the term *collectionism* to refer to this grasping type of behavior (p. 333). If the mess has accumulated so much that access to amenities is compromised, and especially if, in addition, there is a strong odor, and there is excrement around the dwelling, and vermin or insects have invaded, this can be described as severe domestic squalor.

PREVALENCE OF ENVIRONMENTAL NEGLECT

The prevalence of moderate or severe domestic squalor (domestic neglect to a degree where intervention is considered essential) has been estimated to be at least one in 1,000 among people older than 65 years in Sydney, the prevalence being higher among men than women (Snowdon & Halliday, 2011). Of these older people, 41% had never been married (53% of the men, 19% of the women), 27% were widowed, 23% were either divorced or separated, and 9% were still married. Studies have suggested that the numbers of people older than 65 years and of people aged under 65 years living in squalor are nearly the same, meaning that the prevalence among those under 65 years is about one fifth of the rate among older people (McDermott & Gleeson, 2009). Of individuals (mean age 61.9 years) referred to a squalor and hoarding intervention service, 90.7% of the 108 males and 71.3% of the 95 females lived alone (Snowdon, Halliday, & Hunt, 2013).

In their study of 4,627 elderly people (31% White and 69% Black) in a geographically defined population in Chicago, Dong et al. (2012) reported the prevalence of hoarding among White people as 0.9% and of living in unsanitary conditions as just over 0.9%, whereas the rates among the Black population were 6% and 4.6%. The four hoarding items rated were newspapers/magazines, boxes/bags/bottles, trash, and pets. Almost none of the White elderly participants had collected trash, in contrast to 4.6% of the Black participants. The five items assessed when reporting on unsanitary conditions were extremely dirty or cluttered, spoiled or rotten food, many dirty dishes, insect/rodent infestation, and foul odor. The authors noted that a lack of comprehensive measures of socioeconomic status in this study prevented them from commenting on a specific relationship between race and hoarding.

In a later study of Chinese elders living in Chicago, Dong (2014) reported the prevalence rates of moderate or severe hoarding as 3.5% and of unsanitary conditions as 5.4%. The same four items (noted previously) were used in assessing hoarding, but in this later study, the assessed unsanitary conditions were, "filth covering floor, clutter accumulation, spoiled or rotten food, kitchen messiness, insect/rodent infestation, foul odor, inappropriate disposal of urine or feces" (p. 2394). These rates can be compared with an estimated prevalence of hoarding disorder among adults in one part of London of about 1.6% (Nordsletten et al., 2013). We do not have definite information to allow an estimate of what proportion of the occupants in these hoarding disorder cases would be described as living in a situation of environmental neglect. We suspect that fewer than half would be described as living in severe squalor. Some do not live in squalor and their hoarding is well organized, yet they hoard so much that it interferes with how they or other occupants can function in their homes. Whether we should document these latter cases as demonstrating environmental neglect is debatable, and depends on our criteria for defining neglect. We estimate the prevalence of environmental neglect in Sydney to be more than one in 1,000 among older people (squalor), but it could be up to one in 100 if cases of moderate to severe hoarding are included among self-neglect cases.

Dong (2014) reported that the prevalence of self-neglect among a representative elderly population of people from a Chinese background in Chicago was 29.1% (18.2% mild, 10.9% moderate/severe). Of the 310 persons deemed moderate or severe, 153 were reported as living in unsanitary conditions, 100 were reported as hoarding, and 166 (5.8%) were said to live in a house that needed repair. Only 44 (1.4%) were reported as having a personal hygiene problem and 36 (1.3%) lacked heat, food, water, electricity, or provision for food storage. Neither Dong et al. (2012) nor Dong (2014) referred to those who self-neglect by not taking prescribed medication or giving inadequate attention to medical problems. A range of factors have been associated with self-neglect.

CAUSATIVE OR ASSOCIATED FACTORS

Observations during an assessment of the person who lives in a very unclean domestic environment (severe domestic squalor) may point to one of the following as a possible contributor to the apparent environmental neglect:

1. The person may have a mental or physical disorder that makes the person incapable of keeping the home clean, or is unmotivated to do so. A stroke may have left the individual partially paralyzed or weak; frontal lobe damage or developmental disability may have affected his or her appreciation of the need to clean or organize. Neurodegenerative conditions, such as Alzheimer's disease, may have led to a loss of visuospatial skills, planning ability, and judgment. Impaired vision or sense of smell may diminish the individual's ability to recognize the need to throw out or clear away trash, filth, or excrement.

A majority of persons who live in severe domestic squalor, and have been referred to community services for help, have been found to have diagnosable mental disorders (Halliday et al., 2000; Snowdon & Halliday, 2011). Dementia, schizophrenia, and frontal brain disorders (e.g., alcohol-related brain damage) are the most common disorders reported, with abuse of other drugs, personality disorders, developmental disorders, autism spectrum disorders, anxiety, and depression also being listed when considering causation (Halliday et al., 2000; Snowdon & Halliday, 2011). Persons without a mental disorder but with a physical disability may also have problems in keeping their domestic environment clean and clutter-free if they have no help or supports. Review of the various studies (Halliday et al., 2000; Snowdon & Halliday, 2011) suggest that hoarding disorder may account for up to 10% of cases of severe squalor: The fifth edition of the *Diagnostic and Statistical Manual of Mental Disorders* (DSM-5; American Psychiatric Association, 2013) includes a list of criteria that must be fulfilled if a diagnosis of hoarding disorder is to be made. The list is essentially the same as that proposed by Mataix-Cols et al. (2010): (1) persisting reluctance to get rid of material or items, whatever their worth, (2) a belief that the items should be retained, and anguish about throwing them out, (3) resultant accumulation of material, causing interference with their activities of daily living, (4) consequent anguish and interference with their ability to function normally in domestic, social or work situations, and in keeping their dwelling safe for occupants or visitors, or in other significant ways, (5) the hoarding has not resulted from neurological disease or another medical condition, and (6) is not attributable to one of the other mental disorders listed in the *DSM-5*.

2. Personality and cultural factors may affect whether the person recognizes a need to maintain cleanliness in the home. He or she may never have learned the reasons for getting rid of waste or maintaining an organized environment.

3. Access to areas of the home may be limited because of hoarded or accumulated items or material, thus preventing cleaning. As discussed previously, such obstruction may have resulted from the unwillingness to discard items, whether or not attributable to hoarding disorder, cognitive impairment, or other mental or psychological disorders.

An interplay among personality, upbringing, genes, and brain changes may determine how people behave in response to varying circumstances, and whether (for example) they look after themselves and their homes well or not. Physical and emotional factors undoubtedly contribute to the behavior.

Similarly, excessive hoarding is commonly attributable to a complex interplay of factors:

1. A perception that items have sentimental, practical, or intrinsic value, and thus they should be retained. When the desire to retain overrides awareness that there is inadequate space to store the items, hoarding becomes a problem. Culture and upbringing may affect beliefs, the value ascribed to items, and attitudes to waste. Attachment issues may affect a person's ability to do without an item.

2. Genetic factors. There is evidence that obsessional features may be inherited (though they can also be partly determined by upbringing) as can character traits.

3. Aspects of personality, such as perfectionism, a need for security and/or comfort, frugality, and indecisiveness about what to discard or retain.

4. Neurobiological disturbance (e.g., frontal lobe pathology) and problems in attention and categorization.

Various features in cases of severe domestic squalor are also those of frontal lobe dysfunction. Reduction in self-care and personal hygiene, lack of empathy and concern for others, and disinhibition and impaired social skills are reported in dementia of the frontal type (Gregory & Hodges, 1993). Neuroimaging has shown frontal lobe changes in a number of cases of severe domestic squalor and also in cases of hoarding. Describing people with frontotemporal dementia, Lebert (2005) observed both self-neglect and domestic squalor in 28 of the 30 cases studied, although syllogomania (accumulation of waste) was reported in only 15 (50%).

Psychiatric assessment of those living in severe squalor has shown that nearly all have mental illnesses (as mentioned previously), and these can be associated with frontal lobe changes—in particular, schizophrenia, substance-related brain damage (attributable to alcohol or other drugs), and neurodegenerative dementia. Some have developmental disabilities. Lee et al. (2014) provided details concerning 69 patients (two thirds of whom were inpatients) who were reported to be living in squalor, and who underwent detailed neuropsychological testing. This was a selected sample; not all such patients were referred for testing. Almost all were recorded as having frontal executive dysfunction. CT and/or MRI brain scans were obtained from 38 and only three were reported as normal; 63% had vascular changes and 29% showed general or regional atrophy. Of 13 with territorial infarcts, 12 involved the frontal lobes. The mean score of the 52 patients who were tested on the Mini-Mental State Examination was 25.3.

Anderson, Damasio, and Damasio (2005) compared neuroimaging results from nine cases of collectionism (organic hoarding) with those from 54 cases of brain pathology in the absence of hoarding, and found that the maximal region of difference between the two groups was the ventromedial prefrontal cortex, extending back to the anterior cingulate cortex. Other neuroimaging studies of hoarding have implicated a range of frontal and temporal brain regions that may modulate predispositions to acquire and save. Damage to these areas (e.g., by vascular incidents) can lead to hoarding behavior, but fMRI (functional magnetic resonance imaging) studies have shown the same regions being involved even in the absence of known lesions (Slyne & Tolin, 2014, p. 181). Tolin, Stevens, Nave, Villavicencioa, and Morrison (2012) reported MRI results, including frontal abnormalities, from six patients with hoarding disorder. After having cognitive behavioral therapy, their neural activity no longer differed from that of normal controls.

The relevance of considering what factors affect whether people neglect themselves or their domestic environment is that the influence of some of these factors may be modifiable, or their effects may be countered in some way. If the person is neglecting to look after his or her dwelling as a result of psychotic thoughts, ideas, beliefs, or perceptions, it may well be possible to treat the mental disorder and restore good judgment and living skills. This may not be possible in cases of progressive neurodegenerative disorder; in such cases, the main object of treatment may be to remove responsibilities that the person can no longer manage. Neglecting self-care and neglecting to look after one's home are indications that help and support may be needed, but dealing with such situations needs the readiness to examine what is best in the individual case. What will be the best approach when seeing Mrs. LJ, a woman with Alzheimer's disease, who lived in squalor and who appeared to have lost self-care skills (Reyes-Ortiz et al., 2014)? Or Mr. JF, a patient of ours with hoarding disorder, who cannot get into his house in Sydney because it is full (literally) of stuff? In these and all other cases of domestic neglect, whether or not they self-neglect, we need to try to understand them and assess whether they have the capacity to decide for themselves. Then we need to ensure that appropriate support is provided. We should not take over their lives unless it is unarguably necessary.

ASSESSMENT

If health or community service staff members are asked to provide advice or help in cases of environmental neglect, the initial action must be assessment. If the person is willing to have those staff visit his or her dwelling, this allows for assessment of whether the person's living conditions are indeed a cause for concern. If so, why? Does he or she live in a cluttered and/or unclean domestic environment? If so, is there reason to think there could be occupational, health, or safety risks in entering and looking around the dwelling? What sort of safety problems might there be? Before contemplating a visit, those staff members will want to know the details of the case from the referrer, including information about how many people live in the dwelling, and whether the occupant(s) have a known history of mental health problems or aggression.

If the occupant does not wish to allow the staff members to visit, discussion with the referrer is needed to decide what action should be taken. If the dwelling is rented and is the property of a government organization (in Sydney this would most likely be the Department of Housing), officers of that organization need to take responsibility for initiating assessment or intervention. In other circumstances, it may be appropriate to seek the involvement of a community mental health team. The possibilities vary among countries and jurisdictions. Ultimately, what matters is whether the identified person in the dwelling has the capacity to look after himself or herself and the dwelling and whether there is evidence that the dwelling is unsafe for the person to live in—are there risks to health and/or safety?

Supposing that the occupant identified as being responsible for the state of the dwelling does not have the capacity, and/or if the dwelling is deemed to be too unsafe or unhealthy for people to live in, a legal order will need to be sought. Provision for this will vary among countries and jurisdictions. It is inappropriate to discuss how relevant laws in hundreds of jurisdictions vary and can be used, but, as an example, in Sydney, the Local Government Act allows an environmental health officer to seek an order for clearance or cleanup of a dwelling deemed to need it. For a person lacking the capacity to make decisions about whether such action is needed, a guardianship order can be sought, so that a substitute decision-maker can be asked to approve of the proposed actions.

However, if the responsible occupant is willing for a health professional or other authorized person to visit, an assessment can be made by walking through the dwelling. It is important to try to engage the occupant from the beginning so that if cleaning or clearing is needed, the occupant's involvement in decisions about what to do (and when) can be ensured. The health professional will rate the dwelling regarding cleanliness and access, using, for example, in Australia the Environmental Cleanliness and Clutter Scale (ECCS; Halliday & Snowdon, 2009), and could record the degree of hoarding or accumulation of items on the Clutter Image Rating Scale (Frost, Steketee, Tolin, & Renaud, 2008) or other hoarding-assessment tools. A visiting health professional with mental health training will note evidence of mental health problems. Depending on how forthcoming the occupant is, the health professional may be able to develop a formulation concerning

---

BOX 8.1
ASSESSMENT TASKS IN CASES OF ENVIRONMENTAL NEGLECT

1. Obtain information from the referrer: Type of dwelling, home ownership, do any occupants have a history of mental health problems?
2. Consider potential occupational health and safety concerns. Is it safe for the case worker to enter the dwelling? Mold? Dilapidation? Unsafe piles of items? Ease of egress?
3. Schedule a home visit (highly desirable).
4. Rate living conditions (e.g., ECCS, Clutter Image Rating Scale, UCLA Hoarding Severity Scale, Activities of Daily Living in Hoarding, Self-Neglect Severity Scale).
5. Engage the occupant(s).
6. Assess whether there are mental health problems or medical issues that require medical practitioner assessment. Is specific treatment or hospitalization indicated?
7. Ensure interagency coordination with agreement regarding a specific service to take responsibility as case managers.
8. Use local legislation as appropriate (e.g., guardianship, Environmental Health Act).
9. Clean/clear, preferably with involvement of occupant(s).
10. Arrange specialized cognitive behavior therapy, motivational interviewing, group work, web- or manual-based interventions, as appropriate.

ECCS, Environmental Cleanliness and Clutter Scale; UCLA, University of California, Los Angeles.

the issues and factors that may be relevant. There may be evidence pointing to a *DSM-5* diagnosis. A clinical psychologist may be able to recommend a behavioral program if the person is found to be purposely accumulating and retaining too many items, causing impaired access and function around the home. Not everything needs to be done at once. The assessment may extend over two or more meetings.

As indicated previously, the second step in assessment is to consider why the person has so neglected his or her domestic environment that someone (relative, neighbor, or concerned visitor) has made a referral to a service that he or she believes can help deal with the problem. Motives for referral vary. Many refer because they are concerned about the individual or other occupants or the relevant dwelling. Others are concerned for themselves and for the effects of the environmental neglect on them and the community or on the value of their property. Whatever the reason, those in a position to help the person and/or the referrer will want to understand and deal with the cause for concern. Aspects of assessment in cases of environmental neglect are summarized in Box 8.1.

MANAGEMENT ISSUES IN ENVIRONMENTAL NEGLECT

This chapter is focused on the neglect of the domestic environment, but, of course, a prime consideration needs to be the safety and welfare of the occupant(s) of environments rated as risky, unhealthy, and distressing to live in. In addition, the safety and welfare of the neighbors may be of concern.

Commonly, people with hoarding disorder have insight about how their hoarding is affecting their ability to function, both in the home and socially. They may even seek treatment. Specialized cognitive behavioral therapy (CBT) has proved effective in some cases, as has motivational interviewing, but there is a dearth of therapists trained to deal with hoarding. Pharmacotherapy (e.g., serotonin reuptake inhibitors or atypical antipsychotics) can be helpful in some cases (Saxena, 2014). Group CBT, support groups, and web-based interventions are less costly. The Buried in Treasures program has proven effective (Tolin, Frost, & Steketee, 2007), but the workshops are not widely available. However, those whose hoarding is extreme and who live in homes with severely restricted access to amenities (even those with hoarding disorder and no other diagnosed mental disorder) generally do not seek or accept offers of psychological help. They appear to have limited insight about the risks and dangers of their hoarding.

In many cases, people living in squalor (some whose excessive hoarding is a major reason for them not being able to clean their dwelling) decline offers of assessment by clinicians and refuse entry even to those willing to help in cleaning up the mess, garbage, waste, and filth. Two thirds of those living in severe squalor have accumulated excessive amounts of garbage, waste, and an assortment of items of little obvious value—especially when buried/lost at the bottom of a heaped-up pile. Ethical and moral questions may arise in such cases. Do individuals have the right to live in whatever environment they choose, even if that environment is considered by others to be untentable? Is it acceptable to invoke respect for a right to autonomy as an excuse for clinical inaction? Where is the tipping point that makes it necessary to enforce action when a person resists it? Do ratings of degree of uncleanliness or restricted access help us decide?

There is a good reason to agree with Sutherland and Macfarlane's (2014) view that health workers have a responsibility to be proactive. From experience, it is clear that not only health practitioners but local council officers and community services staff commonly shy away from enforcing interventions in squalor and hoarding cases in spite of observed effects of their behavior on neighbors, cohabitants, and pets. Sometimes the necessary applications to courts and tribunals prove too difficult or too expensive. The results of inaction or inadequate responses can be disastrous, as seen in a 2013 fire that engulfed a home in Sydney. The hoard of inflammable material and the nests of rats were well known to the municipal officers, but they did not enforce an order they had obtained under the Local Government Act many months before. In another case, the mold in the house was bad enough to cause illness among staff who entered the place, but the woman who lives there seems to survive as if she is immune to it. The council has not enforced action. Should it? Do we "walk by on the other side of the street"?

Countries and jurisdictions vary in what they do and are able to do in cases of squalor. Health systems and expectations of community services differ. The potential for legal constraints varies among jurisdictions. Legal arrangements and laws differ. There are differences in the type and availability of resources. Some dwellings are more spacious; some have more rooms than others. There are differences in social, domestic, and other arrangements among populations; for example, far higher percentages of elderly persons live alone in some countries (e.g., the United States) than in others (e.g., China). Severe domestic squalor is more commonly a problem in some neighborhoods than in others. Responding to squalor situations may not seem to require so much attention in some jurisdictions as in others. Cleanliness may matter more to some people than it does to others. Nevertheless, certain principles are likely to be applicable to many populations and have been discussed by Snowdon et al. (2012) and others. They commented that, among agencies and people who might be expected to take a lead in initiating interventions in cases of severe domestic squalor, the following list (with a variation in what the various bodies are called) might apply across various states and countries:

1. Municipal councils and their social workers or welfare officers
2. Community health services (aged care, mental health, drug, and alcohol) and primary care doctors

3. Other government-supported community services
4. Not-for-profit caring organizations (including animal welfare organizations)
5. Housing providers
6. Government departments with responsibility for housing and overseeing home care and disability services
7. Guardianship personnel, conservators, substitute decision makers

One of the principles developed by services active in dealing with cases of domestic neglect is that in all cases there should be consultation and coordination among agencies. For example, housing inspectors usually would not deal with a squalor situation in a public housing unit on their own. They would want to link in, as appropriate, with a mental health team, the environmental health officer from the local municipal council, assessors from the fire service, the public guardian, and a cleanup service. In the United States, task forces have been developed in various jurisdictions to ensure effective and coordinated interventions can be initiated (Bratiotis & Woody, 2014). If a person living in an unclean dwelling is happy that various agencies are involved and is able to cooperate with them, the case is likely to have a good outcome.

In all cases, it is desirable that one agency (preferably a designated case manager) take on the leadership role in coordinating services, and that at an early stage there be a case conference, in person or across airwaves, to discuss the roles of the various agencies in each case. The case manager will aim to engage the person—and this may require weeks of establishing confidence and feelings of friendship. Individual problem solving, attention for medical and mental health issues, as well as ensuring that the person has financial and other supports in place will all be part of the business of establishing trust. Clearing away clutter may need to be initiated slowly, with the person involved in decisions about what to discard, but in many cases, special cleaning services may need to be brought in—still with the person's involvement. Expectations by administrators that such cases should, after relatively brief periods, be discharged from the books of the leading agency should be resisted, although it is hoped lengths of time between visits by agency personnel can be progressively increased. Long-term success will require long-term support.

When a person lives in severe domestic squalor in a home he or she owns, it is far more difficult to impel action than if the person lives in public or rented accommodations. If a person has the capacity to make decisions for oneself and is not causing undue harassment to others, it may be difficult to do anything about the state of the home. If he or she has the capacity, but the risk of health problems attributable to the squalor is believed to be considerable, a legal order can be sought to compel change. If the individual does not have the capacity, and it is thought essential to enforce a cleanup or provision of services or a move to residential care or to live with relatives or friends, then a guardianship order should be sought. This, of course, requires reports from qualified practitioners, the acquisition of which may not be so easy if the person refuses to be seen. If the person is deemed to be psychiatrically unwell, an order for psychiatric assessment can be organized. If the person declines assessment but there is adequate evidence that allows the local council to seek entry to the person's dwelling under an order, a decision can be made (following an inspection) on whether a cleanup is vital, and action can be taken even if the person remains unseen. If the person lives in squalor and it is thought that animals in the dwelling are suffering, the country's laws may give right of entry to animal protection staff, who can report on the living conditions in the dwelling.

One of the problems encountered when considering cases of severe domestic squalor is that cleanups, legal actions, and interventions are all costly. Councils may refuse to act because they cannot find the money in their budget. Administrators of services may not be able to fund enough positions to allow for the staff numbers needed to build up intervention strategies. The people who live in squalor commonly cannot pay any of the costs of intervention. So excuses are made for why intervention cannot be initiated. In reply, we would argue that we citizens of our countries do have responsibilities toward our neighbors. In spite of their apparent denial of problems, and their resistance to intervention, we suggest that if service providers have no doubts that persons living in squalor are inflicting or risking considerable harm to themselves or others, they should persist in efforts to guide, persuade, or even force them to accept help. We should not walk past on the other side of the street.

CONCLUSION

We accept that severe domestic squalor is closely related to self-neglect; we argue that neglect of self-care and neglect of care for one's dwelling are linked, but should be considered in tandem, separately. Self-neglect is a broad concept. By concentrating on severe squalor, we avoid the need to discuss the various different forms and features of self-neglect. Whatever the type of squalor, if severe enough, we should facilitate assessment and intervention, preferably by engaging the person and coordinating supporting agencies to help reduce health and safety concerns in a respectful way.

IMPLICATIONS FOR RESEARCH AND PRACTICE

- It is recommended that clinical and research assessments of self-neglecting clients should include separate assessments of capacity, self-care (including personal hygiene), and domestic cleanliness and clutter.
- The ECCS (Halliday & Snowdon, 2009) can be used to rate aspects of domestic squalor and of access within the home. The Clutter Image Rating Scale (Frost et al., 2008) is often used to rate degrees of hoarding.
- There is a need for further studies of the prevalence of different types of self-neglect, examining associations between environmental neglect and self-care deficits. Such studies should clarify their definition of self-neglect. When there is sufficient consensus about the definition of self-neglect, it will be useful to reexamine its prevalence.
- Equally, there is a need for further studies of the prevalence of excessive purposeful hoarding, using *DSM-5* criteria for hoarding disorder; cases in which hoarding is attributable to brain pathology or other mental disorders should be recorded in a different category.
- The prevalence of nonpurposeful accumulation of items or waste (collectionism or organic accumulation, with little resistance to the material being discarded) needs to be examined and recorded.

REFERENCES

American Bar Association Commission on Law and Aging. (2005). *Information on laws related to elder abuse*. Washington, DC: ABA Commission on Law and Aging. Retrieved from http://www.preventelderabuse .org/new/ReportontheNCPEASelf-NeglectSymposium.doc

American Psychiatric Association. (2013). *Diagnostic and statistical manual of mental disorders* (5th ed.). Arlington, VA: American Psychiatric Publishing.

Anderson, S. W., Damasio, H., & Damasio, A.R. (2005). A neural basis for collecting behavior in humans. *Brain, 128*, 201–212.

Bratiotis, C., & Woody, S. (2014). Community interventions for hoarding. In R.O. Frost & G. Steketee (Eds.), *The Oxford handbook of hoarding and acquiring*. Oxford, UK: Oxford University Press.

Burnett, J., Dyer, C. B., Halphen, J. M., Achenbaum, W. A., Green, C. E., Booker, J. G., & Diamond, P. M. (2014). Four types of self-neglect in older adults: Results of a latent class analysis. *Journal of the American Geriatrics Society, 62*, 1127–1132.

Clark, A. N., Mankikar, G. D., & Gray, I. (1975). Diogenes syndrome: A clinical study of gross neglect in old age. *Lancet, 1*, 366–368.

Dong, X. (2014). Elder self-neglect in a community-dwelling U.S. Chinese population: Findings from the Population Study of Chinese Elderly in Chicago (PINE) study. *Journal of the American Geriatrics Society, 62*, 2391–2397.

Dong, X., Simon, M. A., & Evans, D. A. (2012). Prevalence of self-neglect across gender, race, and socioeconomic status: Findings from the Chicago Health and Aging Project. *Gerontology, 58*, 258–268.

Dong, X., Simon, M. A., Wilson, R. S., Mendes de Leon, C. F., Rajan, K. B., & Evans, D. A. (2010). Decline in cognitive function and risk of elder self-neglect: Finding from the Chicago Health Aging Project. *Journal of the American Geriatrics Society, 58*, 2292–2299.

Dyer, C. B., Goodwin, J. S., Pickens-Pace, S., Burnett, J., & Kelly, P. A. (2007). Self-neglect among the elderly: A model based on more than 500 patients seen by a geriatric medicine team. *American Journal of Public Health, 97*, 1671–1676.

Frost, R. O., & Steketee, G. (2010). *Stuff. Compulsive hoarding and the meaning of things*. New York, NY: Houghton Mifflin Harcourt.

Frost, R. O., Steketee, G., Tolin, D. F., & Renaud, S. (2008). Development and validation of the Clutter Image Rating Scale. *Journal of Psychopathology, 30*, 193–203.

Gibbons, S., Lauder, W., & Ludwick, R. (2006). Self-neglect: A proposed new NANDA diagnosis. *International Journal of Nursing Terminologies and Classifications, 17*, 10–18.

Gregory, C. A., & Hodges, J. R. (1993). Dementia of frontal type and the focal lobar atrophies. *International Review of Psychiatry, 5*, 397–406.

Halliday, G., Banerjee, S., Philpot, M., & Macdonald, A. (2000). Community study of people who live in squalor. *Lancet, 355*, 882–886.

Halliday, G., & Snowdon, J. (2009). The Environmental Cleanliness and Clutter Scale (ECCS). *International Psychogeriatrics, 21*, 1041–1050.

Kelly, P. A., Dyer, C. B., Pavlik, V., Doody, R., & Jogerst, G. (2008). Exploring self-neglect in older adults: Preliminary findings of the self-neglect severity scale and next steps. *Journal of the American Geriatrics Society, 56*, S253–S260.

Kirkup, J. (2000). Untitled essay. In P. Bailey (Ed.), *The stately homo: A celebration of the life of Quentin Crisp*. London, UK: Bantam Press.

Lebert, F. (2005). Diogenes syndrome: A clinical presentation of fronto-temporal dementia or not? *International Journal of Geriatric Psychiatry, 20*, 1203–1204.

Lee, S. M., Lewis, M., Leighton, D., Harris, B., Long, B., & Macfarlane, S. (2014). Neuropsychological characteristics of people living in squalor. *International Psychogeriatrics, 26*, 837–844.

Lee, S. M., & LoGiudice, D. (2012). Phenomenology of squalor, hoarding and self-neglect: An Australian aged care perspective. *Internal Medicine Journal, 42*, 98–101.

Lenders, T., Kuster, J., & Bispinck, R. (2015). Management of uninhabitable homes—Investigation of 186 cases of hoarding, domestic neglect and squalor in Dortmund (Germany). *Fortschritte der Neurologie Psychiatrie, 83*, 695–701.

Macmillan, D. (1957). Psychiatric aspects of social breakdown in the elderly. *Royal Society of Health Journal, 77*, 830–836.

Macmillan, D., & Shaw, P. (1966). Senile breakdown in standards of personal and environmental cleanliness. *British Medical Journal, 2*, 1032–1037.

Macquarie Concise Dictionary. (2009). 5th ed. Sydney, Australia: Macquarie.

Maier, T. (2004). On phenomenology and classification of hoarding: A review. *Acta Psychiatrica Scandinavica, 110*, 323–337.

Mataix-Cols, D., Frost, R. O., Pertusa, A., Clark, L. A., Saxena, S., Leckman, J. F., . . . Wilhelm, S. (2010). Hoarding disorder: A new diagnosis for DSM-V? *Depression & Anxiety, 27*(6), 556–572.

McDermott, S. (2008). The devil is in the details: Self-neglect in Australia. *Journal of Elder Abuse & Neglect, 20*, 231–250.

McDermott, S., & Gleeson, R. (2009). *Evaluation of the Severe Domestic Squalor Project: Final report*. Sydney, Australia: Social Policy Research Centre, University of New South Wales.

Norberg, M. M., & Snowdon, J. (2014). Severe domestic squalor. In R. O. Frost & G. Steketee (Eds.), *The Oxford handbook of hoarding and acquiring*. Oxford, UK: Oxford University Press.

Nordsletten, A. E., Reichenberg, A., Hatch, S. L., de la Cruz, L. F., Pertusa, A., Hotopf, M., & Mataix-Cols, D. (2013). Epidemiology of hoarding disorder. *British Journal of Psychiatry, 203*, 445–452.

Pavlou, M. P., & Lachs, M. S. (2008). Self-neglect in older adults: A primer for clinicians. *Journal of General Internal Medicine, 23*, 1841–1846.

Pertusa, A., & Fonseca, A. (2014). Hoarding behavior in other disorders. In R. O. Frost & G. Steketee (Eds.), *The Oxford handbook of hoarding and acquiring*. Oxford, UK: Oxford University Press.

Poythress, E. L., Burnett, J., Naik, A. D., Pickens, S., & Dyer, C. B. (2006). Severe self-neglect: An epidemiological and historical perspective. *Journal of Elder Abuse & Neglect, 18*, 5–12.

Reifler, B. V. (1996). Diogenes syndrome: Of omelettes and soufflés. *Journal of the American Geriatrics Society, 44*, 1484–1485.

Reyes-Ortiz, C. A., Burnett, J., Flores, D. V., Halphen, J. M., & Dyer, C. B. (2014). Medical implications of elder abuse: Self-neglect. *Clinics in Geriatric Medicine, 30*, 807–823.

Roby, J. L., & Sullivan, R. (2000). Adult protection service laws. A comparison of state statutes from definition to case closure. *Journal of Elder Abuse & Neglect, 12*, 17–51.

Saxena, S. (2014). Pharmacotherapy of compulsive hoarding. In R. O. Frost & G. Steketee (Eds.), *The Oxford handbook of hoarding and acquiring*. Oxford, UK: Oxford University Press.

Shaw, P. (1957). The evidence of social breakdown in the elderly. *Journal of the Royal Society for the Promotion of Health, 77*, 823–830.

Slyne, K., & Tolin, D.F. (2014). The neurobiology of hoarding disorder. In R. O. Frost & G. Steketee (Eds.), *The Oxford handbook of hoarding and acquiring*. Oxford, UK: Oxford University Press.

Snowdon, J. (1987). Uncleanliness among persons seen by community health workers. *Hospital and Community Psychiatry, 38*, 491–494.

Snowdon, J. (2015). Accumulating too much stuff: What is hoarding and what is not? *Australasian Psychiatry, 23,* 354–357.

Snowdon, J., & Halliday, G. (2011). A study of severe domestic squalor: 173 cases referred to an old age psychiatry service. *International Psychogeriatrics, 23,* 308–314.

Snowdon, J., Halliday, G., & Banerjee, S. (2012). *Severe domestic squalor.* Cambridge, UK: Cambridge University Press.

Snowdon, J., Halliday, G., & Hunt, G. (2013). Two types of squalor: Findings from a factor analysis of the Environmental Cleanliness and Clutter Scale. *International Psychogeriatrics, 25,* 1191–1198.

Sutherland, A., & Macfarlane, S. (2014). Domestic squalor: Who should take responsibility? *Australian and New Zealand Journal of Psychiatry, 48,* 690.

Tolin, D., Frost, R. O., & Steketee, G. (2007). *Buried in treasures. Help for compulsive acquiring, saving and hoarding.* New York, NY: Oxford University Press.

Tolin, D. F., Stevens, M., Nave, A., Villavicencioa, A. L., & Morrison, S. (2012). Neural mechanisms of cognitive-behavioral therapy response in hoarding disorder: A pilot study. *Journal of Obsessive-Compulsive and Related Disorders, 1,* 180–188.

Wrigley, M., & Cooney, C. (1992). Diogenes syndrome—An Irish series. *Irish Journal of Psychological Medicine, 9,* 37–41.

Wustmann, T., & Brieger, P. (2005). A study of persons living in neglect, filth and squalor or who have a tendency to hoard. *Gesundheitswesen, 67,* 361–368.

CHAPTER 9

SELF-NEGLECT AND DECISION MAKING

Jessica L. Lee

This chapter discusses some of the most widely studied factors involved in elder self-neglect and cognition. The literature review includes 19 studies from 2000 to 2016, with emphasis on elder self-neglect and its association with personality traits, depression, dementia, and executive function. The literature review also includes studies of elder self-neglecters and their decision-making capacity. A section on assessment of decision-making capacity for health care providers is included. A case study of a self-neglecting older adult who was referred by adult protective services (APS) for a capacity evaluation is included and discussed.

Elder self-neglect is a multifactorial syndrome that has a high risk of mortality and has been strongly linked to cognition, including mental health (Hildebrand, Taylor, & Bradway, 2014). More specific, it has been robustly studied in global cognitive impairment, depression, and executive dysfunction. Multiple elder abuse studies have noted that self-neglecters have a higher prevalence of depression and dementia when compared with clients who are referred for other types of elder abuse (Dong et al., 2009; Dyer, Pavlik, Murphy, & Hyman, 2000; Roepke-Buehler, Simon, & Dong, 2015). Subsequent studies found similar increases in the prevalence of depression in elder self-neglecters. However, studies of dementia in elder self-neglecters were less clear. Several studies showed that there are no consistent associations between global cognitive impairment and self-neglect (Dong & Simon, 2015; Dyer, Goodwin, Pickens-Pace, Burnett, & Kelly, 2007; Naik, Pickens, Burnett, Lai, & Dyer, 2006; Pickens et al., 2007; Schillerstrom, Salazar, Regwan, Bonugli, & Royall, 2009). In particular, using certain global cognitive impairment tests, such as the Mini-Mental State Examination (MMSE; Cockrell & Folstein, 1988), was not specific for identifying elder self-neglecters (Dyer et al., 2007; Naik et al., 2006; Naik, Lai, Kunik, & Dyer, 2008; Pickens et al., 2007; Schillerstrom et al., 2009). Health care providers have often seen older adults with normal MMSE scores who are unable to provide for their own basic needs. Further research indicates that problems with executive function, or the cognitive control of behavior, are more correlated with older adults who self-neglect. One explanation for why executive dysfunction may be more commonly identified is because dementia, depression, and other cognitive changes often relate to the frontal lobe, which create and worsen functional decline, exacerbating inadequate physical and social support (Hildebrand et al., 2014).

BACKGROUND LITERATURE

Self-Neglect and Personality Traits

Health care professionals who have worked with self-neglecting older adults have noted that they share certain personality traits such as being unfriendly or suspicious (Dong et al., 2011). In a large cross-sectional study of the Chicago Health Aging Project (CHAP), 1,820 suspected self-neglecters were examined for neuroticism, extraversion, rigidity, and information processing personality traits (Dong et al., 2011). The researchers used some measures from the Neuroticism-Extraversion-Openness Personality Inventory (McCrae & Costa, 1985) and from the Need for Cognition Scale (Osberg, 1987). *Neuroticism* was defined as the "disposition to experience psychological distress" (Dong et al., 2011, p. 745); *extraversion* referred to "the tendency to be outgoing, energetic, and optimistic" (Dong et al., 2011, p. 745); *rigidity* is "the lack of active imagination and intellectual curiosity" (Dong et al., 2011, p. 745); and *information processing* was "the individual's preferred approach to learning and using information" (Dong et al., 2011, p. 745). Despite what was sometimes seen in clinical practice, after adjusting for confounders, these personality traits were not associated with significantly increased risk of elder self-neglect. Therefore, older adults who self-neglect cannot be identified by their personalities alone.

Self-Neglect and Depression

Late-life depression, the most prevalent psychiatric disorder among older adults living in the United States, is present in 15% to 20% of individuals aged 65 and older (Hansen, Flores, Coverdale, & Burnett, 2016). In one of the earliest studies to specifically examine self-neglect and relationship with depression, using a comprehensive geriatric assessment combined with the Geriatric Depression Scale (GDS; Yesavage et al., 1982–1983), it was found that elder self-neglecters had a significantly higher prevalence of depression when compared with older adults who were referred for other forms of abuse (Dyer et al., 2000). In another study of matched case controls, elder self-neglecters were more depressed by the GDS-short form than those who were nonself-neglecters (51% vs. 28%; Burnett, Coverdale, Pickens, & Dyer, 2006). Ninety-one elder self-neglecters who were case matched with 91 community-dwelling older adults also had higher depression scores (Burnett, Regev, et al., 2006). In addition to formal evaluations of depression, one study found that depressive symptoms, such as overall depression and individual factors such as depressed affect, positive affect, and somatic complaints based on a modified version of the Center for Epidemiologic Studies Depression Scale (CES-D; Radloff, 1977), were consistently associated with elder self-neglect (Roepke-Buehler et al., 2015). A recent study found that positive screens for alcohol abuse, lower scores for self-rated health, and higher self-reported pain intensity scores were associated with depression in elder self-neglecters (Hansen et al., 2016).

There have also been several studies based on ethnicity that consider elder self-neglecters and the prevalence of depression. In a study based on the Patient Health Questionnaire (PHQ-9) of Chinese older adults in Chicago, prevalence of mild self-neglect was 22.9% for older adults without any depressive symptoms (Kroenke, Spitzer, & Williams, 2001), whereas those with PHQ-9 scores of 6 or more had a prevalence of 39.3% (Dong & Simon, 2015). In that same study, the prevalence of moderate/severe self-neglect was 9.2% for older adults without any depressive symptoms and 20.2% for those with a

PHQ-9 score of 6 or more. However, in a cross-sectional study of Hispanic and African Americans with elder self-neglect, there was no statistically significant correlation with depressive symptoms as measured by the CES-D (Dong, Simon, Beck, & Evans, 2010).

Although, in general, depression has been associated with increased morbidity and mortality, one study found that elder self-neglecters were specifically more likely to have untreated medical conditions when compared with self-neglecters without depression (Dong et al., 2009). The same study showed elder self-neglecters had an increased risk for neuropsychiatric-related mortality.

Self-Neglect and Cognition

In one of the earliest studies of elder self-neglect and its association with cognitive function, 1,094 elder self-neglecters were assessed for cognitive function based on the MMSE, the Symbol Digit Modalities Test (Lewandowski, 1984) for speed of perception, both the immediate and delayed recall of the East Boston Memory Test (Gfeller & Horn, 1996) for episodic memory (Dong, Wilson, Mendes de Leon, & Evans, 2010), and a summary measure of global cognitive functioning. Self-neglect was associated with lower scores on the sum of all the four tests, as well as the individual measurements. In addition, the lower the scores were on the four tests, the higher were the self-neglect severity scores. Similarly, a study of 4,627 community-dwelling older adults with cognitive impairment based on MMSE scores less than or equal to 20, found rates of self-neglect of 18.8% among men and 13.6% among women (Dong, Simon, Mosqueda, & Evans, 2012). In a longitudinal study of elder self-neglecters, decline in global cognitive function was associated with increased risk of greater self-neglect severity (Dong, Simon, Wilson, et al., 2010). However, MMSE scores and other measures of global cognitive function have not always been found to correlate with self-neglect. There have been several studies on executive function (Dong, Simon, Wilson, et al., 2010; Dyer et al., 2007; Pickens et al., 2007; Schillerstrom et al., 2009), described in the next section, which indicate that executive dysfunction is more common in self-neglecters, even when tests, such as the MMSE, are normal. There seems to be a correlation with lower MMSE score and greater self-neglect severity as indicated by a study that found an increased prevalence of mild self-neglect (34.1%) and moderate/severe self-neglect (14.1%) in those who had lower cognitive function (MMSE scores less than 22) when compared with those with MMSE scores greater than 26 (Dong & Simon, 2015). Thus, more comprehensive cognitive testing is needed, particularly with respect to executive functioning and decision-making capacity.

Self-Neglect and Executive Function

Executive function is maintained by the frontal lobe and specific regions are associated with behaviors, such as motor and impulse control, that are important for maintaining activities of daily living (ADL; Royall, Palmer, Chiodo, & Polk, 2005).When there is damage to the frontal lobes, executive dysfunction occurs, which inhibits appropriate planning, initiation, organization, self-awareness, and execution of tasks, limiting self-care ability (Dong, Simon, Wilson, et al., 2010). Impairment of specific frontal regions, such as the mesiofrontal region, leads to apathy, distractibility, and failure to keep targeted goals (Dyer et al., 2007). When the orbitofrontal region is involved, people display irritability, mood lability, and resistance to care. Lesions in the dorsofrontal region affect planning, hypothesis testing, judgment, and insight. In a study comparing elder self-neglecters with older adults who were seeing an outpatient geriatric psychiatrist, executive dysfunction as measured by the Executive Interview (EXIT 25; Royall, Mahurinm, & Gray, 1992) and the executive Clock-Drawing Task. (CLOX1; Royall, Cordesm, & Polk, 1998), but not global cognitive deficits as measured by the MMSE, was more common in the self-neglecters (Schillerstrom et al., 2009). Similarly, in a cross-sectional comparison of 50 elder self-neglecters matched with 50 community-dwelling elders, self-neglecters with intact cognitive function on MMSE were significantly more likely to fail the Kohlman Evaluation of Living Skills (KELS) test (Kohlman-Thomson, 1992), which has been validated in geriatric populations to assess ADL and instrumental activities of daily living (IADL) and capacity to live independently (Pickens et al., 2007). In another study of over 500 older adults who self-neglected, 50% had abnormal MMSE scores but 58.9% scored less than 2 on the Clock-Drawing Task. (Tuokko, Hadjistavropoulosm, Miller, & Beattie,1992), which is a gross screen for executive function and cognition (Dyer et al., 2007). A separate longitudinal study found that only decline in executive functioning was associated with increased risk of reported and confirmed elder self-neglect, whereas poor global cognition and immediate and delayed recall did not appear related (Dong, Simon, Wilson, et al., 2010). It is important to note that in a group of 182 older adults referred for self-neglect, there was no difference in decision making between the group and matched controls (Naik et al., 2006). There is some thought that the difference between the decision making in those who self-neglect and those who do not is found in the action of carrying out the decision. A model of self-neglect was suggested in which executive dysfunction leads to functional impairment in the setting of inadequate medical and social support (Naik et al., 2006). Whether executive dysfunction is a cause of elder self-neglect or a result is difficult to tell, but leads to important questions about decision-making capacity.

DECISION-MAKING CAPACITY

Decision-making capacity can be defined in many ways, but generally means a person should have an understanding of the basic facts surrounding a decision; an appreciation of the personal impact of the decision, including one's capabilities and limitations; have a reasoning process for comparing the options and predicting the consequences of alternative choices; and the ability to make a choice (Naik et al., 2008). Executive capacity is the ability to execute one's decisions by having a predetermined plan, adapting the plan in response to changing or unexpected circumstances, and delegating these responsibilities to appropriate surrogates when one is physically unable to carry out the plan (Naik et al., 2006). Evaluation of capacity also involves identifying how the decisions fit into the functional domains needed for safe and independent living such as personal needs and hygiene, home environment, management of household affairs, medical self-care, and financial affairs. Unfortunately, there is no standard capacity screening tool or set of procedures for determining decision-making capacity. One study attempted to develop a capacity screening tool to try to identify the potential gaps in the decision-making capacity in vulnerable older adults (Naik et al., 2006). The acronym COMP was used to help the assessors remember the components of the tool, which are: count to 20 forward and backward, name three common objects, test of recall and recent memory, and perceptions of a medical case scenario. The tool was designed to test attention, language, delayed recall, and awareness of risks and benefits with a medical scenario. Interestingly, there were no significant differences between elders referred for self-neglect and matched older adults in screening for decision-making capacity (Naik et al., 2006). Elder self-neglecters were able to describe the risks and benefits associated with the medical scenario and could make appropriate decisions about what should be done in the case. However, there was a discordance between being able to make the appropriate safe choices in a mock scenario and being able to execute similar decisions in their own lives. Yet, health care providers are often asked to assess patients for decision-making capacity. In the United States, these assessments are often used to determine a person's legal competence and whether he or she has the ability to make his or her own decisions per the courts.

Assessing Decision-Making Capacity

Though there are several tools listed in the literature for assessing executive function and self-neglect, such as the EXIT 25 and the KELS, these are not designed to formally assess decision-making capacity. Often health care professionals are asked to determine whether a person is safe to be living on his or her own or whether he or she may need more assistance, even if reluctant to accept help. The idea of autonomy, the individual's right to make his or her own choices, is one of the fundamental ethical principles of medicine, so those making capacity assessments need to be careful about overstepping any boundaries. Figure 9.1 presents a flow diagram for a suggested

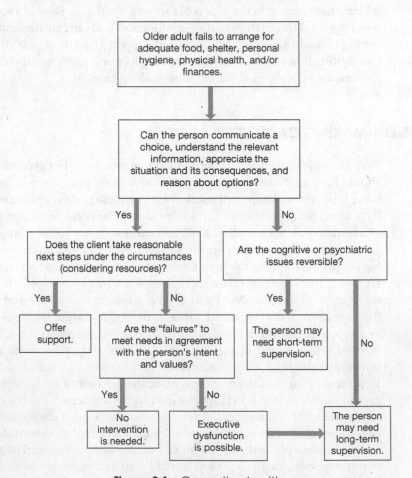

Figure 9.1 Capacity algorithm.

basic capacity assessment. This assessment is subject to individual circumstances and observations but provides a general overview of how a capacity assessment might work. When an older adult begins to manifest problems arranging for his or her own basic needs, the first questions to ask are whether the person can communicate a choice, can understand the relevant information, can appreciate the situation and its consequences, and can reason about options. This helps set the baseline for determining whether the person even understands the circumstances surrounding a decision. If he or she is not able to meet those capacity standards then he or she likely has a cognitive or psychiatric condition impairing the ability to make appropriate decisions. If the condition is reversible, then short-term supervision may be more appropriate, whereas if the condition is irreversible, long-term supervision is likely needed. The capacity issue becomes more confusing if the older adult is able to meet the decisional capacity standards. Further questions about the person taking reasonable next steps need to be determined. If the person is trying to arrange for his or her needs but is limited by things such as finances, offering support through financial or social resources would be reasonable. If the person is not taking the appropriate next steps, then it is important to evaluate whether this "failure" to meet needs is consistent with the person's intent and values. If yes, then respect for the individual's autonomy should be upheld. However, if the answer is no, then there may be some evidence of executive dysfunction, in which case long-term supervision may be needed.

The algorithm in Figure 9.1 provides a framework for examining the case of Mr. X, presented in Case Study 1. Mr. X was seen for a capacity assessment at the request of APS.

CASE STUDY 1: MR. X

Mr. X is a 73-year-old man who was referred to APS because of concerns that he is both neglecting himself and that he is living in a situation in which he is abused and neglected by his companion. APS had been called numerous times by various law enforcement and emergency personnel because Mr. X was repeatedly found living in unsanitary conditions with the companion, who was allegedly physically, emotionally, and verbally abusive. Mr. X's daughter had also tried to intervene previously, but Mr. X refused to sever his relationship with the companion.

Analysis

He Is Failing to Arrange for His Basic Needs

In conversation with Mr. X, he was found to be very articulate and had no difficulties with short- or long-term memory. He has a history of spinal cord injury 10 years earlier, which resulted in multiple surgeries that resulted in lower leg weakness that necessitates the use of a power wheelchair for mobility. He also had a history of chronic kidney disease, diabetes mellitus, coronary artery disease with surgical bypass, and congestive heart failure. He has a box of medications, which he said were "mostly muscle relaxants and pain meds, so I don't really need to take them all of the time anyway." He has a primary care physician at the local veterans' hospital whom he sees regularly and is getting some provider and physical therapy services at home. On physical examination, he was found to be well nourished but had multiple wounds all over his legs. His hair was unkempt and his clothes were dirty. His home was cluttered, with poor lighting, and feces and living insects on the floor. Basic cognitive testing showed that he scored a 27 of 30 on the MMSE, missing points in the areas of orientation, calculation, and design. He scored a 3 out of 5 on the Clock-Drawing Task., missing points because he did not distinguish between the minute and the hour hands and did not put the hands at the right time. He understands that his house is unsanitary and he characterizes his relationship with his companion, not as romantic, but as "someone to provide friendship for a lonely old man."

CASE STUDY (continued)

He Is Able to Communicate a Choice, Understand the Relevant Information, Appreciate the Situation and Its Consequences, and Reason About Options

Due to the unsanitary condition of his home, Mr. X said he was trying to hire more provider services and was working to have his home cleaned by a housekeeping agency. He said he was also looking into moving into an assisted living facility if his companion could live with him. He acknowledged that his companion "had a drinking problem" and had hit him before. However, he insisted that his companion's friendship outweighed the abuse. His companion was completely financially dependent on him but Mr. X did not feel he was being exploited because he was the one who handled the finances.

His "Failure" to Meet Needs Was in Keeping With His Intent and Values

Because Mr. X was assessed as acting in keeping with his intentions, no intervention was indicated. As a follow-up, his companion gave APS more background indicating that Mr. X also often instigated abuse both physically and verbally and that this had characterized their entire relationship. Fortunately, Mr. X did later take steps to hire more provider services and a housekeeper.

CONCLUSION

Evaluation of older adults with self-neglect should always take into account possible cognitive impairments such as dementia or mental health issues such as depression. By the same token, older adults with cognitive impairment or mental health problems should be screened for self-neglect. Although basic cognitive assessment is important in elder self-neglecters, screening for executive function is critical for those who may seem to have normal global cognitive functioning. Assessing basic decision making involves the older adult comprehending the information needed to make the decision, appreciating the risks and benefits of the decision and how it would apply to his or her own situation, having a reasoning process for why he or she is making a decision, and being able to make a choice. Beyond that, the person needs to be able to execute reasonable next steps, taking into account his or her resources, and keeping in mind the person's intent and values. These basic principles can help health care professionals establish capacity in older adults who self-neglect.

IMPLICATIONS FOR RESEARCH AND PRACTICE

- Depression and dementia are more prevalent in older adults who self-neglect.
- Screening for executive dysfunction is important because global cognitive function may not always be affected.
- Decision-making capacity generally involves an understanding of the facts surrounding a decision, appreciation of the personal impact of the decision, having a reasoning process for comparing the options and predicting the consequences, and the ability to make a choice.
- Executive capacity is the ability to execute decisions by having a predetermined plan, adapting the plan in response to changing or unexpected circumstances, and delegating responsibilities to appropriate surrogates if physically unable to carry out the plan.
- Further research is needed to determine whether executive dysfunction is a cause or a result of elder self-neglect.

REFERENCES

Burnett, J., Coverdale, J. H., Pickens, S., & Dyer, C. B. (2006). What is the association between self-neglect, depressive symptoms and untreated medical conditions? *Journal of Elder Abuse & Neglect, 18*(4), 25–34.

Burnett, J., Regev, T., Pickens, S., Prati, L. L., Aung, K., Moore, J., & Dyer, C. B. (2006). Social networks: A profile of the elderly who self-neglect. *Journal of Elder Abuse & Neglect, 18*(4), 35–49.

Cockrell, J. R., & Folstein, M. F. (1988). Mini-Mental State Examination (MMSE). *Psychopharmacology Bulletin, 24*(4), 689–692.

Dong, X., & Simon, M. (2015). Prevalence of elder self-neglect in a Chicago Chinese population: The role of cognitive, physical and mental health. *Geriatrics & Gerontology International, 16*(9), 1051–1062. doi:10.1111/ggi.12598

Dong, X., Simon, M., Beck, T., & Evans, D. (2010). A cross-sectional population-based study of elder self-neglect and psychological, health, and social factors in a biracial community. *Aging & Mental Health, 14*(1), 74–84.

Dong, X., Simon, M., Mendes de Leon, C., Fulmer, T., Herbert, L., Dyer, C., . . . Evans, D. (2009). Elder self-neglect and abuse and mortality risk in a community-dwelling population. *Journal of the American Medical Association, 302*(5), 517–526.

Dong, X., Simon, M. A., Mosqueda, L., & Evans, D. A. (2012). The prevalence of elder self-neglect in a community-dwelling population: Hoarding, hygiene, and environmental hazards. *Journal of Aging and Health, 24*(3), 507–524.

Dong, X., Simon, M., Wilson, R., Beck, T., McKinell, K., & Evans, D. (2011). Association of personality traits with elder self-neglect in a community-dwelling population. *American Journal of Geriatric Psychiatry, 19*(8), 743–751.

Dong, X., Simon, M. A., Wilson, R. S., Mendes de Leon, C. F., Rajan, K. B., & Evans, D. A. (2010). Decline in cognitive function and risk of elder self-neglect: Finding from the Chicago Health Aging Project. *Journal of the American Geriatrics Society, 58*(12), 2292–2299.

Dong, X., Wilson, R. S., Mendes de Leon, C. F., & Evans, D. A. (2010). Self-neglect and cognitive function among community-dwelling older persons. *International Journal of Geriatric Psychiatry, 25*(8), 798–806.

Dyer, C. B., Goodwin, J. S., Pickens-Pace, S., Burnett, J., & Kelly, P. A. (2007). Self-neglect among the elderly: A model based on more than 500 patients seen by a geriatric medicine team. *American Journal of Public Health, 97*(9), 1671–1676.

Dyer, C. B., Pavlik, V. N., Murphy, K. P., & Hyman, D. J. (2000). The high prevalence of depression and dementia in elder abuse or neglect. *Journal of the American Geriatrics Society, 48*(2), 205–208.

Gfeller, J. D., & Horn, G. J. T. (1996). The East Boston Memory Test: A clinical screening measure for memory impairment in the elderly. *Journal of Clinical Psychology, 52*(2), 191–196.

Hansen, M. C., Flores, D. V., Coverdale, J., & Burnett, J. (2016). Correlates of depression in self-neglecting older adults: A cross-sectional study examining the role of alcohol abuse and pain in increasing vulnerability. *Journal of Elder Abuse & Neglect, 28*(1), 41–56.

Hildebrand, C., Taylor, M., & Bradway, C. (2014). Elder self-neglect: The failure of coping because of cognitive and functional impairments. *Journal of the American Association of Nurse Practitioners, 26*(8), 452–462.

Kohlman-Thomson, L. (1992). *Kohlman evaluation of living skills* (3rd ed.). Bethesda, MD: American Occupational Therapy Association.

Kroenke, K., Spitzer, R. L., & Williams, J. B. (2001). The PHQ-9: Validity of a brief depression severity measure. *Journal of General Internal Medicine, 16*(9), 606–613.

Lewandowski, L. J. (1984). The Symbol Digit Modalities Test: A screening instrument for brain-damaged children. *Perceptual and Motor Skills, 59*(2), 615–618.

McCrae, R. R., & Costa, P. T., Jr. (1985). Updating Norman's "adequate taxonomy:" Intelligence and personality dimensions in natural language and in questionnaires. *Journal of Personality and Social Psychology, 49*(3), 710–721.

Naik, A. D., Lai, J. M., Kunik, M. E., & Dyer, C. B. (2008). Assessing capacity in suspected cases of self-neglect. *Geriatrics, 63*(2), 24–31.

Naik, A. D., Pickens, S., Burnett, J., Lai, J. M., & Dyer, C. B. (2006). Assessing capacity in the setting of self-neglect: Development of a novel screening tool for decision-making capacity. *Journal of Elder Abuse & Neglect, 18*(4), 79–91.

Osberg, T. M. (1987). The convergent and discriminant validity of the Need for Cognition Scale. *Journal of Personality Assessment, 51*(3), 441–450.

Pickens, S., Naik, A. D., Burnett, J., Kelly, P. A., Gleason, M., & Dyer, C. B. (2007). The utility of the Kohlman Evaluation of Living Skills test is associated with substantiated cases of elder self-neglect. *Journal of the American Academy of Nurse Practitioners, 19*(3), 137–142.

Radloff, L. S. (1977). The CES-D scale: A self-report depression scale for research in the general population. *Applied Psychological Measurement, 1*, 385–401.

Roepke-Buehler, S. K., Simon, M., & Dong, X. (2015). Association between depressive symptoms, multiple dimensions of depression, and elder abuse: A cross-sectional, population-based analysis of older adults in urban Chicago. *Journal of Aging and Health, 27*(6), 1003–1025.

Royall, D. R., Cordesm, J. A., & Polk, M. (1988). CLOX: An executive clock drawing task. *Journal of Neurology, Neurosurgery & Psychiatry, 64*(5), 588–594.

Royall, D. R., Mahurinm, R. K., & Gray, K. F. (1992). Bedside assessment of executive cognitive impairment: The executive interview. *Journal of the American Geriatrics Society, 40*(12), 1221–1226.

Royall, D. R., Palmer, R., Chiodo, L. K., & Polk, M. J. (2005). Executive control mediates memory's association with change in instrumental activities of daily living: The Freedom House Study. *Journal of the American Geriatrics Society, 53*(1), 11–17. doi:10.1111/j.1532-5415.2005.53004.x

Schillerstrom, J. E., Salazar, R., Regwan, H., Bonugli, R. J., & Royall, D. R. (2009). Executive function in self-neglecting Adult Protective Services referrals compared with elder psychiatric outpatients. *American Journal of Geriatric Psychiatry, 17*(10), 907–910. doi:10.1097/JGP.0b013e3181b4bf64

Tuokko, H., Hadjistavropoulosm, T., Miller, J. A., & Beattie, B. L. (1992). The Clock Test: A sensitive measure to differentiate normal elderly from those with Alzheimer disease. *Journal of the American Geriatrics Society, 40*(6), 579–584. doi:10.1111/j.1532-5415.1992.tb02106.x

Yesavage, J. A., Brink, T. L., Rose, T. L., Lum, O., Huang, V., Adey, M., & Leirer, V.O. (1982–1983). Development and validation of a geriatric depression screening scale: A preliminary report. *Journal of Psychiatric Research, 17*(1), 37–49. doi:10.1016/0022-3956(82)90033-4

THE SERVICE RESPONDS

CHAPTER 10

SELF-NEGLECT: AN ISSUE IN ACUTE CARE

Kieran A. O'Connor

Self-neglect in older adults is a prevalent but often under-recognized problem in acute care settings. It is a complex phenomenon often characterized by inattention to one's health and self-care, typically stemming from the inability or unwillingness to access available services. Medical and psychiatric comorbidities, such as dementia, depression, and alcoholism, are frequently associated causes or contributors to the phenomenon. Overall, there is a scarcity of high-quality epidemiological and controlled studies on self-neglecting behavior. Acute care suffers from an even greater paucity of research evidence than other locations for managing those vulnerable to self-neglect. The complex medical, psychological, and social aspects of self-neglect require a multidimensional and multidisciplinary assessment. Health care professionals in acute care settings should be open to considering self-neglect in vulnerable older patients whose welfare appears compromised. It is important to collaborate with the older persons and with multidisciplinary community services. Many complex cases of self-neglect in acute care will reach a good outcome with a comprehensive assessment, an agreed-upon intervention plan, and an effort to reverse treatable medical causes.

Self-neglect is a largely undiagnosed and an often ignored problem in our society. In their 2003 report, the National Research Council (NRC) defined self-neglect as a "failure of an individual to provide essential services for self as a result of mental or physical inability" (NRC, 2003, p. 39). People who self-neglect are often isolated and hidden in society. Any form of behavior that takes place in a person's own home is by its nature hidden, underreported, and difficult to research (Renzetti & Lee, 1993). Thus, making a determination of prevalence of self-neglect is very difficult (Papaioannou, Räihä, & Kivelä, 2012). From the available epidemiological evidence, self-neglect seems to primarily affect older people, its occurrence increases with advancing age, and it is more common in older men (Dong, Simon, Mosqueda, & Evans, 2012). Elder self-neglect is perhaps the most challenging area to deal with on the spectrum of elder abuse and neglect.

Self-neglect is increasingly being recognized as an important public health issue in community settings (Dong, Simon, & Evans, 2012b). In the United States, self-neglect has been recognized as a form of elder abuse for some time. Most adult protective services (APS) have supported and investigated suspected self-neglect cases. Recent data from the Chicago Health and Aging Project (CHAP) suggest that one out of nine older adults experiences some form of self-neglect in a community setting (Dong, Simon, Mosqueda, et al., 2012). Until recently, safeguarding agencies for older people in Ireland and the United Kingdom did not routinely collect data on the prevalence of self-neglect (Braye, Orr, & Preston-Shoot, 2014; Health Service Executive [HSE], 2012). This is beginning to change with elder self-neglect being the most commonly received report by the APS in the United States (Dong, Simon, & Evans, 2012a). In Ireland, self-neglect cases were the third most common referrals made to senior case workers (HSE, 2014). In Ireland, self-neglect cases now account for 20% of the referrals received by specialist senior case workers who work specifically with elder abuse services (HSE, 2014). Self-neglect is also now recognized as a prominent feature in of the community-based public health nurse caseload (Day, Mulcahy, & Leahy-Warren, 2016).

When the National Health Service was founded in the United Kingdom in 1948, 48% of the population died before the age of 65. Now that figure has fallen to just 14% (Office for National Statistics, 2011). This success story for society and for modern medicine has utterly transformed our health and care needs. Thankfully, many people stay healthy, happy, and independent well into old age. However, as people age, they are progressively more likely to live with complex comorbidities, disability, and frailty. Therefore, it is unsurprising that older people are disproportionately the greater users of the emergency department (ED) and of acute in-hospital care (Blunt, Bardsley, & Dixon, 2010; Oliver, Foot, & Humphries, 2014). Older people are admitted to the hospital more frequently, have a longer length of stay, and occupy more bed-days in acute hospitals compared with other patient groups. As a result of our growing appreciation of the level of self-neglect in the community, we would expect a proportionately higher level of self-neglect cases in acute care, where the population is increasingly older. However, self-neglect in acute care all too often remains unrecognized and underappreciated. The relatively small number of reported cases of self-neglect in acute care is probably only the tip of the iceberg. There remains a myriad of unanswered questions regarding the epidemiology of self-neglect (Gill, 2009; Pavlou & Lachs, 2008). More research is needed so that the size of the issue of self-neglect in acute care can be more precisely defined.

We know that there is considerable evidence of ageism and age discrimination in secondary-care settings, ranging from patronizing attitudes or language, to older people being denied treatment on the grounds of age alone, to common conditions of aging being neglected in service planning, priorities, and training of staff (Centre for Policy on Ageing, 2009). Processes in the hospital not only frequently result in older people being dismissed with labels such as "social admission" or "acopia" (Kee & Rippingale, 2009; Oliver, 2008). Even though all these issues support a view that acute care settings are often neglectful to older people, this is not the focus of this chapter. Instead, this chapter will examine the issue of people presenting to acute care who are experiencing some form of self-neglect within the community. The challenges in identification, assessment, and management of self-neglect in a hospital setting will be explored. The ideas within the chapter are supported by a series of case studies that illustrate some of the types of issues relating to extreme self-neglect encountered in an acute care setting. The case studies are based on actual cases. However, all names are fictitious and the details altered substantially to aid illustration of the issues. In order to maintain client confidentiality, individual cases are not identifiable to a single client, but are a conglomeration of similar themes in a number of cases.

BACKGROUND LITERATURE

Abuse of older people has been recognized for centuries, but has only been reported in the professional literature since the mid-1970s (Baker, 1975; Burston, 1977). Elder abuse has remained the least acknowledged of all the types of human violence and, within this field of elder abuse and neglect, self-neglect remains the least accepted. Self-neglect even continues to occupy an ambivalent position in many adult safeguarding agencies, with some explicitly excluding self-neglect from the remit of their procedures (Braye et al., 2014). Self-neglect receives limited emphasis in medical/gerontological teaching and often still gets a scarce mention in general medical/gerontological textbooks (Fillit, Rockwood, & Woodhouse, 2010).

Self-neglect, as a concept, is hard to define as it is often misinterpreted as purely a choice, a misuse of alcohol, a mental health issue, or simply as being too lazy. Self-neglect is characterized by the inability to perform essential self-care tasks, thereby threatening a person's health and safety (Papaioannou et al., 2012). Self-neglect can manifest itself in an older person as a refusal or inability to provide adequate food, water, clothing, shelter, personal hygiene, or medication when indicated (Day, Mulcahy, Leahy-Warren, & Downey, 2015). Like many other syndromes in the health care of older people, self-neglect is most appropriately viewed along a continuum of severity, rather than in two discrete categories, self-neglect or no self-neglect (Dong & Gorbien, 2005).

Like other syndromes of geriatric medicine practice, self-neglect is multidimensional and complex. It is not only a medical issue, but it is also a social, legal, and ethical one. In the model put forward by Dyer, Goodwin, Burnett, and Kelly (2007), self-neglect often begins with neurodegenerative or mental health issues, followed by executive dysfunction and subsequently impairment in activities of daily living (Dyer et al., 2007; Institute of Medicine [IOM] &NRC, 2014). Self-neglect can result from (coupled with the factors discussed previously) inadequate support services due to lack of capacity for self-care or because of extrinsic issues like poverty or lack of social support (Dyer et al., 2007; IOM & NRC, 2014). The complexities inherent in addressing self-neglect require comprehensive multidisciplinary assessments and interventions. The appropriate management of self-neglect often requires the work of multiple agencies.

SELF-NEGLECTING BEHAVIOR AND THE BURDEN ON ACUTE HOSPITAL CARE

Acute health care, and especially hospitalization, contributes enormously to the cost of health care systems. Preventing disease in the first place is the best way to reduce the need for hospitalization. It is estimated that as much as 70% of premature mortality may be attributable to lifestyle-related diseases (Sullivan, 1990). Over the past century, there have been many advances in preventive medicine. People with self-neglecting behavior often do not access preventive medicine interventions such as vaccinations or cancer screening. Those who self-neglect often manifest behaviors that threaten their health and safety, which predispose them to more encounters with the health care systems. We know that elder self-neglect is associated with a significantly increased risk of 1-year mortality (Dong et al., 2009). However, mortality in self-neglect may not be equal in all groups. Other aspects of culture, access to health care monitoring, and socioeconomic factors might be important also. The CHAP study data have shown that over time the impact of self-neglect on mortality was significantly stronger in Black than in White older adults (Dong, Simon, Fulmer, et al., 2011).

With self-neglecting behavior, people can expose themselves to personal and environmental hazards that negatively contribute to health outcomes. Health care advances have resulted in many pharmacological interventions for disease prevention and treatment. However, we know that medication nonadherence is a prevalent problem among self-neglecting older adults (Turner, Hochschild, Burnett, Zulfiqar, & Dyer, 2012). Self-neglect can sometimes result in extreme nonadherence to medication and treatment plans. Such behavior will almost certainly render disease-prevention activities ineffective or unrealistic, adding to the risk of acute care and hospitalization for potentially preventable illnesses.

Whereas there are the beginnings of more robust data on the community burden of self-neglect (Day et al., 2016; Dong, 2014; Dong et al., 2012b; Dong, Simon, Mosqueda, et al., 2012), the incidence of self-neglect in those presenting to acute services remains less clear. From the CHAP study data, we are beginning to get a picture of the health care utilization of the older people with self-neglect who are known to the APS in the community prior to their presentation to the hospital. In the CHAP study, older people reported to a social service agency have a higher rate of ED use (Dong & Simon, 2013a; Dong, Simon, & Evans, 2011). Greater self-neglect severity has also been associated with a greater increase in ED use (Dong, Simon, & Evans, 2011). Dong and colleagues (2012a) have also found that reported and confirmed elder self-neglect is independently associated with an increased risk of hospitalization compared with those without self-neglect. In addition, greater severity of elder self-neglect is associated with a greater risk of hospitalization (Dong et al., 2012a; Dong & Simon, 2013c). Those with reported self-neglect were nearly 50% more likely to require hospitalization than those without elder self-neglect diagnosis after controlling for socioeconomic conditions, medical comorbidities, cognitive impairment, and physical disability (Dong et al., 2012a).

However, a retrospective case-control study has shown that in the year preceding the involvement of the APS and geriatric medicine teams, self-neglecters had substantially lower rates of health care utilization than their non-self-neglecting counterparts (Franzini & Dyer, 2008). This is not surprising as, by definition, people who self-neglect tend to avoid medical services prior to being identified by health or social services. More interestingly, this study suggested that, once identified, the health care utilization of those with self-neglect was not very different from that of their more medically adherent controls in the year following the involvement of the APS (Franzini & Dyer, 2008).

The acute hospital sector sometimes has to act as a place of safety when care cannot be met in the community. Once individuals in the community are identified with self-neglecting behavior by support or social services, the likelihood of hospital admission increases (Cotton et al., 2007; Dong et al., 2012a; Franzini & Dyer, 2008). Multidisciplinary health professional teams sometimes decide that individuals with self-neglecting behavior may be more readily assessed with 24-hour staff in a hospital rather than in a home setting (Cotton et al., 2007). Even with the involvement of a community-based mental health crisis-resolution team, Cotton et al. (2007) found that self-neglecting individuals needed hospital admission three times more frequently than the entire cohort cared for by community teams. Community and acute care organizations need to provide an integrated structure to support self-neglecting individuals.

We have limited information about those experiencing self-neglect who have not yet been identified by the APS. We have many years of case report evidence of high health care costs among people experiencing gross self-neglect who present acutely with complex needs (Cybulska & Rucinski, 1986; Roe, 1977). All those working in acute geriatric medicine services have anecdotal stories of people with self-neglect who present for the first time with a catastrophic stroke, advanced burrowing basal cell carcinoma of the face, or a gangrenous foot, resulting in substantial health care costs (Lachs, 2008). If these self-neglecting people are identified early and appropriate supports are initiated they may be treated before their self-neglecting behaviors become severe so as to warrant complex and prolonged hospitalization.

The association of elder self-neglect with ED attendance and hospital admissions emphasizes the need to be aware of the issue and to consider screening for self-neglect in acute health care settings. Hospital multidisciplinary teams should contemplate routine screening for self-neglect among older patients who have frequent encounters with hospitals. Further research is required to examine the relationship between self-neglect and acute health care utilization in a comprehensive and systematic way. The role and benefit of screening in acute care settings should also be explored through further research.

ACUTE CARE PRESENTATIONS ASSOCIATED WITH SELF-NEGLECT

The relationship between self-neglect and medical conditions is complex. Self-neglect can potentially be contributed by physical disability, mental health difficulties, or cognitive deficits such as dementia. However, self-neglect is often accompanied by one or more conditions, such as deficits in nutrition and hygiene, elevated social needs, poverty and physical disability, all of which contribute to the development of illness. Self-neglecting behavior is an issue of considerable importance in the exacerbation of pre-existing medical illness (Abrams, Lachs, McAvay, Keohane, & Bruce, 2002). Therefore, it is possible that self-neglect could be both a contributor to acute illness but also contribute to the escalation of pre-existing medical or psychiatric illness.

Unfortunately, doctors in acute hospital settings are often ill prepared to recognize the complexity of a presentation with self-neglect. Whether as a result of inadequate training or biased attitudes, the frail older patient who presents with potential complexities of self-neglecting behavior often does not undergo the same diagnostic rigor offered to other single-organ acute presentations (Oliver, 2008).

Self-neglecting behavior may be the first visible sign of some potential etiological conditions. Risk factors for the development of self-neglect include cognitive impairment, depression, delirium, functional dependence, stressful life events, social isolation, alcohol dependence, or substance abuse (Cocksedge & Flynn, 2014; IOM & NRC, 2014). Particularly for those who live alone, depression or dementia can lead to self-neglecting behavior. Depression can be a factor contributing to one's decision to self-neglect; but neglect can further exacerbate depression, creating a vicious cycle (IOM& NRC, 2014).

Neuropsychiatric diseases, including Alzheimer's disease, vascular dementia, and other dementias, are more common in those who self-neglect than in controls (Abrams et al., 2002; Dyer & Goins, 2000; Krishnan et al., 2005). Mental health disorders are diagnosed more frequently in those with self-neglecting behavior than in hospitalized control groups (Franzini & Dyer, 2008). Franzini and Dyer (2008) showed that diseases of the circulatory system were the most common primary diagnosis in both hospitalized groups with and without self-neglect. Although there was considerable overlap in primary diagnoses of physical disorders in the two groups, mental health disorder was the second most frequent primary diagnosis in those with self-neglect, comprising 15% of diagnoses; it was ranked 12th among controls, with only 3% of primary diagnoses (Franzini & Dyer, 2008).

Those with self-neglecting behavior can often present to acute health care settings with untreated and undiagnosed medical symptoms or with nonadherence to planned management of known medical conditions (Papaioannou et al., 2012; Turner et al., 2012). Self-neglect can affect the individual's physical condition and exacerbate any health concerns. Self-neglecting behavior can result in rashes, pressure sores, or lice infestations (Cornwall, 1981). Malnutrition and dehydration can result in the deterioration of physical ability, thereby increasing the risk of falls and fractures (Papaioannou et al., 2012).

Adverse drug events are responsible for many hospitalizations among older persons each year (Hitzeman & Belsky, 2013). The risk of adverse drug events is increased with the potential overmedication or erratic use of medication in those with self-neglecting behavior (Homeier, 2014). Self-neglecting behavior may exacerbate many existing health conditions that already affect the person's well-being.

Unfortunately, those with self-neglecting behavior may present very late in the course of a disease. Those with self-neglecting behavior can present with extreme manifestations of more common conditions, such as a severely gangrenous foot in peripheral vascular disease or myxedema madness in untreated primary hypothyroidism (Azzopardi, Murfin, Sharda, & De Silva, 2010; Wrenn, 1990). Even for those with advanced life-threatening illnesses, the involvement of health care services may occur much later in the disease course. Elder self-neglect is associated with shorter length of stay in hospice care, and shorter time from hospice admission to death (Dong & Simon, 2013b).

If self-neglecting behaviors are of acute onset, then the probability of an underlying new acute psychiatric or medical problem as the culprit increases. Acute mental health problems, such as the recent onset of schizophrenia or acute mania, can result in bizarre behavior and self-neglect (Ventura, Nuechterlein, Subotnik, Gutkind, & Gilbert, 2000). Delirium is commonly associated with acute illness in frail older people. Delirium results in a serious disturbance in mental abilities causing acutely confused thinking and a reduced awareness of one's environment. Delirium should always be considered in a person presenting with new-onset self-neglecting behavior. The acute stroke syndrome of unilateral posteromedial thalamic infarction can present with an acute neuropsychological disturbance with apathy, poor motivation, and amnesia (De Freitas & Bogousslavsky, 2002). This thalamic dementia can result in a rapid onset of self-neglecting behavior, especially in those living alone or with limited social support. Therefore, anyone presenting with a new onset of strange behavior resulting in self-neglect requires a careful and thorough assessment of possible acute medical or psychiatric conditions.

THE HOSPITAL PHYSICIAN'S ROLE IN MANAGEMENT OF SELF-NEGLECT

All health care disciplines encounter patients with self-neglecting behavior. In acute hospital settings, senior doctors have a specific clinical responsibility for such patients. In the hospital, the medical role tends to be more central to all health care decisions, as compared to community settings. However, in stark contrast to child abuse, where pediatricians play a central role in screening and interventions, physicians have traditionally played a minor role in detecting and reporting cases of elder abuse and neglect. However, physicians in geriatric medicine and psychiatrists for older adults are increasingly expected to develop expertise in the area of self-neglect. As with many of the geriatric syndromes prevalent in older adults, management requires the physician to have expertise that extends beyond medicine. Physicians in this field will often need to coordinate multidisciplinary involvement and expertise to examine medical, social, and legal aspects of care when self-neglect is suspected.

Physicians may occasionally see patients with self-neglecting behavior in ambulatory settings. However, the nature of the condition is such that these individuals often do not attend ambulatory clinics and thus those who self-neglect are far more likely to be encountered by physicians in situations where serious medical sequelae of self-neglecting behaviors have made contact with the acute health care system unavoidable. Physicians without experience in this field who encounter individuals with extreme self-neglect, can be overwhelmed by the multiple medical and social problems they harbor. Cases of extreme self-neglect are often medically complicated and physician involvement is essential. However, appropriate assessment and management usually require a multidisciplinary team rather than a single physician. The foundation of appropriate evaluation of the older self-neglector is a comprehensive geriatric assessment, defined as a multidimensional interdisciplinary diagnostic process focused on determining an older persons' medical, psychological, social, and functional capability (Pavlou & Lachs, 2008; Rubenstein, Stuck, Siu, & Wieland, 1991). The involvement of other disciplines is important not only to access broad expertise, but also to reduce the treatment burden on the primary physician (Reyes-Ortiz, Burnett, Flores, Halphen, & Dyer, 2014).

All physicians working in acute hospitals should be mindful of red flags that may suggest self-neglect. Patients who intentionally neglect chronic medical problems, such as refusing diabetic medication; those with untreated chronic wounds and ulcers; or those with a severe lack of personal hygiene should arouse suspicion. The management of individuals with self-neglecting behavior can be one of the most frustrating experiences for a physician (Pavlou & Lachs, 2008) because of the patients' refusal of interventions. Patients with extreme self-neglect do not present until profoundly ill, and, as a result, may require prolonged and extensive acute care.

If judged only on the rate that they report elder abuse and neglect to the APS, then physicians would seem to see very few cases. However, this may not accurately reflect the actual contribution of physicians (IOM & NRC, 2014). Research on elder abuse and neglect in Ireland ranked physicians as being the eighth reporting source (Clancy, McDaid, O'Neill, & O'Brien, 2011). However, a survey of physicians in geriatric medicine working in Ireland and Scotland by Bartley, O'Neill, Knight, and O'Brien (2011) regarding self-neglect revealed that most had encountered cases in the past year. In Bartley and colleague's study (2011), a refusal of services was a common reason geriatricians were asked to be involved. Dementia, lifelong personality traits, depression, and alcoholism were cited as the most common underlying causes found by geriatricians (Bartley et al., 2011). A similar survey of psychiatrists specializing in care of older people in Ireland revealed over 90% having seen a case of self-neglect in the past year (O'Brien, Cooney, Bartley, & O'Neill, 2013). Personal characteristics, loss of self-care, poor hygiene, medication noncompliance, and hoarding were the most common reasons involvement of these psychiatrists was required (O'Brien et al., 2013).

At least in Ireland, using reports from doctors as an indication of involvement in abuse and neglect may seriously underestimate their contributions. Physicians and psychiatrists working with older people usually work within a multidisciplinary team. When the team is dealing with a case of self-neglect, the doctor has a central role. However, it may be that another team member organizes reporting of the case to the relevant authority, under-representing the role of the physician in reporting data.

COMPREHENSIVE GERIATRIC ASSESSMENT

In the comprehensive geriatric assessment process, a physician in geriatric medicine working with a multidisciplinary team should evaluate medical, cognitive, psychosocial, functional, and environmental factors to address remediable problems and to develop an integrated plan for treatment and long-term follow-up (Rubenstein et al., 1991). This is the appropriate evaluation structure of older persons with suspected self-neglecting behavior presenting within an acute hospital setting (Pavlou & Lachs, 2008).

Self-neglect in vulnerable persons is often not just a personal preference or a behavioral idiosyncrasy. The spectrum of behaviors of self-neglect can be associated with increased morbidity, mortality, and impairments in activities of daily living (Dong et al., 2010; Dyer et al., 2007). Elder self-neglect is associated with an increased risk of 1-year mortality (Dong et al., 2009). Therefore, self-neglect suspicions should be viewed as alerts to potentially serious underlying problems that require evaluation and treatment (Naik, Lai, Kunik, & Dyer, 2008).

When evaluating a suspected case of self-neglect, a clinician will attempt to determine the ways in which one is not taking care of oneself, the cause, and what support would help meet the identified needs. Self-report in these cases is often grossly incorrect and misleading (Burnett, Cully, Achenbaum, Dyer, &Naik, 2011). A broad and inclusive evaluation of a comprehensive geriatric assessment is required to acquire accurate and complete information. Use of a comprehensive geriatric assessment process while in the hospital significantly improves the chances of an older person being alive and in his or her own home a year after an emergency hospital admission (Ellis, Whitehead, O'Neill, Langhorne, & Robinson, 2011).

Self-neglect in older people has many characteristics of other geriatric syndromes (Isaacs, 1976). Its etiology is multifactorial. It shares risk factors with other geriatric syndromes and is associated with increased mortality (Dong et al., 2009). Self-neglect, like other geriatric syndromes, is associated with significant comorbidity, including dementia, delirium, depression, hypertension, diabetes mellitus, arthritis, stroke, and urinary incontinence (Dyer et al., 2007; Reyes-Ortiz et al., 2014). Furthermore, elder self-neglect, like many other geriatric syndromes, is said by many to manifest along a continuum of severity rather than in discrete categories (Dong & Gorbien, 2005; Dong, Simon, Mosqueda, et al., 2012).

The comprehensive geriatric assessment with medical, functional, and social history elements should be considered a best practice in a hospital setting in all those suspected of self-neglecting behavior (Reyes-Ortiz et al., 2014). Within an acute hospital setting, the comprehensive geriatric assessment relies on a core team of physicians in geriatric medicine, nurses, social workers, physiotherapists, and occupational therapists. Other disciplines, such as dietetics, podiatrists, psychologists, speech and language therapists, pharmacists and psychiatrists, are called on to augment the assessment when needed. When added to collateral history from alternative credible sources, the information from a comprehensive geriatric assessment may establish an appreciation of the circumstances contributing to the behavior of a person with self-neglect. Assessment should include screens for depression, delirium, dementia, an assessment of functional abilities, and a physical examination (Dyer, Pavlik, Murphy, & Hyman, 2000). It is also important to recognize that there is a difference between a chosen pattern of behavior and neglect that is instigated by others. Also, neglect can be a result of socioeconomic circumstances that cause deterioration in an older person's condition. An appropriate comprehensive geriatric assessment should reflect these complexities in the evaluation by taking the broad biopsychosocial view of the causes, contributors, and treatment of self-neglect.

INTERVENTIONS IN ACUTE CARE FOR SELF-NEGLECT

The goal in any comprehensive geriatric assessment is to identify a list of potentially reversible or treatable issues, the management of which could potentially improve the quality of life for the individual. The time in acute care is vital in identifying and starting to address the causes of self-neglecting behavior. If a self-neglecting older adult is not identified and is sent home, then the self-neglecting behaviors are likely to continue. It is likely that a vicious cycle will occur, health will deteriorate, and further hospital admissions will be warranted. If it is self-neglecting behavior, such as nonadherence to medication for diabetes mellitus, that is the pivotal issue leading to health problems and necessitating hospital admission, then stabilizing the health deteriorations alone will unlikely change the outcome for the patient. In order to alter the outcome for the patient, the root cause of the self-neglecting behavior must be sought and managed. The CHAP study data show that self-neglect is associated with increased rates of 30-day hospital readmission, with greater self-neglect severity associated with greater increases in the rate of 30-day hospital readmissions (Dong & Simon, 2015). Therefore, identifying and evaluating self-neglect in a timely manner is essential in acute hospital care. It has the potential to improve the health and quality of life of individuals, and it is likely to save hospital costs by reducing readmissions.

Seeking out and treating self-neglecting individuals in acute care is unlikely to unleash an avalanche of health care costs (Franzini & Dyer, 2008). The costly issues of care are usually manifested already when these individuals attend acute care services, but the structures to prevent the next complication are often not put in place. In the long term, there is every reason to believe that early intervention and care planning could avert devastating illness, early readmission, and even the wasting of unnecessary health care costs.

Once self-neglect has been identified and comprehensively assessed, common simple clinical interventions can be targeted at the diagnosed deficits that are fostering vulnerability to neglect in older adults. If the person has decision-making capacity and agrees to more detailed interventions, a plan can be developed in accordance with his or her wishes. There is no standard prescription for intervening in elder self-neglect. The interventions should be worked on and agreed on by the older person (if possible), his or her family (if appropriate), and the multidisciplinary team. This plan should address the issues identified in the comprehensive geriatric assessment and involve collaboration between hospital and community services. Similar to most interventions for vulnerable older people with a geriatric syndrome, a multidisciplinary and multifactorial approach is most likely to be successful (HSE, 2014; Reyes-Ortiz et al., 2014).

If the person has decision-making capacity but refuses services, efforts should be made to negotiate with the person. Sometimes, when time is taken to develop and build rapport and trust, the person will work with the services available. By addressing some contributing factors, this historical reluctance for help may change for the individual. For those working in acute care, it is important to communicate with community services about cases of suspected self-neglect. It is important to continue to monitor the person's well-being after hospital discharge and to offer support again intermittently even if at first refused (HSE, 2014). Family, friends, and community can have a vital role in helping vulnerable people remain safe in the community. Visiting, listening, and volunteering to drive the individual places are examples of ways of reducing isolation.

In the past, many have considered intervention in cases of self-neglect to be impossible and this has led to a nihilistic approach by many in acute care. However, increasing evidence supports the view that we do have the ability to intervene and improve outcomes in this population (Burnett et al., 2014).

ASSESSING DECISION-MAKING CAPACITY

In considering assessment in self-neglect, it is important to recognize that there are occasions when someone chooses a particular lifestyle that others consider to be inappropriate. A person has a right to make decisions that other people may consider unwise (HSE, 2014). The autonomy of the individual must be respected as much as possible. However, in some people, the capacity to identify and extract oneself from harmful situations, circumstances, or relationships may be diminished. A key ethical and clinical issue in identifying older adults at risk for self-neglect, involves determining whether the individual can both make and implement decisions regarding personal needs, health, and safety. Multidisciplinary teams need to be knowledgeable of local policy and legal issues in relation to capacity assessment. There is also a complex interplay among executive functioning, decision-making capacity, social support, and financial resources that should be accounted for in assessment (Dyer et al., 2007; Reyes-Ortiz et al., 2014).

Where decision-making capacity is present, there is a strong professional obligation to support an individual's autonomy in choosing his or her own way of life. Ethical challenges may often arise for the health care provider attempting to balance patient autonomy and safety. Even in circumstances in which a person lacks capacity, it is not appropriate to take a fully paternalistic view, which removes the autonomy of the vulnerable person completely (HSE, 2014). An approach that emphasizes beneficence alone may violate the patients' wishes and, therefore, needs to be avoided. Health care and legal professionals are increasingly required to ensure assistance and support for those with diminished decision-making capacity rather than enlisting someone else to become the decision maker.

In the assessment of a person with self-neglecting behavior decision-making capacity is well understood as a significant factor in determining intervention options. The question of an individual's right to self-neglect is much discussed and it is acknowledged that the decision to self-neglect is related to the right to self-determination and decision-making capacity (IOM & NRC, 2014). However, decision-making capacity is complex and can be challenging to assess in the context of self-neglect. All adults are presumed to have full capacity to live independently; failure to engage with health care professionals is not reason enough to consider a person as having lost that capacity.

Four case studies are presented to illustrate some of the issues relating to self-neglect in acute care. The case studies show some of the diversity in presentation, diagnoses, and outcomes for self-neglect in acute care. All four cases show the benefit of a comprehensive geriatric assessment in acute care to delineate a complete medical, functional, social, and environmental diagnostic list. With this diagnostic list, an individual management plan can be instigated to support and help the individual.

CASE STUDY 1: Paul

Paul's is a typical case of a new, acute trauma that presents to acute care—fall with a fracture—and an existing complex multifactorial extreme case of self-neglect is unmasked. In Paul's case, chronic alcoholism with associated cognitive impairment led to an incapacity for self-care. The addition of social isolation, lack of social supports, and poverty resulted in extreme self-neglect.

Paul is a 65-year-old single man who lives alone. He worked as a construction laborer but has been unemployed for nearly 10 years. Paul has a history of alcohol addiction and continues to drink alcohol excessively. He is a long-term smoker and has medical diagnoses of hypertension and hypercholesterolemia.

Paul was admitted to the hospital after a fall that resulted in a fractured left radius. He has attended the ED four times in the past 2 years related to alcohol-intoxication issues. He has had previous falls but no known fractures. This is his first hospital admission since a work-related injury more than 25 years ago.

Paul's personal hygiene and state of clothing on admission were extremely poor. He was visibly thin. It was suspected he might be suffering from self-neglect. A comprehensive geriatric assessment was employed along with information gathered from his primary care physician in the community, his sister, and his local community public health nurse. Paul had an ataxic gait pattern and significantly reduced balance. He could use a walking stick to mobilize with greater balance. On assessment, he had clear cognitive impairment scoring 15 out of 30 on the Mini-Mental State Examination (MMSE).

Paul has had minimal contact with most of his siblings due to his allegedly "difficult" behavior, which was said to have negatively impacted his family relationships. One of his two sisters is the only sibling who has any meaningful contact with him. Paul had been in denial of any problem at home for a few years despite repeated attempted interventions by his community-based public health nurse and general practitioner. He has been reluctant to accept help and support.

Paul's sister stated that he has had a reluctance to wash himself for a number of years. Hospital nursing staff confirmed Paul's resistance to washing or showering in the ward. He was managing his other personal care activities of daily living on the ward with encouragement and setup assistance. Paul's sister reports that he continues to drink alcohol most days and often goes without eating much food.

His house was reported to be in a very bad state of repair by his sister and the public health nurse. As part of the assessment, a home visit was carried out with Paul's consent. The house was infested with rats and his staircase was partly disintegrated due to roof leaks and dampness. As a result, he was unable to use his bedroom and bathroom, which are both upstairs. Paul had been sleeping in an armchair downstairs and using a bucket in which to urinate and defecate. His downstairs toilet was completely blocked and inhabited by vermin. There was no food visible in his kitchen except beer. There was no refrigerator in his house. The kitchen was unusable, with congealed dirt on the stove and floor.

Diagnostic List After Comprehensive Geriatric Assessment

- Nonsyncopal fall as a result of alcohol intoxication
- Fractured left radius as a result of the fall
- Cerebellar atrophy as a result of alcohol excess with a cerebellar ataxic gait
- Chronic ischemic small vessel cerebrovascular disease from unmanaged multiple vascular risk factors
- Alcohol excess and dependence

(continued)

CASE STUDY (continued)

- Cognitive impairment consistent with dementia, most likely Wernicke–Korsakoff syndrome from chronic alcohol intoxication with malnutrition
- Nonadherence to medication and treatment for hypertension and hypercholesterolemia
- Extreme self-neglect with medical, environmental, and social consequences

Outcome

Paul was deemed to lack decision-making capacity after a comprehensive assessment, including involvement of psychiatric services for older people. Public health and environmental protection services were required to be involved in his home environment. His home was unsuitable for him to return to live independently. He required long-term residential care.

This case study illustrates how a complex case of extreme self-neglect with alcohol addiction and severe cognitive, social, and environmental consequences is first discovered after an acute care presentation.

CASE STUDY 2: Maurice

In this case, an acute hospitalization resulted in the diagnosis of a previously unrecognized psychological illness that was directly contributing to self-neglect and poverty. Maurice was living in a state of severe social isolation. With an integrated management plan between the hospital and community services, Maurice was able to return home with monitoring and support.

Maurice is a 74-year-old single man who lives alone. He has no immediate family. Maurice was admitted to the hospital following a fall at home, where he spent 2 days on the floor before being discovered by a neighbor. At the time of presentation, Maurice was physically unkempt. He was unwashed, with long matted dirty hair, multiple missing and decayed teeth, and very soiled and stained clothing. He is very thin. Maurice has severe generalized osteoarthritis and, as a result, he has reduced mobility, requiring a walking stick to mobilize.

After hospital admission, there were concerns that Maurice had self-neglecting behavior. A multidisciplinary comprehensive geriatric assessment was undertaken. Depression and cognitive assessments revealed no significant deficits. According to a distant relative, Maurice had a long-standing phobia regarding handling rubbish. He was described as reclusive without any close friends. Information was gathered from numerous sources. A case conference between the hospital and the community staff was arranged. A home visit was organized by the social work department.

The visit revealed that Maurice lived in a two-story house. His house was described as being in very poor condition. The kitchen was very dirty and unusable. Maurice's cooker was severely corroded and did not appear to be working. Food was seen left around the living room and in a pot on the cooker. There was a major infestation of insects, described as looking like woodlice, in the kitchen sink. The downstairs toilet was extremely dirty and without a working light. Maurice's bedroom was described as having a strong smell of urine, a wet floor, and a pot full of urine was seen on the floor. The bedclothes were described as "black with the dirt." There was no hot water or central heating working in the house. The telephone was not working. The entire house was very cold with cobwebs everywhere. There were dirty clothes and papers cluttering the rooms.

Diagnostic List After Comprehensive Geriatric Assessment

- Fall at home with prolonged period lying on the floor and unable to arise
- Severe generalized osteoarthritis contributing to fall risk
- Peripheral neuropathy with vitamin B_{12} deficiency contributing to fall risk
- Agoraphobia with long-standing social anxiety
- Avoidant personality traits
- Severe social isolation

CASE STUDY (continued)

- Significant socioeconomic deprivation—welfare entitlements or pension entitlements were not claimed
- Telephone disconnection and lack of heat secondary to failure to pay bills
- Malnutrition with vitamin and nutritional deficits
- Poor oral hygiene and dental caries
- Extreme self-neglect as a result of a combination of psychological, social, and economic issues

Outcome

Maurice had a consistent desire to return home. He was deemed to have maintained decision making. Although somewhat distant and reluctant at first, he agreed to work with the multidisciplinary team to improve safety and care at home. The social workers arranged that he get the support and pension income he was entitled to. His bills were paid. His heating and telephone were restarted. Arrangements and services were organized to have the home environment cleaned up and equipment replaced before Maurice was discharged home. Some new furnishing and bedding were organized by the medical social worker service. The community mental health services got involved in his aftercare. Maurice accepted the help offered to him regarding treatment for his agoraphobia and anxiety. Some home help services and Meals on Wheels services were organized for him. Maurice returned home and has ongoing monitoring by the community social worker services for older people.

This case study demonstrates that significant self-neglect can result from potentially reversible conditions. In this case, psychiatric illness resulted in social isolation and significant socioeconomic deprivation. The broad multidisciplinary assessment in acute care allowed delineation of the underlying causes of self-neglect and the implementation of a successful management plan.

CASE STUDY 3: Jane

Jane was diagnosed with a behavioral variant of frontotemporal dementia during her acute hospital stay. This form of dementia is associated with significant executive dysfunction. Jane's lack of executive function resulted in the inability to self-care and self-protect while at home. The dementia, coupled with her social isolation and solitary home life contributed to Jane suffering from severe self-neglect. Unfortunately, dementia is a progressive condition and Jane was unable to return home to live alone.

Jane is a 68-year-old woman. She was admitted to hospital after being found wandering and confused on the road not far from her house. She lives alone and was never married. Her brother lived with her until he was admitted to a nursing home 2 years ago with advancing dementia. On admission to the hospital, Jane had bronchopneumonia and associated delirium. At the time of presentation, she was extremely thin, weighing only 38 kg (83.5 lbs). Her clothing was dirty and soiled. She had known history of type 2 diabetes mellitus and sarcoidosis.

Information was gathered from her primary care doctor, her public health nurse, and the community pharmacy. It was suspected that Jane might be suffering from self-neglect when she refused offers of support and help in the community. The public health nurse had not been able to gain access to visit her because of the presence of a number of dogs. Her medication had not been renewed in the pharmacy for nearly 6 months.

With her permission, the local police and dog warden entered her property to access her dogs. There were two dogs outside and three dogs kept on the second floor in the house. The police authority reported that the house was not suitable for human living. They reported dog excrement in multiple rooms as well as on the beds. The animals were removed to the dog pound. A social worker home visit revealed a very well kept exterior of the house and gardens. However, the interior of the house had animal feces caked into carpets and flooring. There was paper, waste material, and soiled clothing throughout the house. The kitchen was unusable. The stove and sink were covered in garbage. The inside room where the dogs slept was full of dog feces. In total, 20 garbage bags of dog excrement were eventually removed from this room. There was also evidence of vermin infestation in the home.

(continued)

CASE STUDY (continued)

Jane's acute pneumonia was treated and her delirium settled. A multidisciplinary comprehensive geriatric assessment was undertaken and information was gathered from multiple sources. A cognitive assessment revealed maintained working memory. On the MMSE, Jane scored 26 out of 30. However, the frontal assessment battery revealed frontal dysexecutive functioning. Comprehensive psychology and psychiatry of old-age assessments were organized. Jane had the functional ability to be independent on the ward for personal activities of daily living, but she displayed great disinterest and apathy. She struggled significantly with an occupational therapy kitchen assessment. Even though her short-term memory appeared preserved on assessment, her conversation was limited to few topics. She spoke mainly about her dogs and her garden.

Diagnostic List After Comprehensive Geriatric Assessment

- Acute bronchopneumonia with an associated delirium
- Behavioral variant frontotemporal dementia
- Medication nonadherence
- Malnutrition and weight loss
- Environmental hazards in her home
- Extreme self-neglect

Outcome

Jane was deemed to lack decision-making capacity as a result of her newly diagnosed frontotemporal dementia. There was a requirement for legal advice and a Ward of Court application to help support making future financial and care decisions for her. The social workers organized for environmental cleaning within her home. Most of the internal furnishings and contents of her home were removed. A rodent control company was required to get rid of the rat infestation. She was unable to permanently return to her own home. A long-term nursing home placement was organized. To fulfill Jane's wish, a nursing home with its own dogs was organized for her.

In this case study, a previously undiagnosed frontotemporal dementia was severely affecting executive functioning. There was a lack of social support after her brother was admitted to nursing home care after his own progressive dementia. The combination of lack of executive function and social support resulted in severe self-neglect.

Case Study 4: James

The fourth and final case study outlines the case of James, who presents acutely to the hospital with a recent decline in function. He has some active infection and an associated delirium, which resulted in a recent deterioration in his ability to self-care. There were longer term difficulties with self-neglect secondary to alcohol dependence. His increasing physical frailty, along with severely impaired vision, affected his capacity to care adequately for himself. Complex discharge planning was required for James to return home. Unfortunately, James was subsequently diagnosed with an advanced oral squamous cell carcinoma and admitted to hospice care.

James is an 83-year-old man. He has had recurrent hospital and ED attendances. He lives in a sheltered-living accommodation with his own independent living area, but with an on-site warden. He is known to community social services and to senior case workers (elder protection services) already. He is admitted on this occasion because of concerns raised by the sheltered accommodation warden. The warden felt that James could no longer self-care even with the support structures in place. It appeared he was noncompliant with medication. There were also reports that James was not eating properly and that there was a lot of out-of-date food in his accommodation. His self-care and hygiene were deemed very poor in the weeks prior to admission.

James is divorced. His adult children are estranged from him. He has smoked heavily for many years and he drinks alcohol excessively. He has peripheral vascular disease with a previous amputation of the

CASE STUDY (continued)

left hallux. He has chronic lower limb ulcers. His vision is impaired secondary to age-related macular degeneration. James has known atrial fibrillation and a long history of hypertension.

At the time of presentation to the hospital, he is unkempt with soiled clothing. The dressings on his lower limb ulcers are dirty and the ulcers are infected. On admission, James has an active urinary tract infection and associated delirium. His mobility is reduced and he is struggling to manage personal activities of daily living independently. James is known to have self-neglecting behavior and the acute hospital staff communicated with his community support team. His physical and cognitive functioning is much worse than his usual baseline.

A multidisciplinary comprehensive geriatric assessment was undertaken. After his acute infections are treated, it is decided to arrange a period of inpatient rehabilitation. After 3 months in the rehabilitation unit, his functioning has returned to the baseline level. It is reported that James is recurrently abusive to support staff in his sheltered accommodation. There is also concern that he is very unsafe mobilizing outside with his reduced vision, especially after ingesting alcohol. A case conference is required with the community staff, the hospital multidisciplinary team, and James himself.

Diagnostic List After Comprehensive Geriatric Assessment

- Urosepsis with a coliform urinary tract infection
- Infected lower limb ulcers
- Delirium associated with acute illness, probably accounting for recent deterioration in condition
- Functional decline with acute illness requiring prolonged inpatient period of rehabilitation
- Alcohol dependence and ongoing excessive alcohol intake
- Macular degeneration with severely reduced vision
- Nonadherence to medication and treatment of chronic lower limb ulcers
- Chronic ischemic cerebrovascular disease
- Probable mild dementia secondary to alcohol excess and vascular disease
- Persistent oral ulcer—subsequently diagnosed as metastatic squamous cell carcinoma
- Progressive weight loss
- Socially isolated and estranged from his family
- Recurrent hospitalizations

Outcome

Despite the concerns of the health care professionals involved in his care, James maintained the desire to return home to his sheltered accommodation. After negotiation with those running the sheltered accommodation and James agreeing to work with the alcohol abstinence groups, he returned home. He also agreed to limit his walking outside to the times he would walk with others employed to help and support him. Unfortunately, the oral ulcer identified during his admission turned out to be squamous cell carcinoma of his mouth. There was extensive neck lymphadenopathy from the secondary spread of his carcinoma. James declined further interventions. He was admitted to the hospice 2 months after discharge home and died 10 days later.

This case study shows how chronic self-neglect cases that are known to community social services and the APS can have recurrent and prolonged use of acute care services. The case displays the multiple interactions among medical conditions, alcohol addiction, cognitive impairment, and social issues in self-neglect. In this case, a significant visual impairment coupled with alcohol dependence and cognitive decline were making self-care very challenging. James was eventually diagnosed with oral cancer. Such cancers can be associated with self-neglect and the excessive use of tobacco and alcohol.

CONCLUSION

Self-neglect is a serious and growing challenge in society. It is a complex multidimensional phenomenon that is encountered in acute care settings with increasing frequency. The aging of society is resulting in an increasing number of older frail people requiring acute care, thereby increasing the number of encounters with elder self-neglect in the hospital. Even though comprehensive epidemiological evidence is lacking regarding self-neglect in acute care, those working in EDs and acute in-hospital settings are increasingly likely to come across the challenges of identifying and managing self-neglect. Whether presenting as a medical emergency, as an extreme manifestation of a neglected medical condition, or as an identified indicator of extreme vulnerability, self-neglect poses a significant test to the acute health care system.

Self-neglect is associated with increased mortality and can impose considerable costs on individuals, society, and health services. The mortality related to self-neglect can be interpreted as a failure of the society and the health care system to adequately support the most vulnerable older adults. While awaiting evidence-based answers to the myriad of unanswered questions in acute care regarding self-neglect, we must deal with the challenge and support this vulnerable population as best we can.

First, it is critical that physicians and multidisciplinary teams in acute care remain open to considering the possibility of self-neglect when a vulnerable older person's welfare appears to be compromised. Second, ED staff should consider screening for self-neglect in vulnerable older adults who are recurrently under care. Third, when self-neglect is suspected in acute care, a multidimensional interdisciplinary diagnostic approach focused on the person's medical, psychological, social, and functional capability is necessary. Fourth, hospitals need to establish consistent policies regarding the reporting and management of elder self-neglect. As part of local policies, there must be medical and social service collaborations between acute care and community care in order to optimize continuing care for those with self-neglecting behavior.

This chapter explored the following topics in acute care: self-neglect behavior, burden of hospital care, presentations associated with self-neglect, the role of the hospital physician in self-neglect management, comprehensive geriatric assessment, interventions in acute care, and decision-making capacity assessment. The four case studies further illustrate the complexity of self-neglect and its complex interplay of acute medical illness, socioeconomic factors, psychological functioning, physical ability, and environmental factors. Of great importance is the need for good communication across the interface of acute and community care, and multidisciplinary assessment using various health and social care professionals and agencies based on the individual needs of the patient.

IMPLICATIONS FOR RESEARCH AND PRACTICE

- A comprehensive geriatric assessment by a physician in geriatric medicine working with a multidisciplinary team is an appropriate evaluation structure for an older person with suspected self-neglecting behavior presenting within an acute hospital setting.
- Due to the association of multiple conditions with self-neglect, a multidimensional comprehensive geriatric assessment by an experienced team can help reduce morbidity and mortality.
- If self-neglecting behaviors are of acute onset, then the probability of an underlying acute medical problem as the culprit, such as stroke, delirium, or medications side effects, increases.
- Community and acute care services need to provide an integrated structure to maximally support those who self-neglect.
- The true incidence of self-neglect in those presenting to acute services remains unclear.
- The role and benefit of screening in acute care settings should be explored further in research.
- Research is required to test whether various interventions in cases of severe self-neglect benefit in terms of morbidity or mortality.
- Future research is required to examine the longitudinal relationship between self-neglect and acute health care utilization.

REFERENCES

Abrams, R. C., Lachs, M. S., McAvay, G., Keohane, D. J., & Bruce, M. L. (2002). Predictors of self-neglect in community dwelling elders. *American Journal of Psychiatry, 159*(10), 1724–1730.

Azzopardi, L., Murfin, C., Sharda, A., & De Silva, N. (2010). Myxoedema madness. *BMJ Case Reports*, 2010. doi:10.1136/bcr.03.2010.2841

Baker, A. A. (1975). Granny battering. *Modern Geriatrics, 5*(8), 20–21.

Bartley, M., O'Neill, D., Knight, P., & O'Brien, J. (2011). Self-neglect and elder abuse: Related phenomena. *Journal of the American Geriatrics Society, 59*(11), 2163–2168.

Blunt, I., Bardsley, M., & Dixon, J. (2010). *Trends in emergency admissions in England 2004–2009: Is greater efficiency breeding inefficiency?* London, UK: Nuffield Trust.

Braye, S., Orr, D., & Preston-Shoot, M. (2014). *Self-neglect policy and practice: Building an evidence base for adult social care* (SCIE Report 69). London, UK: Social Care Institute for Excellence.

Burnett, J., Cully, J., Achenbaum, W. A., Dyer, C. B., & Naik, A. D. (2011). Assessing self-efficacy for safe and independent living: A cross-sectional study in vulnerable older adults. *Journal of Applied Gerontology, 30*(3), 390–402.

Burnett, J., Dyer, C. B., Halphen, J. M., Achenbaum, W. A., Green, C. E., Booker, J. G., & Diamond, P. M. (2014). Four subtypes of self-neglect in older adults: Results of a latent class analysis. *Journal of the American Geriatrics Society, 62*(6), 1127–1132.

Burston, G. (1977). Do your elderly relatives live in fear of being battered? *Modern Geriatrics, 7*(5), 54–55.

Centre for Policy on Ageing. (2009). *Ageism and age discrimination in mental health care in the United Kingdom: A review from the literature.* London, UK: Author.

Clancy, M., McDaid, B., O'Neill, D., & O'Brien, J. (2011). National profiling of elder abuse referrals. *Age and Aging, 40*(3), 346–352.

Cocksedge, K. A., & Flynn, A. (2014). Wernicke–Korsakoff syndrome in a patient with self-neglect associated with severe depression. *JRSM Open, 5*(2). doi:10.1177/2042533313518915

Cornwall, J. V. (1981). Filth, squalor and lice. Self-neglect in the elderly. *Nurse Mirror, 153*(10), 48–49.

Cotton, M. A., Johnson, S., Bindman, J., Sandor, A., White, I. R., Thornicroft, G., & Bebbington, P. (2007). An investigation of factors associated with psychiatric hospital admission despite the presence of crisis resolution teams. *BMC Psychiatry, 7*, 52. doi:10.1186/1471-244X-7-52

Cybulska, E., & Rucinski, J. (1986). Gross self-neglect in old age. *British Journal of Hospital Medicine, 36*, 21–25.

Day, M. R., Mulcahy, H., & Leahy-Warren, P. (2016). Prevalence of self-neglect in the caseloads of public health nurses. *British Journal of Community Nursing, 21*(1), 31–35.

Day, M. R., Mulcahy, H., Leahy-Warren, P., & Downey, J. (2015). Self-neglect: A case study and implications for clinical practice. *British Journal of Community Nursing, 20*(3), 110–115.

De Freitas, G. R., & Bogousslavsky, J. (2002). Thalamic infarcts. In G. Donnan, B. Norrving, J. Bamford, & J. Bogousslavsky (Eds.), *Subcortical stroke* (pp. 255–285). Oxford, UK: Oxford University Press.

Dong, X. (2014). Self-neglect in an elderly community-dwelling U.S. Chinese population: Findings from the Population Study of Chinese Elderly in Chicago study. *Journal of the American Geriatrics Society, 62*(12), 2391–2397.

Dong, X., & Gorbien, M. (2005). Decision-making capacity: The core of self-neglect. *Journal of Elder Abuse & Neglect, 17*(3), 19–36.

Dong, X., & Simon, M. A. (2013a). Association between elder abuse and use of ED: Findings from the Chicago Health and Aging Project. *American Journal of Emergency Medicine, 31*(4), 693–698.

Dong, X., & Simon, M. A. (2013b). Association between elder self-neglect and hospice utilization in a community population. *Archives of Gerontology and Geriatrics, 56*(1), 192–198.

Dong, X., & Simon, M. A. (2013c). Elder abuse as a risk factor for hospitalization in older persons. *JAMA Internal Medicine, 173*(10), 911–917.

Dong, X., & Simon, M. A. (2015). Elder self-neglect is associated with increased rate of 30-day hospital readmission: Findings from the Chicago Health and Aging Project. *Gerontology, 61*(1), 41–50.

Dong, X., Simon, M. A., & Evans, D. A. (2011). Prospective study of the elder self-neglect and emergency department use in a community population. *American Journal of Emergency Medicine, 30*, 553–556.

Dong, X., Simon, M. A., & Evans, D. A. (2012a). Elder self-neglect and hospitalization: Findings from the Chicago Health and Aging Project. *Journal of the American Geriatrics Society, 60*(2), 202–209.

Dong, X., Simon, M. A., & Evans, D. A. (2012b). Prevalence of self-neglect across gender, race, and socioeconomic status: Findings from the Chicago Health and Aging Project. *Gerontology, 58*(3), 258–268.

Dong, X., Simon, M. A., Fulmer, T., Mendes de Leon, C. F., Hebert, L. E., Beck, T., . . . Evans, D. A. (2011). A prospective population-based study of differences in elder self-neglect and mortality between black and white older adults. *Journals of Gerontology Series A, Biological Sciences and Medical Sciences, 66*(6), 695–704.

Dong, X., Simon, M., Fulmer, T., Mendes de Leon, C. F., Rajan, B., & Evans, D. A. (2010). Physical function decline and the risk of elder self-neglect in a community-dwelling population. *The Gerontologist, 50*(3), 316–326.

Dong, X., Simon, M., Mendes de Leon, C., Fulmer, T., Beck, T., Hebert, L., . . . Evans, D. (2009). Elder self-neglect and abuse and mortality risk in a community dwelling population. *Journal of the American Medical Association, 302*(5), 517–526.

Dong, X., Simon, M. A., Mosqueda, L., & Evans, D. A. (2012). The prevalence of elder self-neglect in a community-dwelling population: Hoarding, hygiene, and environmental hazards. *Journal of Aging and Health, 24*(3), 507–524.

Dyer, C. B., & Goins, A. M. (2000). The role of the interdisciplinary geriatric assessment in addressing self-neglect of the elderly. *Generations, 24*, 23–27.

Dyer, C. B., Goodwin, J.S., Burnett, J., & Kelly, P. A. (2007). Characterizing self-neglect: A report of over 500 cases of self-neglect seen by a geriatric medicine team. *American Journal of Public Health, 97*(9), 1671–1676.

Dyer, C. B., Pavlik, V. N., Murphy, K. P., & Hyman, D. J. (2000). The high prevalence of depression and dementia in elder abuse or neglect. *Journal of the American Geriatrics Society, 48*(2), 205–208.

Ellis, G., Whitehead, M. A., O'Neill, D., Langhorne, P., & Robinson, D. (2011). Comprehensive geriatric assessment for older adults admitted to hospital. *Cochrane Database of Systematic Reviews, 2011*(7), CD006211.

Fillit, H. M., Rockwood, K., & Woodhouse, K. (2010). *Brocklehurst's textbook of geriatric medicine and gerontology* (7th ed.). Philadelphia, PA: Saunders Elsevier.

Franzini, L., & Dyer, C. (2008). Healthcare costs and utilization of vulnerable elderly people reported to adult protective services for self-neglect. *Journal of the American Geriatrics Society, 56*(4), 667–676.

Gill, T. M. (2009). Elder self-neglect: Medical emergency or marker of extreme vulnerability? *Journal of the American Medical Association, 302*(5), 570–571.

Health Service Executive. (2012). *Policy and procedures for responding to allegations of extreme self-neglect.* Dublin, Ireland: Author.

Health Service Executive. (2014). *Safeguarding vulnerable persons at risk of abuse: National Policy and Procedures.* Dublin, Ireland: Author.

Hitzeman, N., & Belsky, K. (2013). Appropriate use of polypharmacy for older patients. *American Family Physician, 87*, 483–484.

Homeier, D. (2014). Aging—Physiology, disease & abuse. *Clinics in Geriatric Medicine, 30*(4), 671–686.

Institute of Medicine & National Research Council. (2014). *Elder abuse and its prevention: Workshop summary*. Washington, DC: National Academies Press.

Isaacs, B. (1976). *Giants of geriatrics: A study of symptoms in old age*. Birmingham, UK: University of Birmingham Press.

Kee, Y., & Rippingale, C. (2009). The prevalence and characteristics of patients with "acopia." *Age and Ageing, 38*(1), 103–105.

Krishnan, L. L., Petersen, N. J., Snow, A. L., Cully, J. A., Schulz, P. E., Graham, D. P., . . . Kunik, M. E. (2005). Prevalence of dementia among Veterans Affairs medical care system users. *Dementia and Geriatric Cognitive Disorders, 20*(4), 245–253.

Lachs, M. (2008). What does "self-neglect" in older adults really cost? *Journal of the American Geriatrics Society, 56*(4), 757.

Naik, A. D., Lai, J. M., Kunik, M. E., & Dyer, C. B. (2008). Assessing capacity in suspected cases of self-neglect. *Geriatrics, 63*(2), 24–31.

National Research Council. (2003). *Elder mistreatment: Abuse, neglect, and exploitation in an aging America*. Washington, DC: National Academies Press.

O'Brien, J. G., Cooney, C., Bartley, M., & O'Neill, D. (2013). Self-neglect: A survey of old age psychiatrists in Ireland. *International Psychogeriatrics, 25*(12), 2088–2090.

Office for National Statistics. (2011). *Interim life tables, 2008–2010*. Newport, UK: Author.

Oliver, D. (2008). "Acopia" and "social admission" are not diagnoses: Why older people deserve better. *Journal of the Royal Society of Medicine, 101*(4), 168–174.

Oliver, D., Foot, C., & Humphries, R. (2014). *Making our health and care systems fit for an ageing population*. London, UK: The King's Fund.

Papaioannou, E. S., Räihä, I., & Kivelä, S. L. (2012). Self-neglect of the elderly, an overview. *European Journal of General Practice, 18*(3), 187–190.

Pavlou, M. P., & Lachs, M. S. (2008). Self-neglect in older adults: A primer for clinicians. *Journal of General Internal Medicine, 23*(11), 1841–1846.

Renzetti, C. M., & Lee, R. M. (1993). *Researching sensitive topics*. London, UK: Sage.

Reyes-Ortiz, C. A., Burnett, J., Flores, D. V., Halphen, J. M., & Dyer, C. B. (2014). Medical implications of elder abuse: Self-neglect. *Clinical Geriatric Medicine, 30*(4), 807–823.

Roe, P. F. (1977). Self-neglect. *Age and Ageing, 6*, 192–194.

Rubenstein, L. Z., Stuck, A. E., Siu, A. L., & Wieland, J. (1991). Impacts of geriatric evaluation and management programs on defined outcomes: Overview of the evidence. *Journal of the American Geriatrics Society, 39*(9), 8S–16S.

Sullivan, L. W. (1990). Healthy People 2000. *New England Journal of Medicine, 323*, 1065–1067.

Turner, A., Hochschild, A., Burnett, J., Zulfiqar, A., & Dyer, C. B. (2012). High prevalence of medication non-adherence in a sample of community-dwelling older adults with adult protective services-validated self-neglect. *Drugs & Aging, 29*(9), 741–749.

Ventura, J., Nuechterlein, K. H., Subotnik, K. L., Gutkind, D., & Gilbert, E. A. (2000). Symptom dimensions in recent-onset schizophrenia and mania: A principal components analysis of the 24-item Brief Psychiatric Rating Scale. *Psychiatry Research, 97*(3), 129–135.

Wrenn, K. (1990). Foot problems in homeless persons. *Annals of Internal Medicine, 113*(8), 567–569.

CHAPTER 11

MEDICAL PERSPECTIVES OF SELF-NEGLECT: AN ISSUE FOR HEALTH AND SOCIAL CARE

Josephine P. Gomes and James G. O'Brien

Self-neglect is perhaps one of the most challenging and frustrating problems that practitioners in the health care and social services fields encounter. Knowledge of the phenomenon of self-neglect seems to be sadly lacking among many practitioners, particularly in terms of identification, detection, and intervention. Despite the fact that self-neglect constitutes the majority of the cases of elder abuse and neglect reported to official authorities and adult protective services (APS), it continues to receive inadequate attention in terms of developing adequate resources to combat the problem.

The harmful effects of self-neglect extend way beyond harm to the individual and often impacts neighbors, family, friends, medical and social services practitioners, and sometimes the community at large. Efforts to help are frequently rejected, leading to frustration for those trying to help. There is an urgent need for further education, research, improved funding, specific public policy, and expanded resources. Ideally, those who self-neglect need to be evaluated, treated, and followed by an interdisciplinary team.

Self-neglect is perhaps the most challenging of problems encountered in the abuse and neglect arena. Self-neglect is an ancient problem, with accounts dating back as far as ancient Greece. Diogenes, a Greek philosopher from the 4th century BCE, exhibited self-neglect. Despite being the most frequently reported type of abuse and neglect to APS, self-neglect is the least understood within the abuse and neglect spectrum. It results in increased morbidity and mortality and negative consequences, not just for the individual, but frequently for the community. It poses a particular problem for the physicians and other practitioners in the health and social care arena.

There are an estimated 1.2 million older adults who self-neglect annually and this number is steadily increasing (Tatara et al., 1998). Self-neglect accounts for 50% of all reported elder abuse and neglect cases (Naik, Burnett, Pickens-Pace, & Dyer, 2008). Older adults referred to APS for self-neglect are 50% more likely to die within 3 years compared to referrals for other forms of mistreatment (Lachs, Williams, O'Brien, Pillemer, & Charlson, 1998). This increased mortality rate is independent of any result related to the abuse or mistreatment (Fulmer, Paveza, Abraham, & Fairchild, 2000; Lachs et al., 1998). Elder self-neglect was previously believed to affect mainly the rich and the educated. It is now known that this condition crosses all demographic and socioeconomic groups of the aging population without distinction (Mosqueda & Dong, 2011). The aging of the baby boomer population, coupled with a general decline in financial resources, both personal and national, and an increasingly geographically dispersed family structure provide an environment where an increased number of elders are unable to meet their personal and functional needs, leading to an increase in the incidence of elder self-neglect.

BACKGROUND LITERATURE: DEFINING SELF-NEGLECT

Self-neglect is defined by the National Committee for the Prevention of Elder Abuse and the National Adult Protective Services Association (NAPSA) as:

> The result of an adult's inability, due to physical or mental impairment or diminished capacity, to perform essential self-care tasks including (a) obtaining essential food, clothing, shelter, and medical care; (b) obtaining goods and services necessary to maintain physical health, mental health, or general safety; and/or (c) managing one's own financial affairs. (Teaster, Dugar, Mendiodo, & Cecil, 2006, p. 10)

The first documentation of self-neglect in old age in the medical literature appeared in the *British Medical Journal* in 1966 authored by MacMillan and Shaw, who described the syndrome of senile breakdown. Since that time, articles regarding self-neglect appeared sporadically in the medical literature under a variety of other diagnostic labels, including social breakdown syndrome, indirect self-destructive behavior, passive suicide, gross self-neglect, and Diogenes syndrome (O'Brien, 1999).

Reed and Leonard (1989) describe self-neglect as a negative behavior that reduces quality of life and hence warrants attention. They describe characteristic attributes for the diagnosis of self-neglect:

- The behaviors displayed have the potential to be harmful or life threatening.
- There is no specific purpose or clearly identified reason for engaging in the behavior.
- The behavior is not intended to end one's life immediately.
- The effects of the behavior are cumulative and realized over time.
- The behaviors occur in a repetitive pattern that affects self-care needs on multiple dimensions.

Kelly, Dyer, Pavlik, Doody, and Jogerst (2008) further characterize the severity of self-neglect by identifying three domains of self-neglect as indicators:

- Personal hygiene (dirty hair, clothing, unkempt nails, and skin)
- Impaired function (decline in activities of daily living [ADL] and cognition)
- Environmental neglect (unclean house or yard and the inability to manage material goods accumulated over the years)

ETIOLOGY OF SELF-NEGLECT

A clear concept of the etiology of self-neglect is unknown. Self-neglect is a geriatric syndrome and, like other geriatric syndromes, includes a wide array of etiologic factors.

Several theories have been proposed as the possible etiology for elder self-neglect. MacMillan and Shaw (1966) suggested that a presyndrome personality type predisposes one to develop self-neglect. They described a number of recluses whose lack of personal hygiene was mirrored by the filth and dilapidation of their homes and perpetuated by their consistent refusal of assistance. They describe this syndrome as consisting of five personal and 10 home environment characteristics. Refusal of services was encountered frequently. These elders were often described as independent, quarrelsome, unfriendly, stubborn, obstinate, aloof, suspicious, secretive, and aggressive.

Clark, Mankikar, and Gray (1975) coined the term *Diogenes syndrome*. They identified similar traits among those who self-neglect and also showed that many of these individuals have a high IQ, and had been successful in their earlier lives. Patients with Diogenes syndrome have been described as exhibiting a lack of self-respect, social withdrawal, and apathy, having a tendency to hoard rubbish, a willingness to live in domestic squalor, and often a lack of shame. Diogenes syndrome has become a less commonly used description of self-neglect. Others describe self-neglect in more clinical terms and suggest that self-neglect refers to the physically ill individual who intentionally neglects prescribed self-care activities despite available resources and knowledge (Reed & Leonard, 1989). The definition of self-neglect provided by NAPSA contains most of the critical elements of the syndrome. In the late 1980s and 1990s in the United States it became apparent that most cases of abuse and neglect reported to APS were in fact cases of self-neglect (Tatara et al., 1998). Notably, the term self-neglect was excluded from the National Center on Elder Abuse's incidence study (Tatara et al., 1998) and instead the individuals were described as being mentally competent and understanding the consequences of their decisions to engage in acts that threatened their health and safety.

Whitehead (1975) suggested that self-neglect reflected an exaggeration of lifelong standards of poor personal and home hygiene brought on by functional impairments in old age.

Ungvari and Hantz (1991) suggested that self-neglect may represent an atypical adjustment disorder superimposed on long-standing personality abnormalities. In general, there are commonly accepted risk factors for self-neglect, like age, dependency, functional and medical decline, mental health issues, and social factors.

Mental Health and Cognitive Causes

Late-life depression is the most prevalent psychiatric disorder among older adults in the United States, affecting approximately 15% to 20% of adults 65 years of age and older (Geriatric Mental Health Foundation, 2008). Both late-life depression and cognitive impairment are the major predictors of self-neglect in community-dwelling adults (Abram, Lachs, McAvay, Keohane, & Bruce, 2002). Depression is present in approximately 51% to 62% of older adults who self-neglect (Burnett, Coverdale, Pickens, & Dyer, 2006). In spite of depression being readily treatable with medication and psychosocial therapies, less than half of the older adults in need of these therapies access the services. Untreated depression is associated with increased disability, higher health care utilization, and reduced ability to care for oneself (McKenna, Michaud, Murray, & Marks, 2005). Common depressive symptoms associated with elders include apathy, hopelessness, anxiety, isolation from friends and family, and low self-rated health (Dyer, Pavlik, Murphy, & Hyman, 2000). Persons with depression are at risk for self-neglect as they are not motivated to cook meals, to be involved in self-care, or to seek social contacts. Drug and alcohol abuse can be used to mask the depression. Alcohol is also directly associated with self-neglect. The presence of alcohol abuse in self-neglecting older adults is common. Hansen, Flores, Coverdale, and Burnett (2016) found alcohol abuse to be the strongest correlate of depression in their sample of self-neglectors. Alcohol abuse nearly tripled reported rates of depression even with mild increases in the CAGE questionnaire (cut-down, annoyed, guilt, eye-opener).

Premorbid personality traits (aloof, suspicious, quarrelsome), behaviors (reclusive, hoarding), or disorders (obsessive-compulsive, paranoid, schizoid) are described as being associated with elder self-neglect (Clark et al., 1975; Halliday, Banerjee, Philpot, & MacDonald, 2000; Reyes-Ortiz, 2006; Ungvari & Hantz, 1991; Wrigley & Cooney, 1992). Hoarding is considered an important characteristic of the self-neglect syndrome (Halliday et al., 2000; Reyes-Ortiz, 2006; Snowdon, Shah, & Halliday, 2007). Hoarding results in the development of stacks of objects or trash, which then reduces the total living space. Hoarding makes day-to-day activities like cooking, sleeping, and socialization difficult. Older adults who hoard often avoid socialization as they are uncomfortable when people look at, comment on, or touch their possessions. They often refuse home care services for fear of being judged.

As described previously, maladaptive personalities who may have lifelong eccentricities—a reclusive nature, underdeveloped interpersonal skills, and discomfort in social settings—predisposes these individuals to self-neglect in later years. The "at-risk personality" responds maladaptively and differently to common stressors that older adults experience, such as the loss of a loved one, spousal placement, retirement, relocation, or increasing debility (O'Brien, Thibault, Turner, & Laird-Fick, 2000). MacMillan and Shaw (1966) propose self-neglect as an active expression of resentment and withdrawal from the community. Thibault (1984) proposed the concept of self-neglect as an active effort on the part of the individual to regain his or her autonomy and control over choices and circumstances.

Cognitive impairment and depression are independent predictors of elder self-neglect syndrome. Lower levels of cognitive function have been associated with greater morbidity and mortality. Dong et al. (2010) showed a decline in executive function to be independently associated with elder self-neglect. Executive function is often referred to as a frontal lobe function and includes the planning, initiation, organization, and execution of tasks. It involves translating simple tasks to effective behaviors like cooking and dressing oneself. An impairment in executive functioning may make it difficult to participate in regular daily activities like meal preparation, shopping for groceries, or taking medication appropriately (Dyer, Goodwin, Pickens-Pace, Burnett, & Kelly, 2007; Royall, Palmer, Chiodo, & Polk, 2004). Impaired reasoning or formulation may lead to an inability to appreciate the need for use of assistive devices, report a medical condition or change in health, and maintain personal hygiene. The inability to appreciate naturally occurring cues in the environment or perception of hunger can lead to the neglect of eating or drinking to the point of malnourishment and dehydration.

Social Causes

The presence of social support is very important as individuals who self-neglect often live in isolation from others and have medical comorbidities that may impair good cognitive decision making and the ability to care for themselves. Social support has been identified as a critical component in the healing process of individuals with mental and medical illnesses. Dyer et al. (2007) reported that 94% of self-neglecting adults, 65 years of age and older had abnormal levels of social support.

The effects of social relationships on health and mortality show that living with family and maintaining social contacts delayed functional decline, depression, and death. Elders who are involved in various social activities have a better physical and mental health status. A review of the social networks of the elderly has found that elders who self-neglect tend to live in isolation. Even when married, the elderly who self-neglect were significantly less likely to live with their spouses. Living alone even when married could be due to nursing home placement of the spouse or due to separation. Elders who self-neglect are found to have less than weekly contact with their children and siblings, visit less frequently with friends and neighbors, and are less likely to be involved in religious activities (Burnett, Regev, et al., 2006). In addition to an individual's social support network, other social factors that can influence an individual's self-neglect risk are related to external or environmental factors. These could include the quality of the neighborhood where the elder resides (such as the presence of crime or safety of the neighborhood), availability of transportation, community resources, and social support (Paveza, Vanderweerd, & Laumann, 2008)

Lack of transportation can make access to a medical care providers' services difficult. An older adult living alone who is unable to drive may be unable to fill prescriptions or obtain necessary groceries. The individual may avoid asking family and friends for help to maintain autonomy or he or she may have no significant social support. This can put the individual at an increased risk of self-neglect. As a result, the degree to which the lack of transportation increases the likelihood of an individual to become self-neglectful is debatable.

Choi, Kim, and Assef (2009) attributed elder self-neglect to the elders' and their families' inability to pay for essential services. Medicare, a federally funded program in the United States, will only cover home care services for a short period if there is a skilled need (wound care, physical therapy, and intravenous intervention). However, Medicare will not cover the cost of social support services. Older adults are often not able to pay privately for services, such as day programs to avoid social isolation. Some older adults depend on their Social Security checks to cover their living expenditures, that is, they may have to choose among buying medications, food, or utilities. Such financial hardships may make an individual more susceptible to self-neglect.

The family structure has also changed in recent years. Society has become more mobile. Families are more geographically dispersed, with children now living not only in different states from their parents, but also in different countries. Family conflict can lead to situations in which the elder has cut off family attachments, putting the individual at risk for social isolation.

Functional Causes

Naik et al. (2008) showed an association between impairments in ADL and elder self-neglect. Older adults are at risk for self-neglect if they become functionally impaired, especially if they live alone. Many elders are unable to afford to pay privately for assistance with basic daily care. The inability to adequately care for themselves and their homes will eventually lead to poor personal hygiene and an unclean environment. Difficulty or change in mobility may make it harder to take care of daily needs, shopping, and socialization, causing increased social isolation.

Medical Causes

Diabetes, stroke, head trauma, and cardiovascular disease can all contribute to impairment in the frontal lobe and loss of executive function. Turner, Hochschild, Burnett, Zulfiqar, and Dyer (2012) reported that 90% elders who self-neglect were nonadherent to at least one medication, and even more were nonadherent to approximately four medications. Diabetes, hypertension, cardiovascular diseases, nutritional deficiencies, and arthritis not adequately controlled can further impair functional and cognitive functioning. Pickens, Burnett, Naik, Holmes, and Dyer (2006) showed an association between self-reported pain and elder self-neglect. Elders who self-neglect reported significantly higher levels of pain compared with matched control groups even though 93% of the participants in the study had seen their primary care physician in the past 3 months. Mean pain scores between the self-neglect group and controls were statistically significant. This was believed to be related to individuals in the self-neglect group having more conditions associated with pain or receiving less adequate pain control or that these individuals are affected by conditions that impact the perception of pain intensity. Lansbury (2000) showed 25% to 50% of community-dwelling older adults experience significant pain, and pain was the main reason for loss of independence and the need for support services in the elderly. At present, pain is generally underdiagnosed and undertreated in the elderly.

Medical disease can reduce an elder's ability for self-care and self-protection, requiring social, medical, and functional interventions to avoid the onset of self-neglect. Often family members come in and address these deficits and provide the services needed, arrange for such services, or place their loved one in a care facility. Self-neglect occurs when elders fail to recognize their deficits or lack the social support or financial resources to overcome these deficits.

COMMUNITY IMPACT

The impact on the community can be seen in the example provided in Case Study 1 and the analysis provided.

CASE STUDY 1: MR. AND MRS. B

Mr. B, 86, and Mrs. B, 85, were discovered living in absolute squalor in a vermin-infested house with no running water, no toilet, a roof that leaked, and cats and dogs that defecated and urinated indoors. The neighbors noted that the stench was overwhelming, not just inside the house but also in the vicinity. Previous attempts by friends to help were rejected. Finally, the neighbors reported the situation to the Department of Public Health, which condemned the building. APS intervened and Mrs. B, who was severely demented, was placed in a nursing home. Mr. B was admitted to a psychiatric unit for evaluation. It was determined that he had early dementia and was aware of this and of the state of his home, but felt "it was not that bad" and he wanted to remain at home. It was determined that this posed an excessive risk for him and his neighbors so eventually he was placed in the same residential facility as his wife.

Analysis

This case highlights the fact that the individuals who engage in self-neglecting behavior are not the only ones who are affected. The impact is on the neighbors, in this instance, and also on the family, friends, and health care professionals who were trying to help but were frequently rejected. One of the difficulties with self-neglect is that it is a concept that varies in relation to context. Community members can play a crucial role in determining what is tolerated in their neighborhood (May-Chahal & Antrobus, 2012). Self-neglect occurs across a spectrum of neglect from a benign variant of failure to eat properly, exercise, use seatbelts, or failure to comply with medical advice. These behaviors may not result in immediate harm but have long-term consequences. The more malignant form exceeds the threshold, resulting in more immediate harm such as ignoring urgent life-threatening medical conditions or living in extreme squalor in vermin-infested environment.

Everyone self-neglects at different points, ranging from acts like exceeding the speed limit or eating unhealthy foods, hence a certain threshold has to be exceeded before the diagnosis of self-neglect can be determined and an element of subjectivity is added to the assessment process (O'Brien et al., 2000). Often, self-neglect is determined when there is a shift in one's previous standards of home and personal hygiene, which then catches the attention of an observer.

Wrigley and Cooney (1992) suggested that respect for the autonomy of the older person should take priority and caution not to force conformity with regard to standards of cleanliness. Sengstock, Thibault, and Zaranek (1999) find this position untenable and suggest that the rights of the individual be abrogated when the public needs to be protected in situations in which an individual with a communicable disease endangers the lives of others. An individual living in squalor in an apartment infested with vermin and hoarded materials may pose multiple risks to neighbors given the close proximity in which they live, and therefore, requires intervention. Whereas in an isolated rural community there may be no risk to neighbors.

The family, close friends, physicians, home care workers, and other providers may be affected when help is rejected. Family and friends may be unaware of the extent of the behavior such as not taking medications, living in squalor, and refusing access to the home. The threshold for labeling the situation or person as being self-neglectful varies greatly by determinants such as poverty, cultural norms, regional norms, and the perception of the observer.

IDENTIFICATION AND ASSESSMENT

Generally, older adults seek medical care from their primary care providers (PCPs) for the management of their physical or psychological problems. Older adults prefer to avoid mental health settings due to the stigma they associate with psychiatric care and the fact that many psychological problems in older adults manifest as physical symptoms (Arean, Alvidrez, Barrera, Robinson, & Hicks, 2002). Due to their greater contact with these older adults, PCPs have a major role in the identification of elder self-neglect, especially in the early stages, and linking these individuals to appropriate care services.

Despite being in an advantageous position to detect and intervene in cases of self-neglect, the contribution of physicians in this area has been less than expected when compared with, for instance, the contribution pediatricians have made in the area of child abuse and neglect where they have taken the lead in research, detection, intervention, and advocating for public policy to address the problem. When physicians are judged on their ability to report cases of elder abuse they rank lower on the reporting scale than other professionals in the health care field (Tatara et al., 1998). A recent study of elder abuse and neglect in Ireland identified medical doctors as being eighth in rank of reporting incidents of self-neglect (Clancy, McDaid, O'Neill, & O'Brien, 2011).

A comprehensive geriatric assessment (CGA) involving an interdisciplinary team with medical, functional, cognitive, and social history is warranted. This assessment should include information from multiple available resources on the elder's functional abilities and social support. More valuable information is often obtained from previously frequented locations like banks, grocery stores, and pharmacies. Home visits by physicians, public health nurses, or social workers provide much pertinent information regarding elders' living situation and daily functioning in their environment.

A detailed physical examination as well as screening for depression, delirium, dementia, and functional abilities should be performed. Instruments often used in CGA assessments include the 15-item Geriatric Depression Scale (Yesavage et al., 1983), the Mini-Mental State Examination (MMSE; Folstein, Folstein, & McHugh, 1975), Kohlman Evaluation of Living Skills (Thompson, 1992), the CAGE questionnaire (Ewing, 1984), the Confusion Assessment Method (Inouye et al., 1990), and pain assessment scales. It is important to note that the MMSE, a screening tool for cognitive deficits, is usually insensitive to the executive dysfunction needed for decision-making capacity and non-Alzheimer-related dementias. Individuals who pass the MMSE but fail executive measures are more likely to suffer from non-Alzheimer cognitive illness such as subcortical vascular dementia, parkinsonian dementia, and dementias related to metabolic disturbances (Schillerstrom, Salazar, Regwan, Bonguli, & Royall, 2009).

Self-neglecting individuals are prone to nutritional deficiencies, which could contribute to a reversible dementia syndrome. Dong et al. (2010) found no statistically significant association between the MMSE and elder self-neglect. More comprehensive neuropsychiatric testing may be warranted. Tierney, Snow, Charles, Moineddin, and Kiss (2007) found the domains most involved in self-neglect harm were in verbal recognition, memory, executive function, and conceptualization. This indicates that rather than global cognitive impairment, it is the specific domains of impairment that increase self-neglecting behaviors.

There are important questions to be answered when evaluating self-neglect. To live independently without supervision, the self-neglector must be able to perform or arrange for the following needs to be met:

1. ADL (dressing, bathing, toileting, feeding oneself, moving about their home)
2. Instrumental ADL (managing finances, preparing meals, performing housework, using the telephone, shopping, using transportation, taking medications, or managing medical issues)

3. Protection from harm (from strangers or nonstrangers)
4. A reasonably safe and hygienic environment (Lawton & Brody, 1969; Moye, Butz, Marson, Wood, & ABA–APA, 2007)

Physicians struggle with a specific type of self-neglect. In particular, this includes noncompliance with medical recommendations such as failing to fill prescriptions or taking medications as recommended, not complying with diagnostic tests, and failing to keep appointments in situations in which noncompliance results in harm. Noncompliance may be perceived by the physician as intentional, whereas, in fact, the patient may lack the capacity to be compliant as a result of dementia, depression, or extreme poverty. Conversely, the individual may in fact have decisional capacity but chooses not to be compliant and views recommendations as an unwarranted intrusion on his or her life and is willing to suffer the consequences.

A person's decision-making capacity requires the individual has the ability to receive and understand relevant information, reason through the options, communicate a choice, and execute the choice or appreciate the resulting situation. All adults are presumed to have full capacity to live independently. The issue of competence, which is a legal definition, must be preceded by the determination of capacity. If an individual is incompetent, a guardian is then appointed to oversee the patient's needs. It has also been seen that individuals with self-neglect may have decisional capacity and are able to make the right choice but have abnormalities in their execution of the decisions.

A survey of general practitioners in Ireland in 2010 revealed nearly two thirds had encountered cases of abuse and self-neglect with self-neglect being most common; 35.5% of physicians surveyed encountered a case in the past year (O'Brien, Riain, Collins, Long, & O'Neill, 2014). Most cases were detected during a home visit. It is interesting to note that 13% of the physicians had been threatened by a perpetrator or a family member. Seventy-three percent perceived their role as becoming involved beyond medical care and 70% believed the situation for the self-neglecting individual had improved after intervention.

A survey of geriatricians in Ireland and Scotland in 2010 regarding self-neglect revealed most had encountered cases in the past year with personal neglect and refusal of services being common presentations (Bartley, O'Neill, Knight, & O'Brien, 2011). Interestingly, 40% of cases are thought to contain elements of abuse, which is not surprising given the vulnerability of these individuals. Dementia, lifelong personality traits, depression, and alcoholism were cited as the most common underlying causes. Comprehensive geriatric evaluation was identified as the most appropriate intervention. The respondents also identified the need for more education for geriatricians and other health and social care professionals (Bartley et al., 2011).

A survey of psychiatrists specializing in the care of elderly patients in Ireland in 2010 regarding self-neglect revealed significant exposure, with 92% having seen a case in the past year (O'Brien, Cooney, Bartley, & O'Neill, 2013). The most common personal characteristics noted included loss of self-care and poor hygiene. Medication noncompliance and hoarding were the next most common factors. In contrast with geriatricians, 59% of psychiatrists believe the outcome for the patient was unsatisfactory. Nearly three fourths believe the outcome for themselves as psychiatrists was unsatisfactory (O'Brien et al., 2013).

INTERVENTION AND PREVENTION

Self-neglect has a slow insidious progression making it a challenge to identify in its early stages when potentially disastrous outcomes may be avoided (Bartley et al., 2011). The complexities in the unique biopsychosocial profiles of elder self-neglectors limit the effectiveness of standard medical interventions and require a more comprehensive approach. When a concern of elder self-neglect is raised, clinicians should perform a CGA and make a referral to APS. Balancing autonomy and choice cannot win over jeopardizing the community.

Interprofessional teams of health care and social services professionals are recommended for effective treatment and intervention in elder self-neglect. This approach has reported success in reducing self-neglecting behaviors as well as associated risk factors like depression, impairment in ADL, and lack of social support. It is sometimes advantageous to approach self-neglecting adults by "playing to their sense of isolation, their sense of their history, who they are, who they were when they were younger and who they are now" (Longres, 1994, p. 12). Research supports the use of interpersonal therapy, problem-solving therapy, and reminiscence therapy as effective treatment practices in geriatric mental health that may be used in elder self-neglect (Bartels, Haley, & Dums, 2002). In elder self-neglect, it would be a good practice to build a therapeutic relationship and support a patient-centered approach (Day & Leahy-Warren, 2008). It is beneficial to allow the elders to relay their life stories and the reasoning behind their behaviors. Active listening with development of an appropriate behavioral intervention should take precedence over logical persuasion. There will be minimal, if any, benefit if the interventions do not stem from an understanding of the individual's personal choices. Elders usually have a strong desire to maintain control over their lives. In addition to having personal meaning, this control also relates to the individual's perceived sense of independence, dependence, and interdependence. A practice approach to help prevent self-neglect must build on strengths (abilities still intact) rather than deficits (Rathbone-McCuan & Bricker-Jenkins, 1992).

In addition, knowing the specific risk factors of elder self-neglect in an individual can make for more effective intervention. Depression is a known risk factor for elder self-neglect. Appropriate treatment for depression could be facilitated by addressing the contributing factors individually, along with prescribing any necessary medication and psychological therapy as needed. It is also important to address the common associated issues of drug and alcohol abuse. Improved pain control is associated with improvement in coping and self-care. Uncontrolled pain and depression lead to individuals being less motivated and failing to reach out for help, creating increased feelings of loneliness, and worsening depression. A good understanding of the individual's motivation for accepting support and self-perceptions of need for care and health will provide insight into the adult's ability to realize and manage needs on an ongoing basis (Choi et al., 2009).

Elder self-neglectors with executive dysfunction may have impairment in multiple domains. First, it is necessary to determine which factors limit self-care and then to assess whether these findings are due to temporary or permanent causes. Appropriate intervention will be needed to protect the elder from further self-harm. Some self-neglecting elders may have the cognitive capacity but lack the physical ability necessary for managing their health. Medication nonadherence in this population is associated with decreased physical functioning (Turner et al., 2012). Measures aimed at reducing the number of medications and improving physical functioning could lead to better health outcomes and reduced self-neglecting behaviors. An important aspect of care of self-neglecting adults is to create a plan for worst-case scenarios.

Prevention of elder self-neglect is difficult given the complex nature of the condition. At-risk registers are proposed to be used by various professionals as an approach to identify persons as potential self-neglectors at an early stage (O'Brien et al., 2000). For instance, if a PCP is aware that an older male with a past history of alcohol abuse has just lost his spouse and his children live out of state, he should be placed on an at-risk register and referred to an onsite geriatric assessment team to assess his functioning and coping ability and also to identify services that may be needed. Although this may be the correct action, this can be difficult if the person has mental capacity. Other important steps leading to prevention include education on elder self-neglect and providing outreach services for older adults. Publicly subsidized services could be established to assist out-of-area families in helping their older family members avoid becoming at risk for self-neglect. Currently, there are some privately run services such as companion services, transportation, simple ADL assistance, and basic home-repair services. The costs of many of these services are extremely high and out of reach of most older adults.

CONCLUSION

The complexity of elder self-neglect is compounded by the variability in its definition and the lack of valid, reliable, and standardized clinical diagnostic tools to identify elder self-neglect, as well as difficulty identifying when and how to intervene once self-neglect has been identified. Public policy changes are necessary to ensure that older adults have adequate funding for needed services and that more uniform and specific reporting policies regarding self-neglect are developed.

Medical care has become so specialized that caring for an individual involves multiple office visits at multiple locations. Elders are overwhelmed by the complexities of the current medical system. It is evident from the work of Dyer et al. (1999) that the need for a comprehensive interdisciplinary program for assessment and continuing management represents the state-of-the-art approach in managing cases of self-neglect.

IMPLICATIONS FOR RESEARCH AND PRACTICE

- Multidisciplinary teams of health care and social services professionals are recommended for effective treatment and intervention in elder self-neglect.
- A CGA involving an interdisciplinary team that provides medical, functional, cognitive, medication, social network, social history, and home environment status is warranted.
- Further education on elder self-neglect is an important step in the prevention of self-neglect.
- There is an urgent need for research and improved funding to provide scientific evidence on this complex phenomenon.

REFERENCES

Abram, R. C., Lachs, M., McAvay, G., Keohane, D. J., & Bruce, M. L. (2002). Predictors of self-neglect in community dwelling elders. *American Journal of Psychiatry, 159*(10), 1724–1730.

Arean, P. A., Alvidrez, J., Barrera, A., Robinson, G. S., & Hicks, S. (2002). Would older medical patients use psychological services? *The Gerontologist, 42*(3), 392–398.

Bartels, S. J., Haley, W. E., & Dums, A. R. (2002). Implementing evidence based practices in geriatric mental health. *Psychiatric Servies, 53*(11), 1419–1431.

Bartley, M., O'Neill, D., Knight, P., & O'Brien, J. (2011). Self-neglect and elder abuse: Related phenomena. *Journal of the American Geriatrics Society, 59*(11), 2163–2168.

Burnett, J., Coverdale, J. H., Pickens, S., & Dyer, C. B. (2006). What is the association between self-neglect, depressive symptoms and untreaded medical conditions? *Journal of Elder Abuse & Neglect, 18*, 25–34.

Burnett, J., Regev, T., Pickens, S., Prati, L. L., Aung, K., Moore, J., & Dyer, C. B. (2006). Social networks: A profile of the elderly who self-neglect. *Journal of Elder Abuse & Neglect, 18*(4), 35–49.

Choi, N., Kim, J., & Assef, J. (2009). Self neglect and neglect of vulnerable older adults: Reexamination of etiology. *Journal of Gerontological Social Work, 52*(2), 171–187.

Clancy, M., McDaid, B., O'Neill, D., & O'Brien, J. (2011). National profiling of elder abuse referrals. *Age and Aging, 40*(3), 392–398.

Clark, A., Mankikar, G., & Gray, I. (1975). Diogenes syndrome: A clinical study of gross neglect in old age. *Lancet, 1*(7903), 366–368.

Day, M. R., & Leahy-Warren, P. (2008). Self-neglect 2: Nursing assessment and management. *Nursing Times, 104*(25), 28–29.

Dong, X., Simon, M. A., Wilson, R. S., Mendes de Leon, C. F., Rajan, K. B., & Evans, D. A. (2010). Decline in cognitive function and risk of elder self-neglect: Finding from the Chicago Health Aging Project. *Journal of the American Geriatrics Society, 58*(12), 2292–2299.

Dyer, C. B., Gleason, M., Murphy, K., Pavlik, V., Portal, B., Regev, T., & Hyman, D. (1999). Treating elder neglect: Collaboration between a geriatrics assesment team and adult protective services. *Southern Medical Journal, 92*(2), 242–244.

Dyer, C. B., Goodwin, J. S., Pickens-Pace, S., Burnett, J., & Kelly, P. A. (2007). Self-neglect among the elderly: A model based on more than 500 patients seen by a geriatric medicine team. *American Journal of Public Health, 97*(9), 1671–1676.

Dyer, C. B., Pavlik, V. N., Murphy, K. P., & Hyman, D. J. (2000). The high prevalence of depression and dementia in elder abuse or neglect. *Journal of the American Geriatrics Society, 48*(2), 205–208.

Ewing, J. A. (1984). Detecting alcoholism: The CAGE Questionnaire. *Journal of the American Medical Association, 252*, 1905–1907.

Folstein, M., Folstein, S. E., & McHugh, P. R. (1975). "Mini-Mental State." A practical method for grading the cognitive state of patients for the clinician. *Journal of Psychiatric Research, 12*(3), 189–198.

Fulmer, T., Paveza, G., Abraham, L., & Fairchild, S. (2000). Elder self-neglect assessment in the emergency department. *Journal of Emergency Nursing, 26*(5), 436–443.

Geriatric Mental Health Foundation. (2008). Depression late in life: Not a natural part of aging. Retrieved from http://www.aagponline.org/index.php?src=gendocs&ref=depression&category=Foundation

Halliday, G., Banerjee, S., Philpot, M., & MacDonald, A. (2000). Community study of people who live in squalor. *Lancet, 355*, 882–886.

Hansen, M. C., Flores, D. V., Coverdale, J., & Burnett, J. (2016). Correlates of depression in self-neglecting older adults: A cross-sectional study examining the role of alcohol abuse and pain in increasing vulnerability. *Journal of Elder Abuse & Neglect, 28*(1), 41–56.

Inouye, S. K., vanDyck, C. H., Alessi, C. A., Balkin, S., Siegal, A. P., & Horwitz, R. I. (1990). Clarifying confusion: The Confusion Assessment Method. A new method for detection of delirium. *Annals of Internal Medicine, 113*, 941–948.

Kelly, P. A., Dyer, C. B., Pavlik, V., Doody, R., & Jogerst, V. (2008). Exploring self-neglect in older adults: Preliminary findings of the self-neglect severity scale and next steps. *Journal of the American Geriatrics Society, 56*(Suppl. 2), S253–S260.

Lachs, M. S., Williams, C. S., O'Brien, S., Pillemer, K. A., & Charlson, M. E. (1998). The mortality of elder mistreatment. *Journal of the American Medical Association, 280*(5), 428–432.

Lansbury, G. (2000). Chronic pain management: A qualitative study of elderly people's coping strategies and barriers to management. *Journal of Disability and Rehabilitation, 22*(1/2), 2–14.

Lawton, M. P., & Brody, E. M. (1969). Assessment of older people: Self maintaining and instrumental activities of daily living. *The Gerontologist, 9*(3, Pt. 1), 179–186.

Longres, F. (1994). Self-neglect and social control: A modest test of an issue. *Journal of Gerontological Social Work, 22*, 3–20.

MacMillan, D., & Shaw, P. (1966). Senile breakdown in standards of personal and environmental clenliness. *British Medical Journal, 29*(2), 227–229.

May-Chahal, C., & Antrobus, R. (2012). Engaging community support in safeguarding adults from self-neglect. *British Journal of Social Work, 42*(8), 1478–1494.

McKenna, M. T., Michaud, C. M., Murray, C. J., & Marks, J. S. (2005). Assessing the burden of disease in the US using disability adjusted life years. *American Journal of Preventative Medicine, 28*(5), 415–423.

Mosqueda, L., & Dong, X. (2011). Elder abuse and self-neglect: "I don't care anything about going to the doctor, to be honest . . ." *Journal of the American Medical Association, 306*, 532–540.

Moye, J., Butz, S. W., Marson, D. C., Wood, E., & ABA–APA. (2007). A conceptual model and assessment template for capacity evaluation in adult guardianship. *The Gerontologist, 47*(5), 591–603.

Naik, A., Burnett, J., Pickens-Pace, S., & Dyer, C. (2008). Impairment in instrumental activities of daily living and the geriatrics syndrome of self-neglect. *The Gerontologist, 48*, 388–393.

O'Brien, J. G. (1999). *Self-neglect challenges for helping professionals*: New York, NY: Routledge.

O'Brien, J. G., Riain, A. N., Collins, C., Long, V., & O'Neill, D. (2014). Elder abuse and neglect: A survey of Irish general practitioners. *Journal of Elder Abuse & Neglect, 26*(3), 291–299.

O'Brien, J. G., Cooney, C., Bartley, M., & O'Neill, D. (2013). Self-neglect: A survey of old age psychiatrists in Ireland. *International Psychogeriatrics, 25*(12), 2088–2090.

O'Brien, J. G., Thibault, J. M., Turner, L. C., & Laird-Fick, H. S. (2000). Self-neglect: An overview. *Journal of Elder Abuse & Neglect, 11*(2), 1–19.

Paveza, G., Vanderweerd, C., & Laumann, E. (2008). Elder self-neglect: A discussion of a social typology. *Journal of the American Geriatrics Society, 56*(Suppl. 2), S271–S275.

Pickens, S., Burnett, J., Naik, A., Holmes, H., & Dyer, C. (2006). Is pain a significant factor in elder self-neglect? *Journal of Elder Abuse & Neglect, 18*(4), 51–61.

Rathbone-McCuan, E., & Bricker-Jenkins, M. (1992). *A general framework for elder self-neglect*. Westport, CT: Auburn House.

Reed, P., & Leonard, V. (1989). An analysis of the concept of self-neglect. *Advanced Nursing Science, 12*(1), 39–53.

Reyes-Ortiz, C. (2006). Self-neglect as a geriatric syndrome. *Journal of the American Geriatrics Society, 54*(12), 1945–1946.

Royall, D. R., Palmer, R., Chiodo, L. K., & Polk, M. J. (2004). Declining executive control in normal aging predicts change in fuctional status: The Freedom House Study. *Journal of the American Geriatrics Society, 52*(3), 346–352.

Schillerstrom, J. E., Salazar, R., Regwan, H., Bonguli, R. J., & Royall, D. R. (2009). Executive function in self-neglecting adult protective services referrals compared with elder psychiatric outpatients. *American Journal of Geriatric Psychiatry, 17*(10), 907–910.

Sengstock, M. C., Thibault, J. M., & Zaranek, R. (1999). Community dimensions of self-neglect. *Journal of Elder Abuse & Neglect, 11*(2), 77–93.

Snowdon, J., Shah, A., & Halliday, G. (2007). Severe domestic squalor: A review. *International Psychogeriatrics, 19*(1), 37–51.

Tatara, T., Kuzmeskus, L. B., Duckhorn, E., Bivens, L., Thomas, C., Gertig, J., . . . Croos, J. (1998). *The national elder abuse incidence study: Final report.* Washington, DC: National Center on Elder Abuse. Retrieved from http://aoa.gov/AoA_Programs/Elder_Rights/Elder_Abuse/docs/ABuseReport_Full.pdf

Teaster, P. B., Dugar, T., Mendiodo, M. S., & Cecil, K. A. (2006). *The 2004 survey of state adult protective services: abuse of adults 60 years of age and older.* Washington, DC: National Center on Elder Abuse.

Thibault, J. (1984). *The analysis and treatment of indiret self-destructive behaviors in the elderly.* Chicago, IL: University of Chicago.

Thompson, L. K. (1992). *The Kohlman evaluation of living skills* (3rd ed.). Rockville, MD: American Occupational Therapy Association.

Tierney, M. C., Snow, W. G., Charles, J., Moineddin, R., & Kiss, A. (2007). Neuropsychological predictors of self-neglect in cognitively impaired older people who live alone. *American Journal of Geriatric Psychiatry, 15*(2), 140–148.

Turner, A., Hochschild, A., Burnett, J., Zulfiqar, A., & Dyer, C. (2012). High prevalence of medication nonadherence in a sample of community-dwelling older adults with adult protective services validated self neglect. *Drugs Aging, 29*(9), 741–749.

Ungvari, G. S., & Hantz, P. M. (1991). Social breakdown in the elderly: Case studies and management. *Comparative Psychiatry, 32*(5), 440–444.

Whitehead, T. (1975). Diogenes syndrome (Letter). *Lancet, i*(7909), 628.

Wrigley, M., & Cooney, C. (1992). Diogenes syndrome—An Irish series. *Irish Journal of Psychological Medicine, 9*(1), 37–41.

Yesavage, J. A., Brink, T. L., Rose, T. L., Lum, O., Huang, V., Adey, M. B., & Leirer, V. O. (1983). Development and validation of a geriatric depression screening scale: A preliminary report. *Journal of Psychiatric Research, 17,* 37–49.

CHAPTER 12

HOME CARE NURSES AND SELF-NEGLECT

Yvonne O. Johnson

Self-neglect is not a new phenomenon. It is complex, poorly understood, and under-researched. Because self-neglect frequently includes neglecting both self-care and the living environment, home health nurses are perfectly positioned to identify and intervene with these individuals, yet the nurses' voices are virtually silent in self-neglect research reports. The purpose of this qualitative study was to determine how experienced home health nurses perceive elder self-neglect and the steps they employ to intervene when self-neglect is suspected. Semi-structured interviews were conducted with 16 home health nurses. Interviews revealed nurses' perceptions of elder self-neglect, which included clients controlling their territory, clients behaving as if self-neglect was commonly accepted, clients who seclude themselves, and clients who do not conform to common self-care conventions such as maintaining personal hygiene or their living environment. Nurses identified and defined self-neglect based on their observations. Facilitators who intervened in self-neglect cases engaged family members and others on the health care team. Many more barriers to interventions were evident and included a lack of education on self-neglect, protecting client choice, and lack of resources. This is the first study of the U.S. home health nurses' perceptions of elder self-neglect.

Much has been written on the growing population of older adults. The older population of the United States ($\geq$age 65) is expected to approach 84 million (U.S. Census Bureau, 2014) by 2050. It is well known that older adults have more chronic health conditions; are prescribed more medications to treat those conditions; and have greater numbers of hospital, rehabilitation facility, and nursing home admissions (Federal Interagency Forum on Aging-Related Statistics, 2012) compared with other age groups. Less widely discussed is the fact that some older adults fail to take the steps needed to care for themselves (personal care), and, despite increased medical needs, either avoid medical care or fail to adhere to the medical regimen prescribed for them. This phenomenon is known as self-neglect by some authors (Adams & Johnson, 1998; Braye, Orr, & Preston-Shoot, 2011; Burnett, Regev, et al., 2006; Gibbons, 2007; Lauder, 1999a).

Health conditions that could be easily prevented or controlled may be exacerbated when older adults who self-neglect are not identified and treated. Uncontrolled health conditions increase the risk of hospitalizations and the need for rehabilitative services and nursing home admissions, further burdening the health care industry. Improving the understanding of self-neglect should aid the development of a trajectory for worsening self-neglect, which is needed to develop intervention strategies, as well as impact health care spending on potentially preventable health care services. This chapter describes a qualitative study that determined how experienced home health nurses perceive elder self-neglect and the steps they employ to intervene when self-neglect is suspected.

BACKGROUND LITERATURE

In general, self-neglect is characterized by (a) a lack of attention to the basic human physical needs such as nutrition and hygiene, (b) social isolation, and (c) lack of attention to medical needs (Ballard, 2010; Bozinovski, 2000; Braye et al., 2011; Burnett, Regev, et al., 2006; Lauder, Ludwick, Zeller, & Winchell, 2006). This phenomenon lacks clear conceptualization and may be defined differently depending on the perspective of the professional providing care (Lauder, 1999a). Although studies conducted on self-neglect have used similar terms in its definitions, no consistent definition has been adopted (Ballard, 2010; Braye et al., 2011; Dick, 2006; X. Dong, Wilson, Mendes de Leon, & Evans, 2009; Gibbons, Lauder, & Ludwick, 2006; Lauder, Anderson, & Barclay, 2005).

Complicating the lack of understanding of self-neglect is the paucity of research on this phenomenon. This is especially true regarding the perspectives health care professionals have of self-neglect. This lack of evidence to underpin practice decisions translates into the inability to educate health care professionals about self-neglect, and may ultimately contribute to the perpetuation of self-neglect and its sequelae. Given the health consequences of self-neglect, the connection between self-neglect and the elderly population, an increasing elderly population, and the absence of a clear definition for self-neglect used by health care professionals, further research to gain an understanding of self-neglect is crucial in protecting and improving the health of this vulnerable population.

Although self-neglect is glaringly evident in the living environment of the individual (Abrams, Lachs, McAvay, Keohane, & Bruce, 2002; Braye et al., 2011; Macmillan & Shaw, 1966), it may not be noticed when the individual is seen outside of that environment. Practitioners who make home visits, such as nurses and social workers employed by home health agencies, are uniquely positioned to assess for self-neglect; unfortunately, to date, few studies focusing on self-neglect have included nurses (Adams & Johnson, 1998; Ernst & Smith, 2012; Lauder et al., 2006). Published reports of self-neglect have described the experiences of 18 hospital nurses and 10 community health nurses in one study (Adams & Johnson, 1998); 40 public health nurses in another (Lauder et al., 2006), with no distinction of whether those nurses made home visits; and an unknown number of social worker and registered nurse teams in a third study that included nurses (Ernst & Smith, 2012). Although a hallmark consequence of self-neglect is impaired health status, it is surprising that so few studies have included health care practitioners (Adams & Johnson, 1998; Gibbons, 2009; Iris, Ridings, & Conrad, 2009; Lauder, 1999a; Lauder et al., 2005, 2006).

Nurses constitute the largest group of health care personnel, therefore, they have a frontline position in assessing self-neglect where it is most evident, in the home. In spite of this, nurses' voices are virtually silent in the science of self-neglect, as they have been either relatively excluded from self-neglect research or have not developed research on the topic themselves. There remains an inexcusable and perplexing dearth of information regarding nurses' perceptions of and experiences with self-neglect. Including nurses in developing the body of knowledge for this intricate and alarming phenomenon should strengthen the ability to understand the phenomenon, inform public policy decisions, and ultimately improve the care for those impacted by self-neglect.

PURPOSE OF THE STUDY

The purpose of this study was to explore experienced home health nurses' perspectives of self-neglect among the elderly (Johnson, 2014). This exploration focused on (a) definitions for elder self-neglect used by the home health nurse, (b) how elder self-neglect was identified by the home health nurse, and (c) steps usually taken by the home health nurse to address the individual's needs when elder self-neglect was suspected.

DESIGN AND SAMPLE

This qualitative study utilized a naturalistic, descriptive design with semi structured interviews to allow participants to share their personal experiences and perspectives. A senior administrator for the participants' state home health association was instrumental in distributing recruitment materials to all Medicare-certified home health agencies in the state of North Carolina. Purposive snowball sampling provided participants who had experience with self-neglect.

METHODS

The institutional review board for the University of North Carolina at Greensboro provided approval for the study. In addition, each participant provided voluntary consent after receiving an explanation of the study. To protect confidentiality, pseudonyms were assigned alphabetically in order of the sequence of the interviews. Each participant's pseudonym was used for reporting purposes. Transcripts were housed in a password-protected environment.

Interviews were prefaced with an initial global statement: "Tell me about a time that you went into a patient's home to deliver care and felt like the client was self-neglecting." Each participant was encouraged to articulate what he or she envisioned when he or she heard the term *self-neglect*. Specific research questions included: What are home health nurse's perceptions of self-neglect? How do home health nurses identify self-neglect? What actions do home health nurses employ to intervene with self-neglect? What are the facilitators and barriers to identifying self-neglect for home health nurses? What are the facilitators and barriers to intervening with self-neglect for home health nurses? Probing questions were employed to facilitate further discussion and to illicit additional perceptions home health nurses had of self-neglect and the care of elderly clients who exhibit signs of self-neglect. Clarifying questions were asked when the participant's ideas were unclear, or when elaboration on an idea was desired. Field notes of the interviewer's personal feelings regarding the data shared were recorded, and demographic information on the participants was collected.

Data Analysis and Quality

The audio recordings were transcribed into a written document and each document was checked against the recording for accuracy. Member checks with clarifying questions were conducted as needed. Peer scrutiny of the research project and code checking with a second coder were performed. Content analyses of the interview transcripts were conducted. Raw data from each transcript were thoroughly examined for key statements. Significant statements were placed into broad categories based on similarities and differences. These broad categories became the initial codes used for further content analysis and constant comparison, as described by Lincoln and Guba (1985). As statements were placed within the categories each was compared with other statements in that category for best fit. Once the interview data were deconstructed through the process of content analysis, constant comparison was employed to identify major categories present in these interviews. Comparisons were made within the interviews and across interviews. To ensure the credibility of the data, the principal investigator was careful to reflect on and bracket her own perceptions during analysis, to ensure the information from the published literature and her own experiences with elder self-neglect would not contaminate data from this study (Lincoln & Guba, 1985; Sandelowski, 1986). Thus, the perception of self-neglect held by these home health nurses was constructed through an inductive process.

Themes representing home health nurses' perceptions of self-neglect emerged from the interviews and included (a) armor, (b) psychological derivation, (c) seclusion, (d) nonconformity with self-care conventions, and (e) nurses' responses (Johnson, 2014). In addition to the themes, actions taken by home health nurses to intervene with clients who self-neglect, as well as barriers and facilitators to interventions for self-neglect, were evident. Comparisons were made of these data as well and similarities across participants were evident.

FINDINGS

Sixteen experienced registered nurses were interviewed in the summer of 2013. The average age of the nurses in this study was 46 years, consistent with the mean age of registered nurses (RNs) reported by the United States Department of Labor, Bureau of Labor Statistics (2013). Participants had an average of 20.28 years of professional nursing experience (range = 5–41 years), with an average of 11.43 years in home health nursing (range = 2–23 years). The majority (93.75%) held full-time positions in home health nursing and over half (56.25%) practiced in rural areas. Almost half of the nurses (n = 7) were educated at the associate-degree level, whereas another six held baccalaureate degrees in nursing. Three of the participants were diploma graduates. The sample was homogenous, predominately Caucasian (n = 14), with one African American participant, and one participant reporting Caribbean and Thai descent.

Most nurses in this study (75%) reported that elder self-neglect was not a subject taught in their nursing education programs. The only nurse (a diploma graduate) who had some input was taught signs and symptoms used to identify self-neglect and that reporting to adult protective services (APS) might be a requirement. Others stated they were informed that self-neglect was an issue of noncompliance or a symptom associated with mental health disorders such as dementia or depression.

Fifteen of the 16 participants reported they had never heard of a workshop focused on elder self-neglect.

The majority of nurse participants (81.25%) reported using screening tools for home health assessments such as the Geriatric Depression Scale (Yesavage et al., 1983) and the Medicare Outcome and Assessment Information Set (OASIS; Centers for Medicare & Medicaid Services, 2012). All had encountered elder self neglect in practice as a home health nurse, but none reported having used a specific screening tool to determine self-neglect.

Reasons for Home Health Referrals

Most often, home health services were ordered for clients of the participants following hospital discharge for exacerbations of chronic disease processes. Other clients were referred for medication management or wound care. Some were referred for reasons more obscure such as generalized weakness, assessment of home health needs, or post hospitalization teaching. None of the study participants reported clients being referred for home health services due to self-neglect, or even a suspicion of self-neglect. Instead, self-neglect was identified by home health nurses themselves after entering the home and observing the client in the living environment.

Themes Identified

Consistent with Adam and Johnson's research (1998), all nurses interviewed in the current study were able to describe the characteristics used to identify clients who self-neglect. A common perception held by nurses was that individuals who self-neglect exhibit thought patterns and actions that serve to "shield" them: a type of armor that serves to protect the self-neglecter. Three categories within this theme of armor or shielding of self are (a) it's my normal, (b) control of territory, and (c) emotion.

A significant statement reoccurring throughout the interviews related to self-neglect becoming a normal way of life for the individual. Nurses perceived that their clients who self-neglected conducted themselves as if their behaviors and the state of their surroundings were normally accepted practices, and thus, did not give any indication that what was observed by others as odd was anything to be concerned with. Not only did these clients not react as though their situations and surroundings seemed different to others, but they also controlled their territory as part of their armor. This was evident across many interviews and suggests that nurses recognize control is important to these individuals. Display of emotions, such as anger, was reported as one way these individuals controlled their territory, and this was evident to home health nurses in the manner that these clients interacted with them and with others. Some reported clients demonstrated [a need for] control by sending either verbal or nonverbal messages indicating they did not want others intruding into their domain. Diverse emotional responses in individuals ranged from withdrawn or dispassionate, to irate and belligerent. Some nurses described clients as "disconnected." Still other nurses recalled more hostile reactions from clients and related feeling almost attacked when they entered the home.

Maintenance of routines consistently emerged across interviews. Nurses related perceiving that some clients may have been in a pattern of this behavior for so long that it had become who they were, whereas others nurses used the term *control* and identified behaviors such as anger that these clients use to maintain control. The behaviors and the presentation of these clients and their environments served to "shield" the client, making armor an important theme in this study.

The second major theme was psychological derivation. Fourteen out of the 16 nurse participants identified pathological states in their attempts to understand the behaviors exhibited by clients. By viewing the behaviors noted in elders who self-neglect in the context of psychological or cognitive challenges, the nurses could identify steps they needed to take to intervene. Three main categories in this theme were (a) undiagnosed mental illness, (b) depression, and (c) dementia.

Undiagnosed or unidentified mental illness, depression, and dementia were significant constructs identified by nurses. Nurses understood that clients with these conditions often fail to attend to their personal needs such as hygiene and nutrition. Although nurses connected self-neglecting behaviors to mental illness, depression, and dementia, none of the study participants related that their clients actually had a medical diagnosis for any of those conditions.

The third major theme was seclusion. Rationales for seclusion varied and included (a) isolation by choice, (b) isolation by others, and (c) isolation by circumstance. Home health nurses reported sensing that clients isolate themselves by choice and identified elder self-neglecters as "hermits." For example, one participant when speaking on this topic said "It was his choice to live there. . . . He didn't want to go anywhere. . . . It's their home and they do not want to leave that." Others noted that these individuals may have had some element of isolation behavior for years, "I see that more if they are loners or have been loners most of their life." Still others identified actions by these self-neglecters that served to isolate them. Comments shared included, "No, generally speaking the kind of patients that I had to deal with, they shut lots of folks out," and "He still continues to refuse to leave his home."

Abandonment by others was noted as a rationale for seclusion. However, none of the nurses used that term, and instead focused on behaviors noted in elder self-neglecters. For example, one participant commented: "Either because they got . . . excommunicated from their family because they've been so mean to their family and friends that nobody wants anything to do with them." Others noted problematic interactions such as: "And the times that I've seen the adult children come to visit . . . there's not a good relationship."

Isolation also occurred in some clients due to life circumstances; specific life situations such as family moving away, or the lack of any friends or acquaintances. Some participants identified the absence of a support system as problematic in statements such as: "So, it's not like they would have a strong church support system or even a network of friends and I see them as being alone." Another example of a situation that served to isolate was the death of a caregiver. One participant stated: "The biggest majority have very little family support, or no family support."

This lack of conformity with socially accepted self-care conventions was another theme identified and was perhaps the most striking component of self-neglect identified by the home health nurse. These were the actions or behaviors not taken by the individual to ensure his or her own health, comfort, and even survival and included (a) taking medications prescribed, (b) attending to personal hygiene needs, (c) consuming an adequate amount of calories for normal life functions, and (d) attending to the living environment.

Home health nurses identified medication management as one of their key responsibilities and verbalizing medication management as a key behavior in preventing rehospitalization. In spite of the fact that medications for some clients were prescribed for chronic or even life-threatening conditions, study participants identified medication neglect as a common behavior, even when resources were adequate.

Consistent with earlier research describing failure to attend to personal hygiene (Adams & Johnson, 1998; Clark, Mankikar, & Gray, 1975; Dyer et al., 2006; Dyer, Goodwin, Pickens-Pace, Burnett, & Kelly, 2007; Kelly, Dyer, Pavlik, Doody, & Jogerst, 2008; Lauder, 2001; Macmillan & Shaw, 1966; National Center on Elder Abuse [NCEA], 1998; Poythress, Burnett, Naik, Pickens, & Dyer, 2006; Tierney et al., 2004), study participants reported making visits to elders to find the lack of attention to personal cleanliness was so extreme that participants described clients as filthy with a strong smell of body odor, and with no attention to cleaning teeth, hair, or nails. Hygiene problems were noted in all interviews.

Nutrition is a component of the overall assessment of home health patients and is noted as an important element of health maintenance. Reported nutritional problems in those who self-neglect ranged from not eating enough to not eating at all.

One of the most striking components of self-neglect reported was the state of the home environment, often described as cluttered, filthy, infested with bugs and rodents, and even with structural problems that were left unattended. Nurse participants verbalized a sense of disbelief in these living environments, describing them as surreal.

Nurses' Responses to Self-Neglect

The final theme that emerged was nurses' responses to self-neglect. These included both emotional and action responses. Emotional responses included feeling shocked, saddened, and even guilty about their inability to effectively intervene. Feelings of helplessness and frustration were also reported by nurses who verbalized a strong need to help these individuals.

Action responses included utilizing independent nursing actions such as establishing a rapport or trusting relationship and taking nonjudgmental approaches to establish connections with the client. Nurses reported drawing on their foundational nursing education to care for these clients. Nurses prioritized client needs and educated their self-neglecting clients. Nurses even took steps to take clients food from their own cupboards or to stop at fast-food restaurants to purchase food for clients they identified as having nutritional challenges.

In addition to independent nursing actions, the nurses also reported collaborating within their agencies with other nurses and with the interdisciplinary team treating the patient. Medical social work referrals as well as home health aide referrals were reported. When community programs (such as Meals on Wheels) were present, those services were also utilized. As safety threats were identified, the nurses referred clients to the department of social services in their area or to APS agencies.

Facilitators and Barriers to Self-Neglect Intervention

Home health nurses identified many more barriers to self-neglect intervention than facilitators. Facilitators to intervening included collaborating with family members, other nurses, the interdisciplinary team, and, in particular, the medical social workers.

Barriers to self-neglect intervention were readily identified. The ability to persuade clients who self-neglect to change self-neglectful behaviors was nonexistent. Many nurses reported there were no agency protocols for identifying or intervening with elder self-neglect. Other barriers to intervention included limited resources for the elderly. Reimbursement services for home health were being cut, interdisciplinary access was often problematic, and the ethics of patient autonomy and choice sometimes blocked nurses from intervening. When community resources existed, they were often long waiting lists.

Resources for mental health services were identified as limited and necessary. The lack of providers was identified as a huge barrier to mental health care access. One participant said: "So, we have, if you can imagine two counties where the populations are probably 10,000 to 15,000 a piece, and there are two psychiatrists. Who can even serve like that?"

Lack of education on self-neglect was identified. Self-neglect education for health care personnel was reported as virtually nonexistent. Home health nurses related not knowing best practices to care for clients who self-neglect, and therefore having to do the best they could with each situation they encountered. Many nurses referred clients who self-neglect to APS. However, a common refrain across these interviews was that APS would go out for the visits and almost invariably come back with the report that the patient was "in their right mind," "making conscious choices to live as they do," and "the clients have the right to make choices for their lives."

Interdisciplinary access was also a barrier because nurses rarely had direct access to physicians. Instead, when nurses called to give a report to the physician, they either had to leave a lengthy message or speak to a clerical person or medical assistant. In addition, some nurses recalled practices within their agencies of having to communicate with other agency personnel through electronic mail and interdisciplinary notes. Concerns were expressed that written communication methods may not convey the same message that could be transmitted verbally.

Ethical treatment of clients is at the heart of health care and is a core value of nursing. Thus, it is not surprising that nurse participants identified protection of autonomy and choice as a barrier to intervening with self-neglect. Clients did not want to leave their homes, and, as competent adults, have the right to live as they choose. Home health nurses wanted to honor the rights of the individuals, but struggled with not being able to intervene to improve the lives of their clients. One nurse said: "There's really nothing we can do if they're in their right frame of mind. I struggled all the way home yesterday trying to decide . . . maybe this is how she wants to live, maybe this is the way she wants to die, maybe this is her choice."

DISCUSSION

This study highlights self-neglect as a challenging situation for health care professionals. A consensus approach to addressing this complex phenomenon is lacking and complicates the ability of nurses to effectively care for individuals. The diversity in perspectives of self-neglect and the approach to care for those who self-neglect revealed within this study is consistent with the current literature on self-neglect, which also lacks a shared definition for this phenomenon (Braye et al., 2011; National Committee for the Prevention of Elder Abuse [NCPEA], 2008). Despite the diversity in perspectives offered by these nurse participants, they were all keenly aware of behaviors and observations made that reflected self-neglect. Also consistent with Lauder (2001), this study revealed that nurses identify self-neglect based on a constellation of features rather than a single defining attribute.

Because environmental neglect is a cardinal feature of elder self-neglect, the home may be the best place to identify it. Home health nurses often encounter complex cases of self-neglect. A barrier to managing and supporting these individuals includes a lack of education on the topic. Nurses themselves may experience confusion in their attempts to understand the behaviors seen. Frustration also occurs because of the lack of intervention guidelines needed to inform nursing practice. This study represents the first study of self-neglect focused solely on the perspectives of home health nurses in the United States and therefore provides information from the perspective of the health care professionals who may be most likely to identify elder self-neglect.

Five themes emerged from this research: (a) use of "armor," (b) psychological derivation, (c) seclusion, (d) nonconformity with self-care conventions, and (e) nurses' responses (Johnson, 2014). Nurses in this study perceived that elders who self-neglect effectively "shield" themselves from others. This "armor" protects the self-neglecter, but may also serve to further insulate the individual. The effects of self-neglect may be compounded because the individual is shielded from others, and therefore is less likely to be identified. This finding supported Bozinovski's (2000) grounded theory work, which determined that "maintaining customary control" (p. 43) was important to the self-neglecter and that striving for this control compels individuals to exhibit "attitudes and behaviors they hold most comfortable and usual for them" (p. 44).

Psychological derivation was another important theme evident in the data. Nurses attributed self-neglect behaviors to mental health issues, including undiagnosed mental illness, depression, and dementia. It is interesting to note that various types of psychiatric and cognitive disorders can result in labile emotions as well as responses that seem incongruent with an individual's current situation (Alzheimer's Association, 2014) similar to those seen in individuals who self-neglect. None of the self-neglecting clients cared for by these study participants had a diagnosis for any of these types of conditions.

Challenges and behaviors that accompany mental health issues are taught in nursing education; thus, nurses are prepared to care for clients with those issues. It is logical that clients, who are cognitively challenged, have depression, dementia, or mental illness, may lack sound decision making. However, when study participants' clients were referred for determinations of competence, they were not deemed incompetent. This parallels research by Ernst and Smith (2012), who stated that the majority of the elders who self-neglect "are legally competent" (p. 290). Nurse participants expressed frustration with these findings of competence, citing issues of safety arising from these individuals' decisions.

Behaviors noted in some individuals with psychological challenges include failure to attend to basic human needs such as personal care, the living environment, maintaining adequate nutrition, and attending to medical needs. It is interesting to note that these are also salient features of self-neglect. Clients of the nurses in this study were not diagnosed with mental illness. Yet, nurses in this study and in research conducted by Lauder and colleagues (2006) attributed self-neglect behaviors to issues of mental illness. Because nurses are well versed in caring for clients exhibiting challenges in caring for themselves when cognitive deficits or mental illness are present, this may be a plausible reason for nurses associating self-neglecting behaviors with mental illness. Lauder and colleagues (2006) also found that nurses caring for people who self-neglect may "resort to tried and tested cognitive schemata" (p. 285).

Home health nurses reported clients who self-neglect tend to be secluded. Three distinct reasons for that seclusion were given: (a) isolation by choice, (b) isolation by others, and (c) isolation by circumstances. Previous studies on self-neglect have established social isolation as associated with individuals who self-neglect

(Burnett, Coverdale, Pickens, & Dyer, 2006; Burnett, Regev, et al., 2006; Culberson et al., 2011; S. Dong, Simon, Beck, & Evans, 2010; Dyer et al., 2007; Macmillan & Shaw, 1966; Mauk, 2011; Payne & Gainey, 2005). Some researchers have offered possible reasons for the social isolation, but no definitive link has been delineated. Likely the source is multifocal.

Seclusion may compound self-neglect. The elder has no one to interact with and, therefore, eccentricities may become more ingrained than they would if the individual was socially active. This could occur because self-neglecting behaviors go unnoticed and are not addressed in the absence of a caregiver or someone to interact with (Paveza, VandeWeerd, & Laumann, 2008), or just because individuals may not see an urgent need to wash their hair, or change their clothes if no one else is around, as was reported by participants in this study. Social interaction may also improve cognitive function (Glass, Mendes De Leon, Bassuk, & Berkman, 2006; Ristau, 2011). The lack of social interaction may have the opposite effect. Glass and colleagues (2006) found that social engagement had an inverse relationship with depression. This same relationship was reflected in statements from nurse participants in this study who stated that they rarely saw self-neglect in cases in which the elder had a caregiver who was actively involved.

Individuals who self-neglect may fail to conform with any usual manner of attending to self-care, and this failure usually extends over various aspects of self-care. In the present study, that included failure to conform to accepted practices in the areas of (a) medication, (b) hygiene, (c) nutrition, and (d) environment. Nurse participants noted that even though they had questions regarding the competence of these clients, self-neglecters did not react as if there were any differences in the way that they attended to their needs as compared to others. Again, this indifference could be a component of the armor of these individuals.

Older individuals who self-neglect often fail to take their medications as prescribed, even when the medications may be prescribed to treat chronic or even terminal illnesses (Adams & Johnson, 1998; Dyer et al., 2006; Tierney et al., 2004). Many participants in the current study reported the same. Even clients with adequate resources were reported as choosing not to take prescribed medications. Home health nurses reported struggling with attempts to convince these clients to take their medications as prescribed. However, their efforts to educate the client on the value of medication in treating their health conditions, as well as the consequences of not taking the medications as prescribed went unheeded.

Detrimental effects of failing to take medication as prescribed are well known, yet medication nonadherence is widespread. Failing to take medications is not exclusive to self-neglect, as many elderly clients fail to take their medications as prescribed (Berry et al., 2010; Gentil, Vasiliadis, Preville, Bosse, & Berbiche, 2012; Henriques, Costa, & Cabrita, 2012). Nurses are aware that many clients fail to adhere to prescribed medications. What is unknown is whether the cause of failing to adhere in self-neglect is different from other individuals who do not adhere.

Individuals may neglect only one aspect of their care, but often neglect is found in multiple areas of care. Failure to conform to hygiene conventions presents a picture that these nurses reported "never forgetting." Study participants described these individuals and their homes as disheveled, dirty, unkempt, odiferous, and filthy. Yet, nurses reported their attempts to rectify the issues were often rejected by the self-neglecter. These findings are consistent with previous research on self-neglect (Adams & Johnson, 1998; Clark et al., 1975; Dyer et al., 2006, 2007; Kelly et al., 2008; Lauder, 2001; Macmillan & Shaw, 1966; NCEA, 1998; Poythress et al., 2006;

Tierney et al., 2004). Nurses in this study tended to concern themselves with addressing each behavior rather than addressing self-neglect as a whole. Nurses may be overwhelmed by the totality of self-neglect due to the complexity of the issues and the lack of education on this topic. Thus, nurses may focus on what they have experience with, and what they know they have had positive results with in the past.

Home health nurses expressed shock at observing these clients and their homes. They also reported feeling saddened by many aspects of the lives of these individuals and saddened at the deaths of these individuals when they occurred. A feeling of helplessness to do anything effective for these individuals or to impact the choices that these individuals were making was common across interviews. Caring is the core of nursing (National League for Nursing, 2013) and is a concept that nurses value. When nurses are impotent in providing that care, strong emotional responses result.

Action responses in these interviews included nurses relying heavily on interdisciplinary resources such as other members of the health care team, social service agencies, adult protective care agencies, Meals on Wheels, and other community resources. This is consistent with other research (Ernst & Smith, 2012; Schmeidel, Daly, Rosenbaum, Schmuch, & Jogerst, 2012). Although nurses were adept at identifying interdisciplinary resources, employing these resources was not without problems. Some nurses reported communities with excellent resources for elderly clients, although long waiting lists for those programs presented barriers to utilization. Nurses also targeted the lack of health care practitioners to address issues such as self-neglect as a barrier. Studies by the Institute of Medicine (IOM; 2012) corroborate these complaints from nurses, citing few professionals as choosing to specialize in gerontology, and many professionals choosing to "let their credentials in geriatric specialties lapse" (p. 27). The IOM (2012) termed the growing elderly population a "Silver Tsunami" (p. 1) and warned that the current health care workforce is not adequate to address the mental health needs of this population. Nurses in the present study echoed the findings of the IOM (2012), identifying the paucity of education on self-neglect for the health care industry in general, and for nurses in specific, as barriers to self-neglect intervention.

Interdisciplinary access was another barrier evident in this research and extends findings from the U.S. Department of Health and Human Services, Agency for Healthcare Research and Quality (AHRQ; 2013), which cited "poor patient-provider communication" (p. 1). Nurses revealed problematic communication among disciplines when they communicated only through patient records. The ability to convey what the nurse perceives as the client's reality through the written word may be muted. Thus, the problem as perceived by the nurse is not shared as intended with other practitioners. This effectively prepares the other practitioners to enter the patient setting with a skewed picture a priori, and this misunderstanding may interfere with timely and/or effective intervention. In addition to communication barriers within the home health agency, nurse participants identified barriers when communicating with the physician in charge of the client's care. Nurses reported rarely, if ever, getting to speak directly to the physician. If the person taking the message has no experience with self-neglect, he or she may not receive the message as the nurse intended it. In addition, most physicians do not make home visits and therefore may not truly understand the situation of the home.

Although nursing practice is grounded in the ethical treatment of clients (American Nurses Association, 2001), nurses stated that these ethical principles sometimes present barriers to self-neglect intervention. The nursing profession is strongly supportive of client autonomy (Day, Mulcahy, Leahy-Warren, & Downey, 2015; Mauk,

2011) although situations deemed unsafe often caused nurses to question whether intervention should take priority over patient autonomy. Questions of autonomy versus beneficence arose when nurse participants questioned whether they had the right to make choices for these clients when there was no obvious physical impairment, no diagnosed psychiatric or cognitive impairment, and no finding of legal incompetence by APS personnel.

Elder self-neglect presents a conundrum for nurses. In fact, this may extend to disciplines other than nursing as noted by the Agency for Healthcare Research and Quality (2013), which found that health care in the United States is sometimes delivered "without full consideration of a patient's preferences or values" (p. 1). However, it is important for nurses to recognize the role of culture in patient choice (Gibbons, 2007; Lauder, 1999b) and to rigorously seek to protect client choice to every extent possible (Day et al., 2015; Day, Leahy-Warren, & McCarthy, 2016; Gibbons, 2007; Lauder, 1999b; Mauk, 2011). Future research is needed to explore the influence of culture on behaviors in elders who self-neglect.

Elder self-neglect has been proposed as a geriatric syndrome (Pavlou & Lachs, 2006). Indeed, self-neglect is complex and encompasses many behaviors. Lauder (1999b) cautioned against labeling self-neglect as a medical syndrome because the salient features of self-neglect are failure to attend to personal "cleanliness and hygiene" (p. 63) and these are areas open to scrutiny based on cultural values. This study identified self-neglecters as perceiving their behaviors as "normal," which implies a moral judgment of others that these behaviors are not normal. The diversity of constructions of self-neglect in the health care industry may contribute to the lack of understanding of this phenomenon.

LIMITATIONS

The limitations of this study are recognized and are inherent in the sample plan. Convenience sampling provided participants who had experience with self-neglect. In addition, these data were collected in one southeastern state in the United States.

CONCLUSION

This is the first study of self-neglect focused solely on the perceptions of U.S. home health nurses. This is important because home health nurses may be the key individuals to identify self-neglect because they see these clients in their natural environments. Self-neglect may not be evident when these individuals are seen in the physician's office or the hospital. A full understanding of self-neglect continues to elude the health care community. It is only through comprehensively approaching the study of a phenomenon that it can be fully explained. Because home health nurses interact with clients in their natural environments, these nurses are the key to the study of this phenomenon. RNs are professionals who take their jobs very seriously and are dedicated to providing care for their clients. Yet, they are ill equipped to provide this care based on a lack of available information on self-neglect. The key to correcting this situation lies in more research on this poorly understood topic, more education for health care personnel, and more attention to the care of these vulnerable elders. Several studies on self-neglect have been conducted; yet, the voices of home health nurses have remained silent in this research until now.

IMPLICATIONS FOR RESEARCH AND PRACTICE

- Interprofessional education on self-neglect is needed in schools of nursing.
- Increased screening for depression and cognitive issues is warranted.
- Implementation of self-neglect screening tools is vital.
- More nursing research on self-neglect is crucial.
- Comparison studies of nurses and their clients' perspectives may prove illuminating.
- Research to identify antecedents to self-neglect may inform a trajectory for self-neglect.

REFERENCES

Abrams, R. C., Lachs, M., McAvay, G., Keohane, D. J., & Bruce, M. L. (2002). Predictors of self-neglect in community dwelling elders. *American Journal of Psychiatry, 159*(10), 1724–1730.

Adams, J., & Johnson, J. (1998). Nurses' perceptions of gross self-neglect amongst older people living in the community. *Journal of Clinical Nursing, 7,* 547–552.

Alzheimer's Association. (2014). *Aggression and anger.* Alzheimer's and Dementia Caregiver Center. Retrieved from http://www.alz.org/care/alzheimers-dementia-aggression-anger.asp#causes

American Nurses Association. (2001). *Code of ethics for nurses with interpretive statements.* Retrieved from http://nursingworld.org/MainMenuCategories/EthicsStandards/CodeofEthicsforNurses/Code-of-Ethics.pdf

Ballard, J. (2010). Legal implications regarding self-neglecting community-dwelling adults: A practical approach for the community nurse in Ireland. *Public Health Nursing, 29*(2), 181–187. doi:10.111//j.1525-1446.2010.00840.x

Berry, S., Quach, L., Proctor-Gray, E., Kiel, D., Li, W., Samelson, E., . . . Kelsey, J. (2010). Poor adherence to medications may be associated with falls. *Journal of Gerontology: Medical Sciences, 65A*(5), 553–558.

Bozinovski, S. (2000). Older self-neglecters: Interpersonal problems and the maintenance of self-continuity. *Journal of Elder Abuse & Neglect, 12*(1), 37–56.

Braye, S., Orr, D., & Preston-Shoot, M. (2011). Conceptualising and responding to self-neglect: The challenges for adult safeguarding. *Journal of Adult Protection, 13*(4), 182–183. doi:10.1008/14668201111177905

Burnett, J., Coverdale, J. H., Pickens, S., & Dyer, C. B. (2006). What is the association between self-neglect, depressive symptoms and untreated medical conditions? *Journal of Elder Abuse & Neglect, 18*(4), 25–34.

Burnett, J., Regev, T., Pickens, S., Prati, L. L., Aung, K., Moore, J., & Dyer, C. (2006). Social networks: A profile of the elderly who self-neglect. *Journal of Elder Abuse & Neglect, 18*(4), 35–49.

Centers for Medicare & Medicaid Services. (2012). Outcome and assessment information set (OASIS). Retrieved from https://www.cms.gov/Medicare/Quality-Initiatives-Patient-Assessment-Instruments/OASIS/index.html

Clark, A., Mankikar, G., & Gray, I. (1975). Diogenes syndrome: A clinical study of gross neglect in old age. *Lancet, 305*(7903), 366–368.

Culberson, J., Ticker, R., Burnett, J., Marcus, M., Pickens, S., & Dyer, C. (2011). Prescription medication use among self-neglecting elderly. *Journal of Addictions Nursing, 22,* 63–68. doi:10.3109/1088 4602.2010.545089

Day, M. R., Leahy-Warren, P., & McCarthy, G. (2016). Self-neglect: Ethical considerations. *Annual Review of Nursing Research, 34*(1), 89–107.

Day, M. R., Mulcahy, H., Leahy-Warren, P., & Downey, J. (2015). Self-neglect: A case study and implications for clinical practice. *British Journal of Community Nursing, 20*(2), 585–590.

Dick, S. (2006). Self-neglect: Diogenes syndrome and dementia. *Kansas Nurse, 81*(9), 12–13.

Dong, X., Simon, M., Beck, T., & Evans, D. (2010). A cross-sectional population-based study of elder self-neglect and psychological, health, and social factors in a biracial community. *Aging & Mental Health, 14*(1), 74–84.

Dong, X., Wilson, R., Mendes de Leon, C., & Evans, D. (2009). Self-neglect and cognitive function among community-dwelling older persons. *International Journal of Geriatric Psychiatry, 25,* 798–806.

Dyer, C., Kelly, P., Pavlik, V., Lee, J., Doody, R., Regev, T., . . . Smith, S. (2006). The making of a self-neglect severity scale. *Journal of Elder Abuse & Neglect, 18*(4), 13–23. doi:10.1300/J084v18n04_03

Dyer, C. B., Goodwin, J. S., Pickens-Pace, S., Burnett, J., & Kelly, P. A. (2007). Self-neglect among the elderly: A model based on more than 500 patients seen by a geriatric medicine team. *American Journal of Public Health, 97*(9), 1671–1676.

Ernst, J., & Smith, C. (2012). Assessment in adult protective services: Do multidisciplinary teams make a difference? *Journal of Gerontological Social Work, 55,* 21–38. doi:10:1080/01634372.2011.626842

Federal Interagency Forum on Aging-Related Statistics. (2012, June). *Older Americans 2012: Key indicators of well-being.* Federal Interagency Forum on Aging-Related Statistics. Washington, DC: U.S. Government Printing Office.

Gentil, L., Vasiliadis, H., Preville, M., Bosse, C., & Berbiche, D. (2012). Association between depressive and anxiety disorders and adherence to antihypertensive medication in community-living elderly adults. *Journal of the American Geriatrics Society, 60*(12), 2297–2301.

Gibbons, S. (2007). *Characteristics and behaviors of self-neglect among community-dwelling older adults* (Doctoral dissertation). Retrieved from ProQuest UMI. (3246949)

Gibbons, S. (2009). Theory synthesis for self-neglect: A health and social phenomenon. *Nursing Research, 58*(3), 194–200.

Gibbons, S., Lauder, W., & Ludwick, R. (2006). Self-neglect: A proposed new NANDA diagnosis. *International Journal of Nursing Terminologies and Classifications, 17*(1), 10–18.

Glass, T., Mendes De Leon, C., Bassuk, S., & Berkman, L. (2006). Social engagement and depressive symptoms in late life: Longitudinal findings. *Journal of Aging and Health, 18*(4), 604–628.

Henriques, M., Costa, M., & Cabrita, J. (2012). Adherence and medication management by the elderly. *Journal of Clinical Nursing, 21,* 3096–3105. doi:10/1111/j.1365-2702.2012.04144.x

Institute of Medicine. (2012). *The mental health and substance use workforce for older adults: In whose hands?* Washington, DC: National Academies Press. Retrieved from http://www.nap.edu/download.php?record_id=13400

Iris, M., Ridings, J., & Conrad, K. (2009). The development of a conceptual model for understanding self-neglect. *The Gerontologist, 50*(3), 303–315.

Johnson, Y. (2014). *Nurse perceptions of elder self-neglect* (Doctoral dissertation). Available from ProQuest Dissertations and Theses database. (UMI No. 3624201)

Kelly, P., Dyer, C., Pavlik, V., Doody, R., & Jogerst, G. (2008). Exploring self-neglect in older adults: Preliminary findings of the self-neglect severity scale and next steps. *Journal of the American Geriatrics Society, 56,* S253–S260.

Lauder, W. (1999a). Constructions of self-neglect: A multiple case study design. *Nursing Inquiry, 6,* 48–57.

Lauder, W. (1999b). The medical model and other constructions of self-neglect. *International Journal of Nursing Practice, 5,* 58–63.

Lauder, W. (2001). The utility of self-care theory as a theoretical basis for self-neglect. *Journal of Advanced Nursing, 34*(4), 545–551.

Lauder, W., Anderson, I., & Barclay, A. (2005). Housing and self-neglect: The responses of health, social care and environmental health agencies. *Journal of Interprofessional Care, 19*(4), 317–325.

Lauder, W., Ludwick, R., Zeller, R., & Winchell, J. (2006). Factors influencing nurses judgments about self-neglect cases. *Journal of Psychiatric & Mental Health Nursing, 13,* 279–287.

Lincoln, Y., & Guba, E. (1985). *Naturalistic inquiry.* Newberry Park, CA: Sage.

Macmillan, D., & Shaw, P. (1966). Senile breakdown in standards of personal and environmental cleanliness. *British Medical Journal, 2,* 1032–1037.

Mauk, K. (2011). Ethical perspectives on self-neglect among older adults. *Rehabilitation Nursing, 36*(2), 60–65.

National Center on Elder Abuse. (1998). *National elder abuse incidence study.* Retrieved from https://www.acl.gov/sites/default/files/programs/2016-09/ABuseReport_Full.pdf

National Committee for the Prevention of Elder Abuse. (2008). *Symposium on self-neglect: Building a coordinated response.* Retrieved from http://www.google.com/url?sa=t&rct=j&q=&esrc=s&source=web&cd=1&ved=0ahUKEwi2uOS6_tLMAhXB6iYKHQ47AfIQFggcMAA&url=http%3A%2F%2Fwww.preventelderabuse.org%2Fnew%2FReportontheNCPEASelf-NeglectSymposium.doc&usg=AFQjCNE5lPADY0OWsDKHkZOFCBtkl7ehlw&bvm=bv.121658157,d.eWE

National League for Nursing. (2013). About the NLN. Retrieved from http://www.nln.org/about/core-values

Paveza, G., VandeWeerd, C., & Laumann, E. (2008). Elder self-neglect: A discussion of a social typology. *Journal of the American Geriatrics Society, 56,* S271–S275. doi:10.1111/j.1532-5415.2008.01980.x

Pavlou, M., & Lachs, M. (2006). Could self-neglect in older adults be a geriatric syndrome? *Journal of the American Geriatrics Society, 54*(5), 831–842.

Payne, B., & Gainey, R. (2005). Differentiating self-neglect as a type of elder mistreatment: How do these cases compare to traditional types of elder mistreatment? *Journal of Elder Abuse & Neglect, 17*(1), 21–36.

Poythress, E., Burnett, J., Naik, A., Pickens, S., & Dyer, C. (2006). Severe self-neglect: An epidemiological and historical perspective. *Journal of Elder Abuse & Neglect, 18*(4), 5–12. doi:10.1300/J084v18n04_02

Ristau, S. (2011). People do need people: Social interaction boosts brain health in older age. *Generations, 35*(2), 70–76.

Sandelowski, M. (1986). The problem of rigor in qualitative research. *Advances in Nursing Science, 8*(3), 27–37.

Schmeidel, A., Daly, J., Rosenbaum, M., Schmuch, G., & Jogerst, G. (2012). Health care professionals' perspectives on barriers to elder abuse detection and reporting in primary care settings. *Journal of Elder Abuse & Neglect, 24*(1), 17–36.

Tierney, M., Charles, J., Naglie, G., Jaglal, S., Kiss, A., & Fisher, R. (2004). Risk factors for harm in cognitively impaired seniors who live alone: A prospective study. *Journal of the American Geriatrics Society, 52,* 1435–1441.

U.S. Census Bureau. (2014). *An aging nation: The older population in the United States: Population estimates and projections.* Retrieved from http://www.census.gov/prod/2014pubs/p25-1140.pdf

U.S. Department of Health and Human Services, Agency for Healthcare Research and Quality. (2013). *2012 national healthcare disparities report* (AHRQ Publication No. 13-0003). Retrieved from https://archive.ahrq.gov/research/findings/nhqrdr/nhdr12/index.html

U.S. Department of Labor, Bureau of Labor Statistics. (2013). Labor force statistics from the current population survey. Retrieved from http://www.bls.gov/cps

Yesavage, J., Brink, T., Rose, T., Lum, O., Huang, V., Adey, M., & Leirer, V. (1983). Development and validation of a geriatric depression screening scale: A preliminary report. *Journal of Psychiatric Research, 17,* 37–49.

CHAPTER 13

HEALTH AND SOCIAL CARE PROFESSIONALS' PERSPECTIVES OF SELF-NEGLECT

Helen Mulcahy, Patricia Leahy-Warren, and Mary Rose Day

Self-neglect is a serious public health issue that is under-reported and largely hidden. Self-neglect results in cumulative self-care deficits and behaviors, which may include environmental squalor and hoarding. It is more common in older people and in aging populations. As a result, the risk and prevalence of self-neglect will increase in the community. Health and social care professionals, such as community/public health nurses and social workers, are in daily contact with people who self-neglect.

This chapter reports on qualitative findings that explored perceptions of Irish community nurses, public health nurses, and social workers (n = 87) on the phenomenon of self-neglect. Qualitative data were analyzed using the framework method involving a seven-stage process. Findings revealed one overarching theme—fine balance—and four subthemes: complexity of self-neglect, personal response to self-neglect, challenges in managing the case, and recommendations for practice.

The empirical literature on self-neglect suggests it is a global public health issue that is largely hidden and under-reported (Dong, Simon, Mosqueda, & Evans, 2012). The concept of self-neglect is socially, culturally, psychologically, medically, and legally constructed. Self-neglect can present on a continuum of severity and be related to behavioral issues, for example, not taking medication, or living in conditions of squalor where accommodation and environment are extremely neglected (Iris, Ridings, & Conrad, 2010). Environmental factors constitute a major dimension in self-neglect (Day & McCarthy, 2016; Day, Mulcahy, & Leahy-Warren, 2016; Iris, Conrad, & Ridings, 2014; Iris et al., 2010). In Ireland nurses working in the community come from a range of disciplines such as community registered general nurses (CRGNs), public health nurses (PHNs) and community mental health nurses (CMHNs). All nurses' and social care practitioners' work brings them into contact with people who self-neglect (Day, Mulcahy, Leahy-Warren, & Downey, 2015; Doron, Band-Winterstein, & Naim, 2013).

Governance structures need to support effective multidisciplinary working, relationship-centered practice, and collaboration and sharing of information between health and social care professionals across all agencies. Professionals need to have a sound knowledge base on safeguarding vulnerable adults and clear, comprehensive, procedural guidelines (Braye, Orr, & Preston-Shoot, 2015). Perceptions, experiences, and values can influence judgments, decision-making practices, and responses to self-neglect (Bohl, 2010; Gunstone, 2003).

BACKGROUND LITERATURE

A range of research has been conducted with health and social care professionals that has explored characteristics of elder self-neglect (Dyer et al., 2006), judgments and understanding of self-neglect (Lauder, Davidson, Anderson, & Barclay, 2005; Lauder, Ludwick, Zeller, & Winchell, 2006; McDermott, 2008, 2010), perspectives and experiences of self-neglect (Bohl, 2010; Day, McCarthy, & Leahy-Warren, 2012; Dulick, 2010; Gunstone, 2003; Johnson, 2015b), meaning attributed to elder self-neglect (Doron et al., 2013), responding to self-neglect (Lauder, Anderson, & Barclay, 2005), outcomes of self-neglect practice (Braye, Orr, & Preston-Shoot, 2014), and knowledge of self-neglect (Day & McCarthy, 2015; Dulick, 2010).

Health and social care professionals have identified the characteristics of self-neglect as deficiencies in environment, personal hygiene, and cognition (Dyer et al., 2006); poor nutrition; dehydration; falls; noncompliance with medical treatment and medication; visible skin sores (McDermott, 2008; and nonconformity with self-care (Johnson, 2015a, 2015b). Furthermore, it is associated with aspects of elder abuse and neglect (Bartley, Knight, O'Neill, & O'Brien, 2011; Doran et al., 2013).

In Australia, self-neglect is differentiated from squalor in that health professionals are responsible for self-neglect, which is viewed as personal neglect of self, whereas social care workers and community organizations are responsible for environmental squalor situations (McDermott, 2008, 2010). Research with atypical cases of self-neglect by Lauder, Roxburg, Harris, and Law (2009), found that some people who lived in squalor could be fastidious about personal hygiene.

There is no gold standard definition of self-neglect or extreme self-neglect (Day et al., 2012; Gunstone, 2003). This has led to considerable difficulties in practice and research. Comorbidities associated with self-neglect include dementia, depression, delirium, self-harm, psychosis, stroke, alcohol and substance abuse, and reduced physical function (McDermott, 2008, 2010). The ability of the person to cope and meet complex comorbidities and health and social care needs may be a factor (Gibbons, 2009). However, the meaning of self-neglect needs to be seen in the context of each individual's life experiences (Band-Winterstein et al., 2012; Braye et al., 2014; Day, Leahy-Warren, & McCarthy, 2013).

Culture, life history, attitudes, values, and beliefs influence both individuals who self-neglect and health and social care practitioners' views and judgment of self-neglect (Braye et al., 2014; Lauder et al., 2006). Some health and social care practitioners may honor the principle of respect for autonomy and self-determinism, whereas others prioritize the principle of duty of care and promotion of dignity (Braye et al., 2011, 2014). Professional judgments can be influenced by individual agencies policy and procedures (McDermott, 2010). In addition, Lauder et al. (2006) identified that household situations and personal hygiene had a minor part in the judgment of self-neglect. The areas of self-neglect described as most challenging related to high-risk situations in which a person had the mental capacity and refused services (Braye et al., 2014), which escalated perceptions of risk (McDermott, 2010). Evidence found that social care workers valued the rights of self-determinism and autonomy of competent adults to refuse services (Bohl, 2010).

Trying to strike a balance between respecting autonomy and fulfilling duty of care raised many ethical issues (Bohl, 2010). Social care workers' practice is governed by ethical and legal issues and has many gray areas (Bohl, 2010) and is associated with feelings of powerlessness (Day et al., 2012), burnout, and isolation

(Doron et al., 2013). Repeated exposure to self-neglect can result in complacency for health care workers (Gunstone, 2003).

Braye et al. (2014) reported that the most challenging elements of self-neglect related to the clients' capacity and/or refusal/reluctance to engage with services. Additional challenges included the level of risk involved in care of this population, responses and service options, safeguarding policy, and staff training. Key elements to effective practice have been identified as relationship-centered care, a multidisciplinary team approach, and staff who are reliable and compassionate (Braye et al., 2014).

Day and McCarthy (2015), Dulick (2010), and Johnson (2015b) reported gaps in knowledge of health and social care workers. Poor clarity around professional role and responsibilities was evident on self-neglect policy and legislation (Day & McCarthy, 2015). Poor or absent training on self-neglect can obstruct effective management and responses (Braye et al., 2014; Day & McCarthy, 2015; Johnson, 2015a, 2015b). It is essential that practitioners are knowledgeable about legal obligations, legislation, and policy in their jurisdiction (Braye et al., 2014; Day & McCarthy, 2015; Health Service Executive [HSE], 2012, 2014). Training and ongoing supervision for the development of a broad range of skills to support self-neglect practice is essential (Braye et al., 2014). No previous research has explored self-neglect using a diverse sample of community health and social care workers that included community nurses and social workers. The aim of this study was to explore perceptions of health and social care workers on self-neglect.

METHODS

Data Collection

Data were collected during 2013 as part of a larger quantitative descriptive cross-sectional study (see Day & McCarthy, 2015, 2016). Ethical approval was obtained from the Clinical Research Ethics Committee of the Cork Teaching Hospitals. A questionnaire was mailed to a sample of 566 health and social care professionals, of whom 87 (PHN, $n = 53$; CRGN, $n = 11$; CMHN, $n = 11$; social worker [SW], $n = 12$) completed the open-ended responses.

Data Analysis

The framework method was chosen for analyzing the cross-sectional descriptive data. Framework analysis addressed the contextual objective (Ritchie & Lewis, 2003; Ritchie & Spencer, 1994) of enhancing an understanding of the diversity of self-neglect perceptions of the health and social care professionals. This involved a seven-stage process: (1) transcription, (2) familiarization with the interview, (3) coding, (4) developing a working analytical framework, (5) applying the analytical framework, (6) charting data into the framework matrix, and (7) interpreting data (Gale, Heath, Cameron, Rashid, & Redwood, 2013). The framework provided a systematic orderly approach for categorizing and thematically analyzing responses. The analysis was undertaken by an experienced qualitative researcher.

The open-question transcription data with participant labels were exported to an Excel spreadsheet for ease of data management and ensuring links with original sources. Following this familiarization, the initial coding was assisted by drawing on

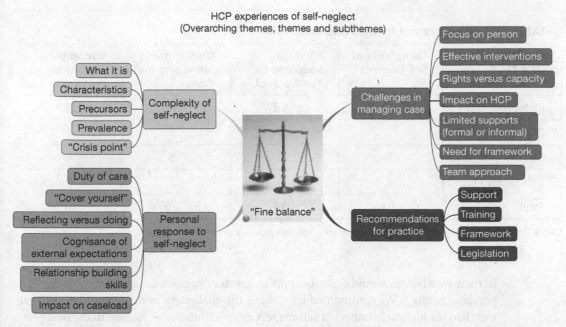

HCP experiences of self-neglect
(Overarching themes, themes and subthemes)

Figure13.1   Mind map diagram illustrates relationships between various themes and categories.

HCP, health care professional.

the a priori questionnaire categories of the person, definitions, challenges in managing case, response, and interventions. The initial indexing of data was primarily descriptive and remained close to these a priori categories. However, as indexing and charting progressed with increasing levels of abstraction and conceptualization, more insightful framework categories, subthemes, and themes emerged (Figure13.1). The analysis was an iterative process enhanced by the depth of participant reflections.

FINDINGS

The majority of the sample was aged 35 to 49 years (56%) and highly experienced, with 61% having 5 to 15 years of clinical experience. In combination, the respondents had involvement in self-neglect cases in the previous year ranging from 0 (17%) to 25 plus (6%), with the median group having three to five cases (33%). Thus, participants were well placed to comment on self-neglect.

Four subthemes emerged from the data: complexity of self-neglect, personal response to self-neglect, challenges in managing the case, and, recommendations for practice. From these themes emerged an overarching theme, which is termed *fine balance* (see Figure 13.1).

As outlined here, the analysis was assisted by a process of charting, which served to organize annotated transcripts. This charting was subjected to successive levels of abstraction until it contained the frequency of themes and was thus useful in terms of comparing theme patterns among different participants (see Table13.1).

As the data analyzed in this chapter were derived from an open question, the charting process illustrates that for all participants, the bulk of commentary relate to the complexity of self-neglect. On a pro-rata basis, it is clear that the complexity of and the personal response to self-neglect provoked the greatest reflection for both PHNs and CRGNs. It is perhaps not surprising that the staff with the most frequent involvement with clients

TABLE 13.1   Frequency of Themes and Patterns

Participants (N = 87)	Complexity of Self-Neglect	Personal Response to Self-Neglect	Challenges in Managing the Case	Recommendations for Practice
PHNs (n = 53)	33	18	14	12
CRGNs (n = 11)	6	9	3	2
CMHNs (n = 12)	6	2	5	4
SWs (n = 11)	6	6	3	6
Total	51	35	25	24

CMHN, community mental health nurse; CRGN, community registered general nurse; PHN, public health nurse; SW, social worker.

in their own homes would describe more or greater experiences, as the response is of a personal nature. SWs commented least about the challenges in managing the case, yet they had the highest numbers of self-neglect cases within their caseload in the past year.

Each of the themes is presented using the participant's own narrative. Participants were anonymized and given the letter codes P for PHNs, C for community CRGNs, M for CMNHs, and S for SWs. A numerical code corresponding to the participant's number is included.

Subthemes

Complexity of Self-Neglect

Participants provided an abundance of descriptions to illustrate their perceptions of the complexity of self-neglect. In particular, they reflected on what they perceived it to be. They described self-neglect as a "catch-all phrase" (S8) and were challenged to distinguish the "world of difference between *self-neglect cases and severe self-neglect*" (S8). More often self-neglect was described in terms of older people and sometimes associated with a "lifestyle choice" (C12) or a person choosing to "live a particular way" (S14). In terms of definitions used, one participant stated that "socially and culturally acceptable standards did not feature" and that they "work more on the ground of (a person's) ability or willingness to avail of services to live safely" (S16). There was also a suggestion that it was a "socially constructed issue" rather than a medical one (S28). Self-neglect was considered difficult to label and classify and described as "complex" (M63) or "borderline" (P69). Furthermore, health and social care professionals were cautioned to be "cognizant of imposing (their own) standards" (P67).

Participant comments are generally indicative of the prevalence of self-neglect, although it may not have been expressed specifically. One participant stated that it is in the nature of community practice to "come into contact with many clients who are self-neglectful" (P22). The extent was variously described as "a huge issue" (P30), "on the increase" (P57), or "becoming more common" (P52), whereas one participant said she "did not come across too many cases" (M35). It was suggested that "statistics need to be accumulated from each area/division to determine the extent of the problem" (M33). The seriousness regarding the extent of self-neglect was borne out by a comment that it accounts for "one case a year of a death" (P11) in her area.

In terms of characteristics of self-neglect one participant described it as "apathy and apparent inability to cope" (C1). Whereas a broader perspective was taken by another participant who described it "as every aspect of [an] individual's life that may not be deemed as safe, or satisfactory . . . as they all constitute the manifestation of self-neglect" (P2). It was also seen as "a symptom of mental health and personal living conditions" (P7). One characteristic related to "single unmarried older men" who "will not spend money on themselves even though they have plenty of it" (P31). Whereas another suggested that "mostly they are women who lived very independent lives, often are childless or widowed/or single and are used to coping alone. When cognitive functioning is impaired this often has a detrimental impact on their coping" (M43). However, there was also caution that "each client has individual characteristics and it is difficult to generalize" (C36). The specific characteristics described are isolation; lack of insight; risky behaviors; vulnerability; poor standards of hygiene, both in the house and general environment as well as personal hygiene and appearance.

Precursors described the underlying factors, which were considered to be "poor emotional well-being and instability" (C1), "depression, which is largely underdiagnosed and often easily treated" (P10), "mental health problems or alcohol abuse (where) the family have pulled away" (P11). One participant suggested the there was no consideration of "Asperger's syndrome or undiagnosed intellectual challenges that can seriously hamper a person's ability to cope—often undiagnosed in an adult population in Ireland" (S14).

In terms of crisis point as a theme, participants described cases that "could bubble along for years" (P3). This point was often perceived to "snowball" in a "very short amount of time" (S4), obviously requiring a response from the professional involved.

Personal Response to Self-Neglect

Personal response to self-neglect captures the personal challenges that participants' experienced from reflections of working with particular individual clients. A number of participants described feeling "a duty of care to self-neglecting clients" (C36) or "feeling responsible for them as they are under our care" (P54). This caused great concern and one participant stated that "the area PHN carries a responsibility to this client and is unable to close the case as other disciplines can" (P67). Another participant described the need to "cover yourself" by making reports to SWs (P3). There were implications that a case could deteriorate to the extent that there would be legal ramifications or some sort of media attention.

Self-neglect was described as having an impact on caseload "I find this (self-neglect) aspect of my caseload challenging . . . if the client is deemed to have capacity there is little to be done" (P67). There was also the personal impact of a case in that it "causes a lot of worry for staff" (C65) or makes the "job . . . extremely difficult and stressful" (P15). Participants were personally challenged in reflecting versus doing, which was a theme found to describe instances in which there was personal conflict in relation to how to proceed: "How far can or should the health professionals go in assisting the client and when can they say they did all they could?" (C20). The following quote from a participant reflects his/her personal struggle "self-determination, empowerment, participation, fulfillment, and independence of the client needs to be pivotal, even if individual professionals and services struggle with their fears and accountability, which can lead to, or risk eroding the rights, fundamental freedom and entitlements of service users" (S14). At the core of many narratives was a cognizance of external expectations. Participants had a perception that others wanted them to intervene, but this was not always considered the best course of action as articulated here:

> Self-neglect is a very challenging area to deal with . . . others such as family and neighbors expect us to be able to have a positive impact on "helping" the person change and live within their understanding of the "norm." Other health professionals are inclined to pass their concerns on to the PHN for "divine intervention." (P18)

Participants spoke about the importance of building relationships as: "The importance of relationship building over time cannot be underestimated" (P6). Furthermore, professional/client relations were seen as a key to managing self-neglect: "building up and maintaining trusting relationships and seeking consent and permission to make changes in their lives" (S8).

Challenges in Managing the Case

This theme differed from the previous in that here there was a focus on the person. One participant stated that "All . . . need to take cognizance of the sensitivities, complexities, resistances, and strengths of the older person including a measure of happiness" (S14). It is clear that participants had a real affinity with their clients: "sometimes I think nobody cares or has any concern about these people" (M50).

The elements of effective interventions were described as:

> in many instances appropriate interventions can greatly enhance self-care and reduce risk—however, this is not a tick box job—starting where the person is at, to try to establish what small thing can initiate small change with the view to forming an alliance with the person to address the issues. A supported team work approach is essential. The language we use needs to respect differences and seek understanding. (M25)

However, one participant observed that there are challenges in balancing rights versus capacity and stated:

> There seems to be a major obstacle around consent and capacity where a patient's behavior impacts on their wellbeing but no intervention can be pursued. In one case of ours, an involuntary admission took place but was revoked by the commission on Mental Health. This patient continues to live in terrible conditions, self-neglecting, malnourished. (P27)

Challenges exist in managing cases in order to achieve positive outcomes:

> It is usually at this point (crisis) that efforts are made to intervene and "improve" the older person's situation. It is important to note that our interventions are not always seen or experienced by the older person as positive. Self-neglect is an area that poses huge challenges for frontline staff. (P80)

Further challenges articulated were limited supports, both formal and informal. From the initial assessment, the presence or absence of family in the form of informal supports is important. All too often, family ties were described as lost and as a consequence "Family members estranged from individuals who self-neglect and do not feature much in self-neglect cases" (P37). However, the value in terms of effective interventions was well recognized with one participant stating that "Forging links with neighbor/family key members is vital to making any difference in these cases (if available)" (C61).

In terms of formal supports, SWs were mentioned numerous times as valuable assets in managing self-neglecting clients. The unavailability of this professional group within the multidisciplinary team was considered a major deficiency. Psychiatric services came in for criticism with one participant, albeit from within that service, stating the services were "not very helpful in supporting these clients, and are quick to discharge them from their services" (M50).

Participants expressed a need for a framework to guide interventions: "I would welcome a framework to complement and underpin care plans for self-neglect" (P6) and the strongly held belief that a team approach was vital to success. One participant succinctly outlined the approach used by her in collaboration with the multidisciplinary team:

> I would aim to build up a rapport/trust with the client. Once the client has agreed I would link with other team members, e.g., GP [general practitioner], Community Psychiatric Nurse, Social Worker, Psychiatrist, Saint Vincent De Paul [nongovernmental organizations], Physiotherapy, Occupational Therapy, corporation [Housing agencies] etc., and use a team approach. I feel the priority at initial assessment is to assess mental/cognitive status of the individual and identify immediate hazards/safety issues. If client's cognitive status is deemed by the GP/Psychiatrist as okay then the other issues, e.g., clothing, hygiene, medications, housing, food etc. can be addressed at the clients [*sic*] pace. (M40)

This approach demonstrated a very pragmatic yet sensitive approach to managing a case. A number of participants highlighted that teams and thus their effectiveness were limited by the unavailability or lack of input from mental health services.

Recommendations for Practice

Many recommendations for practice were described. These included support, training, need for a framework, and legislation. Participants were concerned about the lack of support for professionals dealing with clients and recommended that support as the key for practice. Not only is line managerial support vital but the role of the "social worker for protection of older people is much valued in supporting the PHNs team" (P2). Recommendations also related to better integration as "supporting services can be disjointed with poor communication with secondary services" (C20) especially in relation to a lack of "feedback from referrals" (P57).

Many participants expressed a need for training: "particularly hoarding behavior and its management" (P84). This tied in very clearly with an expressed need "for an assessment tool and guidelines to support nursing staff" (P6). Participants were regularly faced with "deciding where the responsibility lie [*sic*] . . . the impact of the cognitive ability of the client . . . and legal standing?" (C20). Another perceived that practice challenges were compounded by a "lack of legislation to ensure older persons who cannot care for themselves/lack capacity to make decisions regarding their daily care" (S19). This clearly was a matter of concern for staff who worried about the welfare of clients.

Fine Balance

For each of the four themes presented previously, an overall theme of "fine balance" was identified. In the theme "complexity of self-neglect," participants suggested there was a borderline between a life choice and a definitive pathology. The analysis of data revealed an overarching theme of "fine balance" to describe the perceptions of participants. One participant observed that "it is a fine balance between respecting the right to self-neglect and determining capacity of the client to decide same" (P6). In terms of personal response to self-neglect, there was a conflict between duty of care and covering one's self. Whereas the principle of self-determinism versus capacity and person-centeredness versus box ticking were features described in the theme—challenges in managing the case. Ultimately, however, the recommendations for practice indicated the desire to mobilize the supports necessary to assist the person in the context of an unusually large multidisciplinary input.

DISCUSSION

From this study, it is evident that health and social care professionals are grappling with the phenomenon of self-neglect in the community. Participants described and articulated key characteristics and precursors of self-neglect; however, professionals were challenged to define and classify self-neglect, which may be compounded by the lack of a self-neglect assessment instrument. Subjectivity and absence of valid and reliable assessment criteria can result in missed opportunities to reduce the negative health outcomes associated with self-neglect (Burnett et al., 2012).

Cognitive impairment and mental health issues are present in people who self-neglect (Dong & Simon, 2015). Coping with everyday life, multiple comorbidities, impaired physical function, and cognition have been linked to self-neglect (Gibbons, 2009; Hildebrand, Taylor, & Bradway, 2014). Failure of self-neglecting adults to spend money on maintaining their environment was seen as a factor by participants.

In responding to self-neglect cases, participants in this research were trying to balance their personal responses around duty of care, moral obligation, and external expectations. Although Braye et al. (2011, 2014) found duty of care and promotion of dignity to be prioritized by some community professionals and Doran et al. (2013) found burnout of staff, this study further demonstrates the moral stress associated with self-neglect for health and social care professionals. Participants strive to balance the fine line between respecting and understanding the person, self-determinism and capacity, health and safety, and duty of care. This concurs with Doron et al.'s (2013) and Day et al.'s (2012) findings that significant ethical, personal, and professional challenges are associated with self-neglect cases. The challenges in managing self-neglect cases begin with knowing the individual, his or her life experiences, and strengths as articulated by participants in this study. Similar challenges were identified by Doran et al. (2013), Day et al. (2013), and Braye et al. (2014). However, this study further illustrates the importance of shared risk taking, multidisciplinary teamwork, and person-centered responses in managing self-neglect cases. However, the unavailability or lack of input from mental health professionals and services were limitations of this study.

Setting goals with clients to engage in formal and informal supports, including working with families, neighbors, and communities, is paramount. In this study, participants articulated the need for further training and education in regard to self-neglect, hoarding, and legislation, similar to findings from previous research (Braye et al., 2014; Johnson, 2015b). In Ireland, self-neglect holds an ambivalent position in that exceptional cases are recognized for referral in relation to Safeguarding Vulnerable Adult Policy (HSE, 2012, 2014), whereas other less severe cases are overlooked. At the time of this writing, a *Practitioners Handbook* is in development, Safeguarding Vulnerable Adult Policy is being reviewed, and legislation on assisted decision-making capacity (Department of Justice, Equality & Law Reform, 2015) is being operationalized.

CONCLUSION

Health and social care professionals in this study clearly identified the fine balance that self-neglect work presented to them. The challenges were personal and professional, but participants were able to articulate effective solutions in dealing with the challenges. These include knowing and understanding the client, fostering relationship-building skills, using a multidisciplinary team approach, clinical supervision, and training.

IMPLICATIONS FOR RESEARCH AND PRACTICE

- Self-neglect is a complex and multidimensional phenomenon that requires multidisciplinary staff training, including use of an objective measure of self-neglect.
- Supervision and support for all members of the multidisciplinary team dealing with self-neglect are vital.
- Case studies and serious cases reviews can provide opportunities for problem-based learning and shared decision making.
- Research is required to examine moral distress and to practice wisdom of self-neglect.

REFERENCES

Band-Winterstein, T., Doron, I. I., & Naim, S. (2012). Elder self-neglect: A geriatric syndrome or a life course story? *Journal of Aging Studies, 26*(2), 109–118.

Bartley, M., Knight, P. V., O'Neill, D., & O'Brien, J. G. (2011). Self-neglect and elder abuse: Related phenomena? *Journal of the American Geriatrics Society, 59*(11), 2163–2168.

Bohl, W. B. (2010). *Investigating elder self-neglect: Interviews with adult protective service workers.* Columbus: The Ohio State University.

Braye, S., Orr, D., & Preston-Shoot, M. (2011). Conceptualizing and responding to self-neglect: The challenges for adult safeguarding. *Journal of Adult Protection, 13*(4), 182–193.

Braye, S., Orr, D., & Preston-Shoot, M. (2014). *Self-neglect policy and practice: Building an evidence base for adult social care.* London, UK: Social Care Institute for Excellence.

Braye, S., Orr, D., & Preston-Shoot, M. (2015).Serious case review findings on the challenges of self-neglect: Indicators for good practice. *Journal of Adult Protection, 17*(2), 75–87.

Burnett, J., Achenbaum, W. A., Hayes, L., Flores, D. V., Hochschild, A. E., Kao, D., . . . Dyer, C. B. (2012). Increasing surveillance and prevention efforts for elder self-neglect in clinical settings. *Aging Health, 8*(6), 647–655. doi:10.2217/ahe.12.67

Day, M. R., Leahy-Warren, P., & McCarthy, G. (2013). Perceptions and views of self-neglect: A client-centered perspective. *Journal of Elder Abuse & Neglect, 25*(1), 76–94.

Day, M. R., & McCarthy, G. (2015). A national cross-sectional study of community nurses and social workers knowledge of self-neglect. *Age and Ageing, 44*(4), 717–720. doi:10.1093/ageing/afv025

Day, M. R., & McCarthy, G. (2016). Self-neglect: Development and evaluation of a self-neglect (SN-37) measurement instrument. *Archives of Psychiatric Nursing, 30*(4), 480–485. doi:10.1016/j.apnu.2016.02.004

Day, M. R., McCarthy, G., & Leahy-Warren, P. (2012). Professional social workers views on self-neglect: An exploratory study. *British Journal of Social Work, 42*(4), 717–720. doi:10.1093/bjsw/bcr082

Day, M. R., Mulcahy, H., & Leahy-Warren, P. (2016). Prevalence of self-neglect on public health nurses caseloads. *British Journal of Community Nursing, 21*(1), 31–35.

Day, M. R., Mulcahy, H., Leahy-Warren, P., & Downey, J. (2015). Self-neglect: A case study and implications for clinical practice. *British Journal of Community Nursing, 20*(3), 110–115. doi:10.12968/bjcn.2015.20.3.110

Department of Justice, Equality & Law Reform. (2015). *Assisted Decision-Making (Capacity) Act.* Dublin, Ireland: House of the Oireachtas.

Dong, X., & Simon, M. (2015). Prevalence of elder self-neglect in a Chicago Chinese population: The role of cognitive physical and mental health. *Geriatrics & Gerontology International, 16*(9), 1051–1062. doi:10.1111/ggi.12598

Dong, X., Simon, M. A., Mosqueda, L., & Evans, D. A. (2012). The prevalence of elder self-neglect in a community-dwelling population: Hoarding, hygiene and environmental hazards. *Journal of Aging and Health, 24*(3), 507–524.

Doron, I. I., Band-Winterstein, T., & Naim, S. (2013). The meaning of elder self-neglect: Social workers' perspective. *International Journal of Aging and Human Development, 77*(1), 17–36. doi:10.2190/AG.77.1.b

Dulick, K. C. (2010). *Self-neglect among the elderly: Knowledge and perceptions of MSW students* (Unpublished master's thesis). Department of Social Work, California State University, Long Beach, CA.

Dyer, C. B., Toronjo, C., Cunningham, M., Festa, N. A., Pavlik, V. N., Hyman, D. J., . . . Searle, N. S. (2006). The key elements of elder neglect: A survey of adult protective service workers. *Journal of Elder Abuse & Neglect, 17*(4), 1–10.

Gale, N. K., Heath, G., Cameron, E., Rashid, S., & Redwood, S. (2013). Using the framework method for the analysis of qualitative data in multi-disciplinary health research. *BMC Medical Research Methodology, 13*, 117. doi:10.1186/1471-2288-13-117

Gibbons, S. W. (2009). Theory synthesis for self-neglect: A health and social phenomenon. *Nursing Research, 58*(3), 194–200.

Gunstone, S. (2003). Risk assessment and management of patients who self-neglect: A "grey area" for mental health workers. *Journal of Psychiatric and Mental Health Nursing, 10*(3), 287–296.

Health Service Executive. (2012). *HSE policy and procedures for responding to allegations of extreme self-neglect.* Kildare, Ireland: Author. Retrieved from http://bit.ly/1SPIbxA

Health Service Executive. (2014). *Safeguarding vulnerable persons at risk of abuse: National policy and procedures.* Dublin, Ireland: HSE, Social Care Division.

Hildebrand, C., Taylor, M., & Bradway, C. (2014). Elder self-neglect: The failure of coping because of cognitive and functional impairments. *Journal of the American Association of Nurse Practitioners, 26*(8), 452–462. doi:10.1002/2327-6924.12045

Iris, M., Conrad, K. J., & Ridings, J. (2014). Observational measure of elder self-neglect. *Journal Elder Abuse Neglect, 26*(4), 365–397. doi:10.1080/08946566.2013.801818

Iris, M., Ridings, J. W., & Conrad, K. (2010). The development of a conceptual model for understanding elder self-neglect. *The Gerontologist, 50*, 303–315.

Johnson, Y. O. C. (2015a). Elder self-neglect: Education is needed. *Home Healthcare Now, 33*(8), 421–424.

Johnson, Y. O. C. (2015b). Home care nurses' experiences with and perceptions of elder self-neglect. *Home Healthcare Now, 33*(1), 31–37.

Lauder, W., Anderson, I., & Barclay, A. (2005). Housing and self-neglect: The responses of health, social care and environmental health agencies. *Journal of Interprofessional Care, 19*(4), 317–325.

Lauder, W., Davidson, G., Anderson, I., & Barclay, A. (2005). Self-neglect: The role of judgements and applied ethics. *Nursing Standard, 19*(18), 45–51.

Lauder, W., Ludwick, R., Zeller, R., & Winchell, J. (2006). Factors influencing nurses' judgements about self-neglect cases. *Journal of Psychiatric and Mental Health Nursing, 13*(3), 279–287.

Lauder, W., Roxburgh, M., Harris, J., & Law, J. (2009). Developing self-neglect theory: Analysis of related and atypical cases of people identified as self-neglecting. *Journal of Psychiatric and Mental Health Nursing, 16*(5), 447–445.

McDermott, S. (2008). The devil is in the details: Self-neglect in Australia. *Journal of Elder Abuse & Neglect, 20*(3), 231–250. doi:10.1080/08946560801973077

McDermott, S. (2010). Professional judgements of risk and capacity in situations of self-neglect among older people. *Ageing & Society, 30*(6), 1055–1072. doi:10.1017/S0144686X10000139

Ritchie, J., & Lewis, J. (Eds.). (2003). *Qualitative research practice: A guide for social science students and researchers*. London, UK: Sage.

Richie, J., & Spenser, L. (1994). Qualitative data analysis for applied policy research. In A. Bryman & R. G. Burgess (Eds.), *Analyzing qualitative data* (pp.173–194). London, UK: Routledge.

CHAPTER 14

ADULT SAFEGUARDING AND SELF-NEGLECT: EMERGENT LESSONS FROM ENGLAND

Suzy Braye, David Orr, and Michael Preston-Shoot

Changes in legal and policy context in England have broadened the remit of adult safe-guarding and protection services to include self-neglect. Yet, self-neglect is one of the most challenging aspects of adult social care; and there is ample evidence of practice failures, from serious case reviews conducted, where an adult has died. As a consequence, interest in the evidence base on effective practice has grown. This chapter reports on "what goes wrong" and "what goes right" in self-neglect work, drawing on two studies conducted in the English context. Themes emerging from serious case reviews are followed by findings from in-depth interviews with adult protection managers, practitioners, and service users, which sought to identify approaches that produced positive outcomes. Effective practice required relationships built through sensitive, patient, and concerned curiosity about the unique lived experience of self-neglect, and an integration of knowledge, personal quali-ties, and professional judgment to create proportionate and consensual risk-reduction strategies. Such approaches required an organizational infrastructure that supported relationship-based practice and effective joint working between practitioners from dif-ferent disciplines and agency contexts.

In the English policy context, the term *self-neglect* covers "a wide range of behavior neglecting to care for one's personal hygiene, health or surroundings, and includes behavior such as hoarding" (Department of Health [DH], 2016, para. 14.17). Such a definition can be applied to self-neglect of differing degrees, and it is often a risk (to the individual or to other people) to place a particular set of circumstances above a threshold at which professional concern is triggered, particularly when allied with a refusal on the part of the individual to accept services that would mediate that risk.

Self-neglect has occupied a varied position in the U.K. adult safeguarding legislation and social policy. In Wales, it was included in the original adult protection statutory guidance (Welsh Government, 2000) and is now contained within the adult safeguarding provisions of the Social Services and Well-being (Wales) Act 2014. In Scotland, self-neglect is included within the code of practice (Scottish Executive, 2014) that supports the implementation of the Adult Support and Protection (Scotland) Act 2007.

In England, however, over the same period, self-neglect was specifically excluded from adult protection statutory guidance (DH, 2000). In the review of that guid-ance as part of the adult social care policy making process that resulted in the Care

Act 2014, it was recommended that self-neglect be included in the new adult safeguarding provisions (Law Commission, 2011). The initial statutory guidance that supported the implementation of the 2014 legislation (DH, 2014) included self-neglect in the types of abuse and neglect for which Safeguarding Adults Boards (SABs)[1] must develop policies and procedures and, in certain circumstances, must commission Safeguarding Adults Reviews. Updated statutory guidance (DH, 2016) has also now included self-neglect in the principles and standards for the promotion of well-being and for care and support, as well as in adult safeguarding practice.

This varied position is mirrored in the different approaches taken by other countries. In Australia, self-neglect has not been legislated for specifically (Carter-Anand et al., 2013; McDermott, 2008), but in most of the United States it is a significant component of adult protection work (Hildebrand, Taylor, & Bradway, 2014) as a result of the Older Americans Act of 1965 (amended 2006). The Republic of Ireland's definition of elder abuse excludes self-neglect (Carter-Anand et al., 2013). This variability perhaps betrays anxieties about how to strike a policy and legislative balance between a duty of protective care owed to individuals and concerns to safeguard people's rights to autonomy and self-determination.

This balance is also struck variously with respect to mandatory reporting and intervention powers in adult safeguarding. The Social Services and Well-Being (Wales) Act 2014 places a duty on local authority partners to report an adult at risk and has a provision for an adult protection and support order that would give social workers a power of entry to a dwelling to interview an adult at risk. The Adult Support and Protection (Scotland) Act 2007 contains a similar power to enter a premises to visit and interview an adult at risk and also creates three specific protection powers—assessment, removal, and banning orders. None of these provisions exist within the Care Act 2014 for England, where the statutory duty (section 42, Care Act 2014) is merely to "make inquiries" without any accompanying powers of intervention. Moreover, mandatory reporting of adults at risk (including those who self-neglect) exists in many U.S. states, but not in Australia (McDermott, Linahan, & Squires, 2009). Such variability exposes the equivocal nature of the evidence base on the effectiveness of mandatory reporting but also how law-making is a confluence of research-based policies, diverse ethical perspectives on human rights, and political ideologies.

In a U.K. context, adult safeguarding is about more than adult protection. It involves prevention of risk, abuse and harm, early intervention, the provision of information and advice, as well as the provision of advocacy and measures to raise awareness. Adult safeguarding operates along two axes. The first is a continuum from individual to community engagement. The second is a continuum from preventive approaches to reactive, protective interventions (Braye, Orr, & Preston-Shoot, 2011b). Thus, working with adults who self-neglect is not the preserve of any single agency or profession. Nor is it simply about protecting individuals from risk and harm. It must also include raising awareness about the lack of self-care, living in squalor, and hoarding, behaviors that are often subsumed within the concept of self-neglect, and enlisting familial and community supports to prevent the escalation of concerns.

---

[1]Safeguarding Adults Boards (SABs) are multiagency committees with a core membership comprising the local authority, the police, and the National Health Service. Their statutory function (section 43, Care Act 2014) is to help and protect adults with care and support needs who are experiencing or at risk of abuse and neglect and who, as a result of their care and support needs, are unable to protect themselves.

At the time of this writing, policy makers and practitioners in England remain in a state of adjustment to the new legal framework and with familiarizing themselves with the implications of self-neglect being included as an adult safeguarding issue. In this context, research carried out by the present authors during the period 2010 to 2014 has been influential at both the national and local policy levels, and for practitioners it provides a strong evidence base about the challenges of self-neglect practice and the approaches that are likely to produce positive outcomes. This chapter, having opened with an overview of the legal and policy context, first considers evidence on intervention from the literature, then presents key findings from the authors' own research to draw out messages on good practice in responding and intervening with self-neglect.

LITERATURE REVIEW

The literature identifies a range of risks to which self-neglect can give rise, through its effects on health, hygiene, and safety. In the United States, Dong et al. (2009) identified a significant increase in mortality for older adults living in the community who were self-neglecting. Equivalent data are not available for other countries, but it is clear everywhere that the implications of self-neglect for health and well-being can be severe (Braye, Orr, & Preston-Shoot, 2011a, 2015a, 2015b; Day, Leahy-Warren, & McCarthy, 2013). Less easy to measure, but also of huge significance, are the potentially negative effects not only of conditions of self-neglect themselves but also of practitioner responses, which are experienced as disempowering, restrictive, or at variance with the person's wishes. Although it is sometimes necessary to take protective measures without the person's agreement (e.g., in some situations in which individuals lack mental capacity to decide on their care), practitioners should take care that this does not occur at the expense of due consideration for the individuals' right to autonomy in deciding about their own lives (Braye et al., 2011a; Braye, Orr, & Preston-Shoot, 2013). By the same token, respect for autonomy should not preclude exploring with the person concerned the reasoning behind his or her choices and the influences that may bear on them (Bergeron, 2006; Preston-Shoot, 2016).

A growing number of qualitative studies have explored the perspectives of people who self-neglect and of practitioners who work with them on the situations in which they find themselves. Study findings are of considerable relevance to thinking about how best to work with self-neglect, whether within or outside formal safeguarding procedures. Although the studies took place across different countries and with individuals who presented varying profiles with respect to their patterns of self-neglect, certain common themes emerged in the discussion of their experiences. Many service users spoke to the researchers about "turning points" in their lives and the major events that had contributed to their current situations, which included childhood physical and sexual abuse, traumatic wartime experiences, abandonment, broken relationships, and loss (Band-Winterstein, Doron, & Naim, 2012; Bozinovski, 2000; Olson, Pavlou, Reid, Lee, & Lachs, 2007). Lauder and colleagues noted the "fractured personal biographies" of the interviewees they spoke to (Lauder, Roxburgh, Harris, & Law, 2009, p. 451), for whom combinations of comorbid serious health problems, histories of substance misuse, and periods of homelessness had led to lives characterized by instability and a long-term slide into self-neglect; the researchers described their interviewees as "atypical" in their age profiles (age range 24–73 years) compared with the older client groups that self-neglect research has generally focused on, but point out how their research supports the view that self-neglect develops across the life course, not exclusively in old age. A study from Israel reinforces this point, demonstrating how the life experiences of the people they interviewed had been such that "preserving a normative lifestyle [had become] an inappropriate and impossible option" (Band-Winterstein et al., 2012, p. 116) for them; what others saw as "self-neglect" was for them a reasonable response to losses and suffering that recalibrated their sense of what was important in life. In Bozinovski's (2000) research, in which she interviewed 30 adult protection service clients in the United States, it was found that self-neglect often arose as a reflection of individuals' needs to maintain continuity of self-perception and to feel that they retained control over their lives. Often they saw themselves as people who could cope capably and independently, and were resistant to challenges to this self-image, particularly when this might involve accepting support that implied renouncing a degree of control. Seen in this light, behaviors generally viewed as "self-neglect" became an aspect or a consequence of the ways they actively managed their identity and self-worth.

When the meaning and purpose that self-neglectful behavior might hold for individuals were not taken into account by services, interviewees' stories made clear how problems frequently occurred. Service users in Ireland often refused services at least in part because of their past experiences of not having had their choices respected (Day et al., 2013), and in Israel and the United States they clearly conveyed how the label of "self-neglect" in itself frequently failed to capture the complexities and histories of their situations (Band-Winterstein et al., 2012; Kutame, 2007). Band-Winterstein et al. (2012) identified the ambivalence that many service users felt when services offered did not speak to what they felt their needs to be, even though they accepted they might be in need of some form of assistance; Lauder and colleagues similarly noted how the structure and approach of agencies in Scotland was often experienced as off-putting for self-neglecting clients (Lauder, Anderson, & Barclay, 2005b). Fundamental differences in how services and clients understood the situation at times combined with such factors as clients' distrust of others' motives, difficulties in perspective taking to be able to grasp how others might perceive things, social isolation, or concerns about the financial implications of service involvement to hinder the search for a way forward (Bozinovski, 2000; Day et al., 2013; Lauder et al., 2009).

Studies with practitioners have consistently reported that they commonly face challenges in successfully getting access to and engagement with clients (Day et al., 2013; Doron, Band-Winterstein, & Naim, 2013; Lauder et al., 2005b). Challenges noted for practitioners include the characteristic complexity of self-neglect cases in which multiple comorbidities, functional capabilities, social context, and individual motivations and histories, among other factors, may be in mutual interaction and must all be grasped if effective assessment and intervention are to take place. Difficulties in achieving consistency of practice in assessment, response thresholds, and coordinated working can also be challenging. In addition, negotiating a balance between legal and policy mandates for action, the duty of care to work toward the health and safety of the client, and the need to respect the client's autonomy to make their own decisions are also important (Braye et al., 2011a, 2013; Day et al., 2013; Doron et al., 2013; Gunstone, 2003; McDermott, 2010).

To date, there have been no prospective studies in outcomes of intervention in self-neglect (Mosqueda & Dong, 2011), with the existing body of research concentrating overwhelmingly on prevalence, associated risk factors, and screening measures

(Braye et al., 2011a). Despite this last focus, there is still no "gold standard" array of assessment tools for use with self-neglect. Although some advances have been made in the United States toward developing standardized assessments, for the most part these have primarily focused on a single dimension of self-neglect, such as executive function or daily-living skills, rather than approaching the phenomenon holistically, or have failed to show consistent validity across diverse populations (Hildebrand et al., 2014). Generally, there has been more progress with assessment measures for hoarding than those for self-neglect (Grisham & Williams, 2014).

The lack of a generally adopted self-neglect measure with which to quantify change has been one factor impeding the development of robust outcomes studies. In its absence, however, there are nonetheless some consistent messages coming from the existing literature. There is overwhelming support for working to prioritize consensus and persuasion rather than imposing measures on the individual, not only for ethical and legal reasons, but on the pragmatic grounds that this approach is more likely to support the success of interventions (Braye et al., 2011a; Lauder, Anderson, & Barclay,2005a; Payne & Gainey, 2005). Solid understanding of the legal frameworks that apply to self-neglect within the relevant jurisdiction is important to undergird a carefully considered support plan (Braye et al., 2011a). Because of the need for different practitioners to work closely together in addressing the multidimensionality of self-neglect, care is required in reaching a shared understanding among workers of what the needs are and how they will be met (Braye et al., 2011a; Lauder et al., 2005b). And finally, the research literature reiterates the point with which this section began: Self-neglect can only be satisfactorily resolved by engaging closely with the person in order to understand better how his or her current circumstances have arisen and what his or her perspective on them is (Braye et al., 2011a).

METHODS

The research findings drawn on in this chapter are taken from two projects. The first was a study of Serious Case Reviews (SCRs) to learn lessons from the cases, which may have seen safeguarding failures. The second study used a national survey and interviews to identify the challenges and examples of good practice in working with self-neglect.

SCRs (renamed Safeguarding Adults Reviews by the Care Act, 2014) are carried out in England when an adult dies as a result of, or experiences, serious abuse or neglect, and concerns exist that the relevant partner agencies did not work as effectively as they could have to protect that person. As they are not consolidated through any central repository, to bring together the lessons they hold for safeguarding practice it was necessary to carry out a bespoke search. All 152 Local Authority (LA) and SAB websites in England were searched to identify review summaries that referred, directly or indirectly, to self-neglect. Additional SCRs that did not appear on the Internet were identified by contacting independent chairs of SABs to see whether they were aware of others. This search process produced 32 SCRs that could be accessed; eight further reviews were identified, but could not be obtained either because they had not yet been completed or because they had not been made publicly available. Thematic analysis was carried out on the 32 SCRs to map the key issues highlighted. The analysis was structured at four levels: the self-neglecting individual, the team working with the individual, the organization(s) within which the team worked, and the direction provided by the SAB. Additional details regarding methods can be found in Braye et al. (2015b). This study of SCRs was initiated as part of a larger study on workforce development needs for self-neglect work (Braye et al., 2013).

The second study set out to determine what policy and practice approaches were associated with perceived positive outcomes in cases of self-neglect. A survey questionnaire inquiring about the volume of, and responses to, self-neglect cases was distributed to all LAs in England. The response rate was 34.9%. The most striking finding from the survey was how little data LAs collected about self-neglect outcomes at that time (2013–14, before the Care Act 2014; Braye, Orr, & Preston-Shoot, 2014). The findings reported here, therefore, draw primarily from the semi structured interviews that were carried out, which were intended to complement the larger scale survey with a more in-depth exploration of practice experience and policy implementation than the study permitted. Twenty managers with either strategic or operational responsibility for safeguarding, 42 practitioners (mainly social workers and social care staff), and 29 service users across 10 different LAs were recruited using purposive sampling. These participated in interviews, which in broad terms focused on their experiences of self-neglect work, its challenges, and how they had found those challenges could be overcome to secure outcomes that were experienced as positive by those involved. The interviews were recorded and transcribed where possible, but when permission for this was withheld, written notes were taken with the consent of the interviewee. Interviews with service users took place only when the interviewee was judged to have the mental capacity to consent to take part. Framework analysis (Ritchie & Lewis, 2003) was used to analyze the interview data and extract relevant themes. A fuller account of the methods used can be found in Braye et al. (2014).

FINDINGS

Insights From SCRs

The SCRs brought together for the study form a catalog of challenging situations and practice responses. Sometimes aspects of the work of practitioners and agencies were undeniably good, but often the overall panorama was inadequate to meet the needs of the person who was self-neglecting, with very serious consequences. Because specific issues tend to recur across several SCRs, consideration of what they identified as having gone wrong can be instructive in thinking about how to improve practice with self-neglect in the future. Though SCRs may have their own blind spots (Preston-Shoot, 2016), the detailed scrutiny they afford to specific case studies offers lessons that can have application beyond the local context.

Many of the SCRs identified ways in which practitioners had lost sight of or never adequately engaged with the self-neglecting individual at the heart of the case. This was shown by failures of understanding, empathy, or actions in one or more aspects of the work. Examples included failures to engage with the person as a unique individual, failure to understand decision making by the person, failure to engage correctly with the family members and social networks around the person, and failure to understand the person as someone whose situation changes over time.

Engaging With the Person as a Unique Individual

The SCRs sometimes found a lack of evidence that practitioners had put in the required efforts to establish a trust-based relationship with the individual. Often this meant that there had been a failure to explore with the person what his or her interests and reasons were for acting in the way he or she did. Windows of opportunity were missed when it might have been possible to build a connection with the person's core concerns. These concerns frequently differed from what services were most concerned about, but could have served as a bridge to address those issues as trust developed. Moreover, exploring their concerns could have given practitioners much clearer insights into the person's motivations, goals, and values. Assumptions about, and over emphasis on, the individual's impairments occasionally reflected a focus on "deficits" and "problem behaviors" that made it harder to find common ground and a positive way forward.

Understanding Decision Making by the Person

Although the first principle of the Mental Capacity Act 2005 places practitioners under the obligation to start from the assumption that an individual has the mental capacity to make a specific decision unless demonstrated otherwise, in some SCRs this axiom had become an end point as well as a starting point. Even when individuals had made decisions that exposed them to considerable risk or harm, their decision-making capacity was not questioned and no assessments were recorded. It was often noted that the individuals concerned had not been offered support in making their decisions; noone had explored the different options with them or ensured that information was supplied about the implications of the different choices they could make. Although some of these individuals were noted to be "hard to engage," there was a view that this had sometimes led practitioners to give up the attempt to explore decisions and decision-making capacity too easily.

Engaging Correctly With the Family Members and Social Networks Around the Person

Practitioners sometimes failed to separate out the person as a unique individual from the web of relationships within which they lived. Other people, instead of being consulted and brought into deliberations alongside the individual, were allowed to speak for them, with the result that the self-neglecting individual's views were subsumed within those of the caregivers. At times, respect for family members' views became excessive, with practitioners deferring to them rather than fulfilling their responsibility to make their own assessments and consultations. The converse of this was also identified in some reviews, where concerns about the individual's confidentiality led practitioners to exclude family members, losing valuable additional perspectives and a potential resource in intervening effectively with the person.

Understanding the Person's Situation Over Time

Too often, practitioners found themselves responding to self-neglect cases "in the moment." Work was reactive rather than proactive, dealing with crisis situations as they came up rather than looking ahead to agree on a proactive plan to serve as the basis for a constructive response over a longer period. Insufficient consideration was given to how the person's needs might change so that measures could be put in place to follow this and services could respond appropriately if the person decided at a later date that he or she would accept help or if his or her ability to manage the situation deteriorated. Failure to look ahead to the future was sometimes mirrored in failures to consider the past, with practitioners not picking up on elements of the case history that could have enabled fuller understanding. The result was that they did not identify patterns in the events that occurred in the person's life.

Flaws were found by the SCRs, not only in how practitioners worked with self-neglecting individuals, but also in how they worked with each other. A common theme was that there was poor coordination among agencies, giving rise to a lack of clarity over roles and responsibilities. Decisions were sometimes made by one agency without input from or communication with the others involved. When professionals did work with each other, they sometimes tended to defer to a practitioner seen as authoritative rather than to question, falling into groupthink instead of ensuring that planning benefited from robust, constructive challenge. Difficulties in working together were exacerbated when systems were not in place, or were not used, to facilitate collaboration. This was the case when information sharing happened erratically or not at all, with there being no clarity on how and when it should occur. Risk assessments were sometimes not done or done patchily, and some practitioners displayed a lack of knowledge of mental capacity assessment, safeguarding procedures, and legal frameworks that might have been considered.

The SCRs sometimes pointed to the role of organizational culture or management failings in contributing to the weaknesses in practice. Practitioners were sometimes left unsupported by managers or were expected to prioritize other concerns. When managers did not recognize their inexperience or the risks that the case presented, they could be left to deal with challenges that they should not have had to.

By showing in painstaking detail what went wrong in some very tragic cases, the SCR findings emphasize what must be done in order to achieve more positive outcomes with self-neglect. It is important to make every effort to build a relationship with the individual that facilitates real understanding of the situation. Equally, effective interprofessional and interagency collaboration is vital, along with management recognizing what is required by the situation and supporting staff to do it.

Findings on Practice and Policy

The second study that informs this chapter took a deliberately different approach, seeking evidence on "what goes right" rather than "what goes wrong." The findings reinforce the message that good practice in self-neglect relies upon a whole-systems approach in which there is synergy between the broad legal and policy mandates (discussed earlier), the organizational approaches that implement them, and the quality of the individual/professional interaction that is at the heart of the work.

The Quality of the Individual–Professional Interaction

Our findings show that effective direct work in self-neglect demands an integration of three domains of professional practice: a sound knowledge base, a range of personal and professional qualities, and proportionate intervention derived from the exercise of carefully balanced professional judgment.

"Knowing" requires first that practitioners have a sound understanding of an individual's self-neglect trajectory. As indicated earlier, the literature provides only a broad-brush understanding of the possible factors associated with self-neglect rather than any clear model or pattern of causation. For this reason, there is no substitute for seeking a personalized understanding of each and every individual's own perspective and story. The narratives of the service users in our study cast light on the experiences that can culminate in a picture of self-neglect. A number of themes emerged from the analysis of their narratives.

Many of those who were neglectful of their personal care experienced a strong sense of demotivation, arising from features of their lives that made self-care meaningless. This could be associated with chronic health conditions, loss of someone important or of a valued role, social isolation, or adverse living circumstances:

> I'm drinking, I'm not washing, I wouldn't say I'm losing the will to live, that's a bit strong but . . . I don't care, I just don't care. If I wake up smelling, so what, I'm not going to find a girlfriend or a job cause I ain't got nowhere to live, why do I care? But I do morally, but . . . day-to-day life, so what? I try my best but . . .

Negative self-image could both contribute to and arise from such demotivation, with embedded feelings of worthlessness and even despair: "I would sit here and not even have a wash. I got it in my head that I'm unimportant, so it doesn't matter what I look like or what I smell like."

Demotivation was sometimes associated with self-care becoming a challenge as a result of significant practical obstacles such as illness or homelessness:

> It [homelessness] would lower . . . your esteem, everything about you, you lose your way, your jeans are dirty, you have to buy crap jeans, so now you're lessening yourself as the way you dress, so now you're demeaning yourself as the person you knew you were and then in the end, it's the physical neglect. You can't wash because there's nowhere to wash, you can't be nice and tidy because you look like shit because you're literally sleeping in what you're sleeping in, how do you get someone out of that?

Social standards affect people in different ways. Some explained their self-neglect by expressing a disregard for social appearances, or a degree of indifference to societal standards: "I wouldn't say I let my standards slip; I didn't have much standards to start with." But others emphasized their attempts to keep up appearances: "I try my best, really do [. . .] I could walk down the street now and people would never know that I was homeless unless I took my clothes off." For some, priorities other than norms of self-care had taken over: "I wouldn't bother to wash and no, I haven't this morning either. [. . .] I don't bother washing up, I'm out [of the flat], me. And these other priorities sometimes involved care for other people, demonstrating that social isolation was not always a feature of their lives: "Everyone else to me came first and I think that's what—I kind of neglected myself on and off for 10 years, putting what I wanted on the back burner."

Those who were neglectful of their domestic environment often talked about the influence of the past on their behavior. Hoarding was presented as a continuation or intensification of long-established patterns of collecting, or as a response to parental influence and childhood experiences:

> When I was a little boy, the war had just started, everything had a value [. . .] everything in my eyes then and indeed now, has potential use.

> The only way I kept toys was hiding them.

Collected materials often had a positive value, whether that was aesthetic, monetary, psychological, or instrumental:

> We—people who self-neglect—we cling onto our triumphs . . . it was a work of art, all chopped up (referring to a bookcase he had made, which was removed by the clearance team).

> It's mainly photocopies, books, newspapers, and I don't have time to make a note of everything in the paper that has an interest to me and so I'm very fearful of throwing something away.

> I want things that belonged to people so that they have a connection to me.

> People know I might have things that they are short of, so I feel needed.

Neglect of one's environment was often presented as being beyond the person's control, perhaps due to practical issues such as shortage of space or physical problems, perhaps due to hearing voices or feeling compelled: "The distress of not collecting is more than the distress of doing it."

The lived experience of self-neglect was very painful and clearly affected emotional health. For one individual even his wartime experiences had not been nearly as terrifying as the fear of what he termed his "mess" coming to the attention of others. Another felt:

> just lost, you just feel worthless, no self-worth, there's absolutely nothing inside you, there's no focus to doing anything, your whole shell's just collapsed and it doesn't necessarily have to be drink or drugs, you just give in mentally and physically. The life's drained out of you, you see no hope and you just deteriorate, mentally and physically.

Knowledge of the complex mix of factors affecting an individual's experience of self-neglect is thus an essential component of practice, and indeed the practitioners' accounts of their interventions showed how carefully they inquired into each individual's personal journey and experience to build knowledge of the person.

The second aspect of knowing is the need to bring together wide-ranging sources of professional knowledge, in particular, understandings of human development, mental health and mental capacity, and sound knowledge of theories of intervention. Given the findings from SCRs, a particular priority should be knowledge of the legal rules that permit and, in some cases require, intervention. In the English context, these include the Care Act 2014 and the Mental Capacity Act 2005, each providing powers and duties in relation to the assessment of need and of mental capacity, and the provision of care and support. Knowledge of the Human Rights Act 1998, incorporating the European Convention on Human Rights within the domestic legal framework, is vital, too. Article 2 (the right to life), article 3 (the right to protection from inhuman and degrading treatment), article 5 (the right to liberty and security of the person), and article 8 (the right to respect for private and family life) may all be engaged, and the principle of proportionality must underpin all interventions—that where a convention right is interfered with, this must be for a legitimate aim, done according to law, and involving the use of suitable, necessary and reasonable measures.

When intervention may need to be imposed rather than care and support being negotiated with consent, additional legal rules are engaged. These include:

- The Mental Health Act 1983, permitting compulsory admission to psychiatric hospital
- Environmental and public health legislation permitting enforced clearance of materials or cleaning of filthy and infested premises
- Housing legislation permitting eviction on grounds of breach of tenancy or intervention to make unsafe premises safe
- Antisocial behavior legislation permitting injunctions to prevent nuisance and annoyance to others
- Animal welfare legislation permitting intervention to ensure that animals are appropriately treated

Practitioners who facilitated positive outcomes demonstrated sound levels of legal literacy, with knowledge of the legal rules well integrated within their thinking about options for intervention:

We would be regularly exploring the law to make sure that we'd done everything we could around supporting her within her home, and exploring what life would be like if we moved her as well . . . we'd hypothesize a lot and then see, based on how we knew her, what impact that would have on her life and would that be worse or better?

The second element affecting the quality of the individual/professional interaction is "being." "Being" required the professional use of a range of personal qualities that enabled a practitioner to engage effectively with someone who may be reluctant to build a relationship of trust. This relationship became the vehicle through which other interventions could be delivered because it enabled consensus to be slowly built about what needed to happen. In some cases, it became an intervention in itself, providing a positive regard that could gradually and gently challenge negative cognition: "She got it into my head that I am important, that I am on this earth for a reason."

"Being" included qualities of patience and perseverance, which were often needed in order to overcome the shame and embarrassment that often lay behind an individual's reluctance to engage. Refusal to be shocked on the first encounter was important. Unless risks were so acute that they needed immediate action, the persistent expression of concerned curiosity was the approach used to establish rapport over time. Practitioners felt it a priority to establish some kind of a personal connection, some common ground, such as shared knowledge of a particular place, or love of music or books, that was not about self-neglect:

> I like gardening and so we used to go out into the garden and potter around, put a few plants in.

Of all the visits probably only 20% of the time we spent with her would probably be trying to have a conversation about her care needs; just by sitting and chatting and looking at her photographs and all of that, I did come to understand her life.

Honesty about the substance of concerns was also important, but service users valued a person-centered, non-directive approach to this dialogue:

> The idea is not to get too pushy about it; people start getting panicky then, you know? "You're interfering in my life," that kinda thing.

> With me, if you're too bossy, I will put my feet down and go like a stubborn mule; I will just sit and just fester.

They greatly valued practitioners who showed compassion and empathy about the experience of self-neglect, recognizing the emotional literacy that enabled practitioners to convey a sense of common humanity: "He has been human, that's the word I can use. He has been human." For practitioners too, authenticity of approach was an important feature: "If you're genuine and genuinely want to help the person, they can tell I think." They emphasized the value of shared humanity: "I cajoled him into soaking his hands in this warm water; I cut his fingernails and do you know, he was so appreciative of that, I really do think, that human touch."

Practitioners also emphasized the importance of their own personal resilience. Self-neglect work was experienced as highly stressful, frustrating, and often distressing: "It does have an emotional impact . . . at weekends, because you never really switch off, I revisit scenarios from every angle and I think 'what more could be done?' Organizational responses to this will be discussed later but in terms of qualities of "being," personal resilience featured high on the list.

The third important element for the quality of interaction is "doing." "Doing" related to the skills and approaches that practitioners brought to their intervention. Holistic assessment and the ability to weigh different options that arose from that assessment were the key focus. The nature and extent of, and the risks arising from self-neglect may be evident, but identifying the underlying reasons and understanding the individual's own life history and perspective, could entail an extended and iteraive process.

Determining what to do about an individual's self-neglect involved establishing a careful and morally reasoned balance between respect for autonomy, and fulfilling a duty of care and protection. These two considerations were often experienced as competing imperatives in situations in which apparent choices exercised by the individual resulted in living circumstances that constituted an affront to human dignity and triggered societal expectations that "something should be done." Where a practitioner positioned herself or himself on the spectrum between them could influence the balance struck between "hands-on" and "hands-off" approaches, with the former sometimes becoming necessary when the latter did not secure sufficient reduction of risk, but was seen very much as a last resort: "I'm very strong on human rights, autonomy and free will. . . . But . . . it's just that human thing, can you leave someone? Do we leave people in society? You're sort of battling with the level of morality as well."

Mental capacity was a key consideration in the practitioners' decision making and required careful assessment. Under the Mental Capacity Act 2005 in England, mental capacity is a decision-specific question—an individual may have the capacity to make simple decisions, for example, but lack the capacity to engage in more complex questions. Thus the key consideration for practitioners was to determine the extent to which the self-neglect resulted from explicit decision making on the part of the individual, and whether he or she had the capacity to make the decisions involved in self-care or in the care of their environment. Although the Act establishes a right for a person with the capacity to make a decision that others might consider unwise, if someone lacks capacity anyone who makes a decision on his or her behalf must act in the individual's best interests, taking account of his or her wishes, feelings, beliefs and values, and the views of others close to them. Intervention in these circumstances must be proportionate, however. Although it could involve removing an individual from a high-risk environment to the one in which the self-neglect could be monitored and moderated, it need not necessarily intrude on his or her life to such an extent. The research findings included examples of "best-interest" interventions that involved the provision of care and support at home, just sufficient to manage risk rather than remove it altogether.

Interventions described in the narratives of practitioners and service users showed a number of common features: they were flexible, constructed from understanding an individual's unique circumstances; they required extensive negotiation to establish a degree of consensus, sometimes starting with small steps that could be agreed while waiting longer for the trust that would facilitate more major changes; they focused on risk reduction rather than "symptom" reduction. So, positive outcomes were achieved by interventions such as simply remaining in contact, sufficient to identify small changes in motivation over time that could widen possibilities for change. Small practical tokens of support were valued—items of kitchen equipment, repairs, welfare benefits, help to secure medical appointments—and risk could sometimes be reduced through the provision of equipment such as smoke detectors and fire-retardant furniture. Practitioners made use of specific approaches such as motivational interviewing, seeking to engage with the ambivalence that characterized some individuals' thinking about his or her situation. Sometimes small support packages or partial clearing or cleaning could be agreed on, and family members were often instrumental in such negotiations. Occasionally, therapeutic inputs, such as psychotherapy or counseling, might be helpful in engaging with deep-seated needs and finding ways of replacing what was being given up through the removal of valued collections through the acceptance of care and support. Where solutions had to be imposed, perhaps through the use of legal powers on grounds of environmental health, even then practitioners found ways of remaining alongside the person, providing emotional support and maximizing choices where possible. Throughout, relationship was the central feature; as one service user commented:

> I think the only thing that will help that is concern, another human being connecting with you that's got a little bit more strength than you that pulls you through those forms of depression, that's what keeps you alive.

Multidisciplinary approaches to interventions were very evident in the practitioners' narratives about "doing." The complexity of an individual's journey into self-neglect, and the diverse influences that contribute to each unique picture, engage a wide range of professional and disciplinary expertise. Mental capacity assessment, for example, sometimes required the joint involvement of medical and social care professionals, for example, in situations in which a suspected loss of executive brain function was implicated in the self-neglect. Fire-service involvement was often crucial to successful intervention to minimize fire risk from hoarded materials. Equally, the involvement of family and community networks could provide persuasive leverage or a tailored solution that stemmed from long-standing knowledge of an individual's motivators and preferences.

His granddaughter had visited his home and was in tears—"Oh, you've got to get rid of these." Usually a person's hoard is stronger than his or her relationship with the family, but something about his relationship with her made him give us a little window of opportunity.

Organizational Approaches That Facilitate Positive Outcomes

Beyond the domain of interaction between the professionals and the individuals, lies the organizational domain—the second key set of findings from the study reported here (Braye et al., 2014). The relationship-based approaches to practice outlined previously take time, and often it is time that practitioners do not have unless local authorities make adjustments in how the workflow is managed. Since the early 1990s, adult social care has been dominated by models of care management characterized by short-term, task-focused involvement, moving rapidly through the predetermined stages of assessment, care planning, delivery of care and support packages, and periodic review—each with its own allocated time frame. Practitioners reported pressure to close even high-risk cases in which individuals refused support and no "progress" could be reported—what one manager referred to as the "they've got capacity, walk away" approach. The pressure to do so, in the context of a waiting list of new referrals and intensifying resource shortage, was strong:

> The combination of people who are either terrified of losing their independence or terrified of losing their relationships, or terrified of state intervention, together with a state process that is desperate to apply eligibility criteria and find reasons not to support people, is just lethal . . . it was just like "oh you're saying it's all fine, thank goodness, we can go away.

This contrasted with what was frequently termed "good old-fashioned social work," which takes time to build rapport, and then to move from rapport to a relationship of a kind so valued by the service user respondents in this study:

So to have a chance of having any sort of rapport or relationship, trying to achieve everything in two or three visits is just not going to work . . . it's like winning points with someone until they realize that you're on their side.

The study provided examples of the imaginative use of staffing resources to create dedicated time for some practitioners to engage in longer term, in-depth work in the most complex and high-risk cases:

> What we're trying to do is give a framework to workers, to support their practice, and to make decisions and judgments on when to escalate difficult cases and thus make the process robust. It's no good just saying those people have got capacity so they can live like that. We have to make some judgments and we have to be in a position to support the workers, in terms of when they need to escalate those cases for different reasons, to make the whole process robust.

Staff training, supervision, and support needs were recognized by many of the managers and practitioners interviewed. They placed emphasis on the importance of supervision that could engage with the stressful and sometimes distressing lived experience of self-neglect practice: "So supervision is essential, good reflective time to unpick, and slow it down if you can . . . so helping people hold that level of discomfort and emotion." Equally important were supervisory challenges to counteract possible complacency and desensitization to risk, and supervisory support for imaginative and creative practice: "My manager is brilliant, she . . . gives me lots of space to try out new ideas and . . . she always comes out with an idea that I haven't thought of."

The approaches that produced positive outcomes also required strong interagency ownership at the strategic level. Self-neglect had historically been neglected within the interagency safeguarding governance mechanism of SAB: "Well that's the worst one, 'somebody else's business' actually, isn't it? Obviously, we are trying to make it 'everybody's business.'" Given the changes introduced by the Care Act 2014, SABs now play a key role in the multiagency governance of self-neglect work, ensuring that the respective roles of different agencies are well understood, that referral routes are clear, and that mechanisms for shared decision making are in place. Practitioners who had access to multiagency high-risk panels or discussions experienced these as helpful in reviewing options for intervention, securing commitments from other agencies, or even just receiving reassurance that their approach was sound and justifiable.

CONCLUSION

Achieving positive outcomes in individuals who self-neglect requires imaginative and creative approaches to practice that match the complexity of self-neglect itself. Changes in the legal context in England have created a policy environment that facilitates positive engagement with the challenges of self-neglect by a range of agencies and supports safeguarding systems used to address the barriers to good interagency collaboration. Individual organizations have shown they can find the latitude to create space and support for practitioners to engage proactively with people whose lives are often disturbed, disturbing, and highly risky, both for themselves and for others. The evidence base on direct practice emerging from the research reported in this chapter adds to the increasingly rich picture drawn in the international literature and shows that at the heart of good practice are relationships built through sensitive, patient, and concerned curiosity about the unique lived experiences of self-neglect.

IMPLICATIONS FOR RESEARCH AND PRACTICE

- The experience of self-neglect arises from a personal constellation of factors in an individual's life; practitioners who engage with an individual's story and perspective will be better placed to shape an intervention that can achieve satisfactory resolution.
- The range of needs experienced by an individual who self-neglects, and the often deep-seated complexity of the factors that give rise to them, require health and social care agencies to work closely together to provide multidisciplinary expertise.
- There is strong evidence for the value of negotiated interventions based on consensus and persuasion, rather than imposed measures.

REFERENCES

Band-Winterstein, T., Doron, I., & Naim, S. (2012). Elder self-neglect: A geriatric syndrome or a life course story? *Journal of Aging Studies, 26*, 109–118.

Bergeron, L. R. (2006). Self-determination and elder abuse: Do we know enough? *Journal of Gerontological Social Work, 46*(3), 81–102.

Bozinovski, S. D. (2000). Older self-neglecters: Interpersonal problems and the maintenance of self-continuity. *Journal of Elder Abuse & Neglect, 12*(1), 37–56.

Braye, S., Orr, D., & Preston-Shoot, M. (2011a). Conceptualizing and responding to self-neglect: The challenges for adult safeguarding. *Journal of Adult Protection, 13*(4), 182–193.

Braye, S., Orr, D., & Preston-Shoot, M. (2011b). *The governance of adult safeguarding: Findings from research into Safeguarding Adults Boards.* London, UK: Social Care Institute for Excellence.

Braye, S., Orr, D., & Preston-Shoot, M. (2013). *A scoping study of workforce development for self-neglect work.* Leeds, UK: Skills for Care.

Braye, S., Orr, D., & Preston-Shoot, M. (2014). *Self-neglect policy and practice: Building an evidence base for adult social care.* London, UK: Social Care Institute for Excellence.

Braye, S., Orr, D., & Preston-Shoot, M. (2015a). Learning lessons about self-neglect? An analysis of serious case reviews. *Journal of Adult Protection, 17*(1), 3–18.

Braye, S., Orr, D., & Preston-Shoot, M. (2015b). Serious case review findings on the challenges of self-neglect: Indicators for good practice. *Journal of Adult Protection, 17*(2), 75–87.

Carter-Anand, J., Taylor, B., Montgomery, L., Bakircioglu, O., Harper, C., Devaney, J., . . . Nejbir, D. (2013). *A review of elder abuse in Northern Ireland and a review of adult protection legislation across the UK, Ireland and internationally.* Research Report for the Commissioner for Older People for Northern Ireland. Belfast, Ireland: Queens University Belfast and University of Ulster.

Day, M. R., Leahy-Warren, P., & McCarthy, G. (2013). Perceptions and views of self-neglect: A client-centred perspective. *Journal of Elder Abuse & Neglect, 25*(1), 76–94.

Department of Health. (2000). *No secrets: Guidance on developing and implementing multi-agency policies and procedures to protect vulnerable adults from abuse.* London, UK: The Stationery Office.

Department of Health. (2014). *Care and support statutory guidance: Issued under the Care Act 2014.* London, UK: The Stationery Office.

Dong, X., Simon, M., Mendes de Leon, C., Fulmer, T., Beck, T., Hebert, L., . . . Evans, D. (2009). Elder self-neglect and abuse and mortality risk in a community-dwelling population. *Journal of the American Medical Association, 302*(5), 517–526.

Doron, I., Band-Winterstein, T., & Naim, S. (2013). The meaning of elder self-neglect: Social workers' perspective. *International Journal of Aging and Human Development, 77*(1), 17–36.

Grisham, J. R., & Williams, A. D. (2014). Assessing hoarding and related phenomena. In R. O. Frost & G. Steketee (Eds.), *The Oxford handbook of hoarding and acquiring* (pp. 235–246). Oxford, UK: Oxford University Press.

Gunstone, S. (2003). Risk assessment and management of patients who self-neglect: A 'grey area' for mental health workers. *Journal of Psychiatric and Mental Health Nursing, 10*, 287–296.

Hildebrand, C., Taylor, M., & Bradway, C. (2014). Elder self-neglect: The failure of coping because of cognitive and functional impairments. *Journal of the American Association of Nurse Practitioners, 26*, 452–462.

Kutame, M. M. (2007).*Understanding self-neglect from the older person's perspective* (Unpublished doctoral dissertation). Ohio State University, Columbus, OH.

Lauder, W., Anderson, I., & Barclay, A. (2005a). A framework for good practice in interagency interventions with cases of self-neglect. *Journal of Psychiatric and Mental Health Nursing, 12*(2), 192–198.

Lauder, W., Anderson, I., & Barclay, A. (2005b). Housing and self-neglect: The responses of health, social care and environmental health agencies. *Journal of Interprofessional Care, 19*(4), 317–325.

Lauder, W., Roxburgh, M., Harris, J., & Law, J. (2009). Developing self-neglect theory: Analysis of related and atypical cases of people identified as self-neglecting. *Journal of Psychiatric and Mental Health Nursing, 16*, 447–454.

Law Commission. (2011). *Adult social care* (Paper 326). London, UK: The Stationery Office.

McDermott, S. (2008). The devil is in the details: Self-neglect in Australia. *Journal of Elder Abuse & Neglect, 20*(3), 231–250.

McDermott, S. (2010). Professional judgments of risk and capacity in situations of self-neglect among older people. *Ageing and Society, 30*(6), 1055–1072.

McDermott, S., Linahan, K., & Squires, B. J. (2009). Older people living in squalor: Ethical and practical dilemmas. *Australian Social Work, 62*(2), 245–257.

Mosqueda, L., & Dong, X. (2011). Elder abuse and self-neglect: "I don't care anything about going to the doctor, to be honest . . . " *Journal of the American Medical Association, 306*(5), 532–540.

Olson, A. C., Pavlou, M. P., Reid, C., Lee, F., & Lachs, S. (2007). Stories of self-neglect in New York City. *Journal of the American Geriatrics Society, 55*(Suppl. 4), S123–S124.

Payne, B., & Gainey, R. (2005). Differentiating self-neglect as a type of elder mistreatment: How do these cases compare to traditional types of elder mistreatment? *Journal of Elder Abuse & Neglect, 17*(1), 21–36.

Preston-Shoot, M. (2016). Towards explanations for the findings of serious case reviews: Understanding what happens in self-neglect work. *Journal of Adult Protection, 18*(3), 131–148.

Ritchie, J., & Lewis, J. (2003).*Qualitative research practice: A guide for social science students and researchers*. London, UK: Sage.

Scottish Executive. (2014). *Adult Support and Protection (Scotland) Act 2007: Code of Practice*. Edinburgh, UK: Scottish Government.

Welsh Government. (2000). *In safe hands: Implementing adult protection procedures in Wales*. Cardiff, UK: National Assembly for Wales.

CHAPTER 15

PRACTICE WISDOM: PROFESSIONAL RESPONSES TO SELF-NEGLECT IN ISRAEL

Toya Band-Winterstein, Israel Doron, and Sigal Naim

Self-neglect among older adults is a social and health phenomenon that has attracted increasing research interest in recent years. Very little empirical attention has been devoted to evaluating intervention programs in the field of self-neglect among older adults. The aim of this study is to explore the meaning attributed to the phenomenon of elder self-neglect by social workers in their encounters with self-neglecting elders. A qualitative phenomenological study was conducted using a sample of 16 certified social workers. Data collection was performed through in-depth semi structured interviews, followed by content analysis. Four key scenarios emerged: (a) immediate threat to life, (b) potential future threat to life, (c) avoiding deterioration in the absence of imminent risk, and (d) addressing environmental nuisance. The complexity of the self-neglect phenomenon is experienced not only on the personal level, but also on the interpersonal, societal, and professional levels. The findings of this research show that social workers developed intervention strategies based on the tension and the need for balance between preserving autonomy, protecting human rights, and respecting the older persons' wishes versus paternalism and client safety.

Practice wisdom is knowledge gained from practice, "knowledge at hand," which goes beyond theoretical and scientific knowledge. This knowledge is acquired through direct experience with social phenomena and with people representing them. It is heuristically derived through personal reflection and deliberation and is used in the process of identifying, detecting, explaining, and intervening with relevant issues, problems, and social phenomena. Practice wisdom mediates between intervention theory and practice experience (Chu & Tsui, 2008).

This chapter applies a "practice wisdom" model in the context of older adults engaged in self-neglectful behavior. Self-neglect among older adults is a social phenomenon that has attracted increasing research interest in recent years (Burnes, Pillemer, & Lasch, 2016). The phenomenon usually manifests through unwillingness to receive basic medical attention and a lack of concern for one's basic life needs, or through the choice of a lifestyle that includes neglected appearance, poor health and nutrition, hoarding and squalid living conditions (Burnett et al., 2006; Poythress, Burnett, Naik, Pickens, & Dyer, 2007). In specific, this phenomenon has received attention in the Israeli context, and questions, such as the adequacy of existing legal remedies, have been raised (Doron, Alon, & Nissim, 2005; Doron, Band-Winterstein, & Kornfield, 2016).

Despite the growing knowledge and interest in studying this phenomenon, some "blind spots" in knowledge still exist. Thus, this chapter describes and adds a better understanding of the interventions that professionals apply in their encounters with older adults who are engaged in self-neglectful behavior. More specific, in the context of growing awareness of the need for evidence-based practice, very little empirical attention has been devoted to evaluating intervention programs in the field of self-neglect among older adults. Based on our study findings, we developed an integrative heuristic model of interventions for different scenarios. The scenarios and interventions emerged from the experience and practice of all professionals (i.e., social workers working in the field) in Israel.

BACKGROUND LITERATURE

Israel as a Contextual Case Study

Israel is a mixed society, which includes very religious and traditional Jewish and non-Jewish minority groups, who live alongside the large majority of the modern, secular society. Moreover, both the religious and the secular sectors are characterized by their multiculturalism and diversity. It is widely agreed that, over the years, Israel has transformed from a communal and traditional society to a more liberal and individualistic society and that these changes are still in process (Al-Haj, 1988, 2004). Therefore, it is very difficult to characterize Israeli society as a whole. This difficulty manifests specifically, for example, in the field of abuse and neglect of older adults on the one hand—as part of the Jewish and Muslim traditions, a general culture of respect for older persons is prevalent—but on the other hand, empirical data reveal high levels of ageism and abuse of older adults (Lowenstein & Doron, 2008).

From a legal perspective, throughout its history Israel has developed a broad range of legislative instruments to address cases of elder abuse and neglect (Doron et al., 2005). No less than four different "generations" of laws have been enacted—starting from "social welfare" legislation of the 1960s, providing intervention authority to social welfare officers; moving to adding a whole new chapter in Israel's criminal code in the 1980s, which specifically defines abuse, and neglect of helpless older persons, establishing mandatory reporting of such cases. In the 1990s, specific legislation that covers family violence and abuse, along with protective and therapeutic orders, was established. Finally, in the early 21st century, laws specifically addressing and empowering older persons and professionals with specific references to identifying and providing care and information to victims of elder abuse and neglect were implemented (Lowenstein & Doron, 2008). Nevertheless, despite this rich body of legal development, the specific issue of elder self-neglect was left "neglected" within the legal system (Alon & Doron, 2009).

The unique mixture of values and cultures in Israeli society is reflected also in its social work profession, which has also experienced significant changes over the years. It can be said that social work has slowly transformed from a communal and paternalistic-based profession to a more liberal, human-rights and value-based profession (Mautner, 1993; Weiss & Welbourne, 2007).

In this context, the different aspects of encountering self-neglect have been well known in Israel for many years. Nevertheless, the visibility and awareness of the phenomenon were exposed only when abuse and neglect of older adults were recognized as a social problem. At the same time, despite its prevalence (Abrams, Lachs, McAvay, Keohane, & Bruce, 2002), there are those who claim that self-neglect is overlooked both in the literature and in practice, where attention is focused mainly on abuse of older adults (Payne & Gainey, 2005). In this context, when social workers were asked about the phenomenon, although it appeared to be recognized, it was still an unsolved riddle, for which they lacked the conceptual knowledge and a theoretical framework to fully understand (Doron, Band-Winterstein, & Naim, 2013).

Interactions Between Professionals and Older Adults

In the research literature, a relatively large amount of attention has been devoted to how health and welfare professionals perceive their encounters with family violence and abuse of older adults (Anetzberger, 2005; Bell, 2003; Dekel & Peled, 2000; Goldblatt, 2009; Iliffe & Steed, 2000; Slattery & Goodman, 2009; Trevitt & Gallagher, 1996).

A wide array of reactions are noted, ranging from repulsion, distancing from, and blaming the victim (Anetzberger, 2005) to a sense of helplessness (Trevitt & Gallagher, 1996). Other reactions are countertransference, secondary traumatization, stress and burnout, which influence the workers' functioning in the professional and personal domains (Bell, 2003; Campbell & Wasco, 2005; Dekel & Peled, 2000; Dutton, 1992; Figley, 1995; Iliffe & Steed, 2000; Jenkins & Baird, 2002; McCann & Pearlman, 1990; Miller, 1998; Slattery & Goodman, 2009; Trippany, White Kress, & Wilcoxon, 2004; Walker, 2004; Way, VanDeusen, Martin, Applegate, & Jandle, 2004). Nevertheless, these encounters have also been found to provide opportunities for growth (Linley & Joseph, 2006).

The professional encounter with self-neglect among older adults has attracted little research attention. Self-neglect includes two content categories that have the potential to influence the professionals. The first relates to self-neglect as a way of life, the characteristics of which can appear threatening to the professionals' attitudes, emotions, and personal lifestyle (Goldblatt & Buchbinder, 2003; Goldblatt, Buchbinder, Eisikovits, & Arizon-Messinger, 2009). The second deals with old age and its uniqueness, as associated with illness, reduced functioning, the end of life, and death. These components are manifest also in ageist attitudes toward older adults (Rees, King, & Schmitz, 2009) through feelings such as fear of isolation and death, helplessness, repulsion, and recoil (Bar-Tur & Hantman, 2010). Specifically, a qualitative study about professionals' judgment of self-neglect (McDermott, 2010) found that professionals focus on risk and capacity, which influences their interventions.

In light of the literature review described previously, it is evident that there is room to broaden the scope of understanding of the phenomenon of self-neglect among older adults through the lens of the social workers' practice wisdom. Using case scenarios social workers plan interventions. Practice wisdom is knowledge gained from practice and it goes beyond theoretical and scientific knowledge. The practice knowledge is acquired by professionals through direct experiences with social phenomena and the people who represent it (Band-Winterstein & Alon, 2015).

METHODS

In light of the complexity of the phenomenon of self-neglect, one of the most significant challenges in the research reported here was designing the study method. The aim of this study was to explore the meaning attributed to the phenomenon of elder self-neglect by social workers in their encounters with the self-neglecting elders. The qualitative, phenomenological research method was chosen, which enabled in-depth description and examination of all aspects, perceptions, and meanings of the self-neglect phenomenon among older adults (Patton, 2002). Sixteen professionals in this field were purposefully selected (Patton, 2002) by criterion sampling to obtain the widest information possible within the phenomenon. All were Israeli certified social workers, who were employed in the welfare departments and in the senior citizens day centers, including 15 women and one man. The sample criteria were working as professionals in a service for senior citizens. The experience range was between at least 2 years ($n = 1$) to more than 20 years of experience ($n = 6$) in the field of aging, and were in ongoing, daily contact with this population. The sample included a geriatrician ($n = 1$), social welfare officers ($n = 9$), social workers ($n = 5$), and an assistant ($n = 1$). The final number of participants was determined by a theoretical saturation that was reached during content analysis, at the stage when no additional content areas were found (Morse, 2000).

Data collection involved in-depth interviews and was based on an interview guide (Kvale, 1996) that included four content areas. In the first of these, professional encounter with the self-neglect phenomenon, participants were asked questions, such as: What are the first three things that come to mind when talking about self-neglect among older adults? For the second content area, interaction between the professionals and the self-neglectful older adults, participants were asked to describe this interaction. The third area concerned personal (and nonprofessional) encounters with the self-neglect phenomenon and participants were asked questions such as: Which emotions does the older adult engaged in self-neglectful behavior evoke within you? The final content area concerned retrospective and future perspectives, in this context, the participants were asked questions such as: In your opinion, what is the right way to treat the self-neglect phenomenon?

Content analysis of the transcribed interviews was performed by a team of researchers who were experienced in qualitative methodology, using grounded theory methodology (Strauss & Corbin, 1997). As an initial step, transcripts were read from a phenomenological perspective allowing in-depth acquaintance with the text. Second, the data were coded and grouped according to meanings relevant to the study aim (i.e., the meaning attributed to the phenomenon by social workers in their encounter with the self-neglecting elders) and conceptualized into unique theoretical categories. Each unit of meaning and category included several quotes that expressed the participants' experiences and perceptions of the subject. Third, the major themes were organized by a transition from the theoretical to the interpretative level. Several units of meaning that have similar content were connected and unified to create a distinct and organized theme that incorporates patterns of human experience. Finally, the interactions between themes were described constructing a theory, a narrative, or a typology at a higher level of abstraction to understand the essence of the experience through the creation of links, understandings, and meanings between the themes (Creswell, 2007; Moustakas, 1994).

The research team conducted face-to-face in-depth interviews with all the professionals as previously detailed. The team comprised the two head researchers, (a woman and a man, both with PhDs in gerontology and experience in qualitative research) and the research coordinator (a graduate gerontology student with experience in qualitative research). The interviews took place at locations chosen by the participants—in most cases, in their offices. All the participants were informed in advance of the proposed recording and transcription, but they were assured that the interviews would be kept confidential and would be used only for purposes of the study. In addition, the interview transcriptions and quotes would not include any details that might expose their identities and the names of all the participants were changed (all names hereinafter are pseudonyms). Finally, the study was approved by the Ethics Committee of the University of Haifa. The data analysis was performed according to the accepted methods for qualitative data analysis, as described previously (Lincoln & Guba, 1985).

FINDINGS

The interventions described by the professionals included three different domains: the first related to four different intervention scenarios, the second focused on intervention strategies, and the third addressed maintaining continuity of treatment and the attributed importance to information dissemination and raising awareness of the phenomenon.

"Intervention Scenarios": When to Intervene

In their own words, the participants described different types of professional interventions, according to the four possible intervention scenarios. Each of the scenarios focused on different types of potential situations of self-neglect, ranging from life-threatening situations demanding active intervention and involvement of a social welfare officer, through cases that involved a potential threat to life, to less imminent cases of self-neglect that were more of an environmental nuisance, to the mild cases that posed neither a genuine risk or a nuisance (Table 15.1). Each type was allocated a different intervention scenario, which will be described in the following.

Scenario A: Immediate Threat to Life

Scenario A focuses on a life-threatening situation in which the professionals have identified and assessed an immediate risk to the older person. Accordingly, they described the order of the actions that they planned to take. This is illustrated by Ehud, who described how he makes contact with the older adults engaged in self-neglectful behavior in such cases:

> When I see neglect, it is my obligation to make professional contact, and to urge him [the self-neglectful older adult] to care for himself. It doesn't always work. I don't always succeed in influencing him. I have the legal option; if a person can't take care of himself and refuses medical treatment for implausible reasons and medical evidence indicates a risk to his physical or mental health, I can apply to the court to enforce things.
>
> (Ehud, 32 years in the profession)

TABLE 15.1 Intervention Scripts

Script	Characteristics	Professional's Response	Outcome
Script A: Immediate threat to life	In need of quick medical intervention or long-term 24-hour care, health risk	Immediate medical and/or psychogeriatric diagnosis along with enforcement of legal authority through courts	Forceful legal intervention (e.g., forcing medical treatment; removal from home to nursing home)
Script B: Potential future threat to life	No immediate intervention needed but potential future risk alongside cognitive deterioration, health risk	Attempts to persuade the older person to accept treatment and/or move out of home, attempts to involve family members, psychiatric diagnosis, bringing the case before professional committees	Depends on the diagnosis and level of cooperation and can vary from agreeing to move from home to receiving different types of assistance
Script C: Preventing deterioration in the absence of imminent risk	Independent—no risk, refuses offers of help, continues life of self-neglect	Offers varied means of assistance; negotiates provision of services, including cleaning and/or renovating the home	Continuation of life in self-neglect situation, occasional control/ follow-up by professionals
Script D: Environmental nuisance	Either independent or with physical health disability but with no health threat, yet living in environmental-nuisance conditions	Works together with public health authorities, offers a variety of assistance, via sanitation bylaws and Nursing Care Law criteria or providing help despite not meeting the criteria	Provision of environmental interventions (e.g., cleaning the house; removal of waste and dangerous materials) and, if necessary, using public health laws

Ehud described his professional obligation, which motivates him to act in situations of self-neglect. The action might be simple: a conversation in which he attempts to make an impact on the person, to convince him to improve his living conditions. As Ehud described, he does not always succeed in influencing the self-neglectful older adult, which "forces" him to turn to the alternative path available in such a case—the legal system, which can enforce the necessary treatment even without the person's consent. This is the last resort and is used in cases of immediate risk when a person is behaving in an irrational or unreasonable way and when the concern for his or her physical or mental welfare is validated by medical authorities.

Inbal illustrated how she acts when evaluating a situation that is potentially life-threatening to the self-neglectful older adult:

> If I evaluate risk and neglect, I automatically go directly to the family physician. [I ask him or her to] write me a letter [whether], in your opinion, there is a risk. Is this being an acute situation under the Law for the Protection of the Helpless? What is the urgency of medical treatment? How dangerous is it? I don't make the decision about whether she is at risk, even though the Law for the Protection of the Helpless allows me to work a bit, but I have never acted without getting a medical opinion. So, first of all, a medical opinion; after that, a psychiatric opinion as to whether or not judgment is intact, because people who are of sound mind have the right to die at home. In absolutely all cases, without exception, we consult the family physician about whether it is self-neglect. I will not decide on my own that someone is self-neglectful.
>
> (Inbal, 12 years in the profession)

When Inbal has evaluated a risk to the self-neglectful person's life, her first automatic act was to obtain medical documentation by requesting a letter from the family physician, which confirms and assesses the risk. In other words, she turns to a professional medical authority to endorse her recommendation, which she will use when applying for legal intervention under a court order. It should be kept in mind that under Israel's Law for the Protection of the Helpless social welfare officers cannot act autonomously without a court order. Therefore, whenever they do not receive the cooperation of the older person, and there is a real and serious threat to his or her physical or mental health—they will apply for court orders. Inbal described the additional step of also requesting information from a psychiatrist regarding the person's judgment and decision-making capability. In other words, she relieves herself of the responsibility to make the decision: "I will not decide on my own that someone is self-neglectful." However, if the medical opinions reflect both significant health risk as well as a lack of decision-making capacity, she will use the legal power of immediate and forceful intervention through the court order.

Scenario B: Potential Threat to Life

Scenario B describes a situation in which the self-neglectful older adult does not pose an immediate threat to the self, but demands intervention to prevent future risks. This is illustrated in the following scenario:

> I knew an old man with diabetes. He had dreadful sores on his legs and he didn't want to go for medical treatment. They looked and smelled terrible and the bandages were filthy and he didn't understand [either because of cognitive decline or because of lack of awareness]. So I try to persuade him and try to explain, sometimes involving other colleagues. I often manage to enlist another social worker, someone with a relationship of trust, whether it's a family member, a caregiver, anyone who I know goes in there and has some kind of good attitude toward him. And of course, if that doesn't work, then there is no choice but to use the law.
>
> (Sima, 19 years in the profession)

Sima described a state of neglect that has led to gangrene and putrefaction. Such a situation, in which the sores might become infected as a result of neglect, although not posing an immediate life-threatening situation, might become life threatening to the older person if no action is taken, even though the self-neglecting person does not appreciate the danger. In this type of scenario Sima, the social worker, described how she first tries to gain cooperation and appeals to the older person's common sense, talking to him to persuade him and explaining his dangerous condition. Furthermore, she tries to recruit other relevant persons to convince him, mainly people with whom the older person has an ongoing, trusting relationship. She does not rush to decide whether to resort to legal measures or to receive the necessary medical expert evaluations. However, at a certain point, the boundaries of this scenario touch and meet those of the previous scenarios: when all options are exhausted, when the potential threat to life increases significantly, her only possibility is to use the law.

Scenario C: Preventing Deterioration in the Absence of Immediate Risk

Scenario C deals with self-neglect situations among older adults with health issues who are cognitively competent and do not pose a danger to themselves or to the environment. In these cases, the scenario is different, as illustrated by Tamar:

> [In these cases] you don't need to go and change their lifestyle. If I see that he is really functioning properly with the self-neglect, never mind the dirt and the bad smell, I see that he is managing to function and is okay, then I keep in touch with him and nothing more. . . . Why do I need to do anything about it? After all, if he wants to live in squalor, then let him.
>
> (Tamar, 12 years in the profession)

Tamar described how she acts in the case of an older person who is functioning well despite self-neglect and poses neither an immediate threat nor a near-future threat to himself or to others. In this instance, the treatment can take the form of ongoing contact with no application to the legal system or to medical opinions.

The next quote illustrates how this ongoing contact can also involve an ongoing negotiation process for improving the self-neglectful older adult's living conditions:

> The man undoubtedly needs treatment, so he gets himself all kinds of carers, but it can't be on a permanent basis. He receives a stipend for special services but is not willing to exchange it for a nursing benefit. He is refusing treatment, as it were. I try to find all sorts of alternative solutions. I thought of maybe going down the legal path, but that's apparently no good, because he is completely mentally competent. I thought of exchanging the special services for a nursing benefit, and he told me that it's impossible. Now I want to check out a day center that could provide him with meals and showers. I also try to get along with him through humor. He comes with a request for a computer because he thinks that will make things easier for him. If he is able to type that might enable me to get other things for him. On the one hand, to humor him, and on the other hand, to introduce more services to which he is entitled.
>
> (Adi, 13 years in the profession)

Adi, the social worker, encounters an independent person who is not suffering from cognitive deterioration, but is in need of help. She negotiates with him about the various available services that could make his life easier. The older person is interested in a specific type of assistance and, in return, the social worker tries to persuade him to accept assistance for his neglect, satisfying his needs and his desires. She feels that by acting according to his wishes (in obtaining a computer), or even through the use of humor, she might succeed in introducing additional services that could assist him.

Scenario D: Environmental Nuisance

Scenario D describes self-neglect cases in which the core issue seems to be a nuisance to the environment (for example, hoarding, collecting garbage, or housing cats or dogs without any regard to personal or public hygiene or safety). In these cases, the self-neglectful older adult is of sound mind, without a clear health issue that needs medical intervention, but poses a nuisance to the surrounding environment. In such cases, Israel's legislation has a different (and general) set of laws that address cases of public nuisance (without any specific or necessary reference to elder self-neglect as such). Such laws are found not only in Israel's general torts law, but also in municipal bylaws, which differ from locality to locality. As described by Aliza, in such cases, the intervention takes the following form:

> In general, if there is neglect, in certain cases, we might need to make use of the nuisance law, like the Public Health Regulations. In these cases, we don't usually work alone, but with other authorities like the municipal sanitation authority. They need to go to the municipal court that deals with the sanitation bylaws, to obtain legal orders. We always go in "good ways" [i.e., without involuntary enforcement mechanisms], whether informally, in the "shadow" of the law, or formally and according to the law, in order to try to resolve the nuisance. In some places, we receive the authority of the social welfare officer because sometimes we need to see if they are putting themselves or their neighbors at risk and when we think [so], then we need to intervene, sometimes even via the law.
>
> (Aliza, 23 years in the profession)

As described by Aliza, sometimes the focus of the self-neglect is on its aspect as a public health nuisance. In such cases of a sanitation or health risk alongside an environmental nuisance, she must apply to the sanitation department at the local municipality, and together, they will try to resolve the case. Before formally using the public health legislation (which, unlike the Law for the Protection of the Helpless that focuses on the helpless person and intervention in his or her life, focuses on the environment and on the surrounding health conditions), she tries to use the law informally, or as she described it, as working "in the shadow of the law" (i.e., convincing the person to cooperate with the social worker under the understanding/threat that if he or she will not cooperate, the social worker will force the cooperation under a court order). Only if working informally does not produce results do the social workers then take formal measures ("in the light of the law") and use the law for the benefit of the older person and the environment (for example, enforced cleaning of the apartment or removal of hazardous materials). The aforementioned intervention scenarios are summarized in Table 15.1.

As can be seen in Table 15.1, the two key areas for assessment and attention are the severity of the older person's self-neglect, and the risk and harm to others and/or to the home environment. The outcome of the various interactions between these areas takes the form of whether to use the force of the law or to prefer softer negotiation and cooperation-based intervention. The preferable response and intervention will be negotiation, a clinical-therapeutic approach building relationships with older persons; however, some case scenarios necessitate a legal response.

Approaches and Intervention on an Individual Level

As reflected in the experience of the participants, the issue is not only when and how to intervene, but also to decide which intervention approach to adopt. In the encounter with the self-neglect phenomenon, the social workers in this research chose a variety of intervention approaches on the individual level, including clinical therapeutic, problem focused, integrative, and follow-up.

Clinical-Therapeutic Approach

Social workers who chose the clinical-therapeutic approach attributed importance to acknowledging the self-neglectful older adult's history in the context of tailoring the intervention and treatment, as illustrated by Sima:

> Whoever falls into the self-neglect category seems to have started from some point of crisis [turning point], and it is ongoing. It is not usually something that they can improve by themselves. . . . We make the connection, have one or two conversations, and gradually, after that, we make a home visit. That is, it's a relationship that is built very slowly. I look for certain points, some kind of strength, and through their strengths, I try to get them to cooperate. I think that, all in all, the therapeutic approach is good.
> (Sima, 19 years in the profession)

Sima described a situation in which the source of the self-neglect is not always clear, but she attributes importance to knowing the self-neglectful persons' history and to knowing about a crisis to which she can relate their situation. In the process that she initiates, she expresses the clinical-therapeutic approach to coping with self-neglect. The process includes establishing a long-term relationship of bonding and trust, in the hope of bringing about a change. During the process, the social worker tries to find and enlist "strengths" that might help achieve cooperation for change. These steps are designed to prevent the situation by which the social worker is perceived as an intruder or as threatening the older person. From the social worker's perspective, this slow, ongoing process is a vehicle for change. In other words, as part of the clinical-therapeutic approach, she tries to establish trust and lead a mutual process that will help the older person to find the inner strength for change.

Problem-Focused Approach

As opposed to the clinical-therapeutic approach, the problem-focused approach focuses on resolving the current situation of self-neglect, regardless of the life history of the self-neglectful older adults, as illustrated in the following quote:

> I know a lot about the [non-self-neglectful] older people whom I sit with once a week and do a broad intake [an extensive assessment of the client]. I have an

hour a week with them and a whole month where I might get to know them and hear their life story, and afterward, I sit with them for a year or a year and a half or 2 years of treatment, and I learn about their world. [However, in cases of self-neglect] I don't start learning about the world of the person suffering from self-neglect; I get specifics, I ask for a diagnosis, I ask for medical tests, I see the condition of the house, I check if there are any children to whom I can say that A, B, and C bother me. The intervention is much more specific, short term, it's not a therapy.

(Amalya, 6 years in the profession)

Unlike the clinical-therapeutic approach, which is based on regular meetings, Amalya described an approach that advocates a much more focused and short-term intervention. In the interviews, she was undecided as to whether to refer to this approach as therapy. It differs from what she perceives as the classic approach, which she uses with her non-self-neglectful clients. She focuses on the problem and the speedy diagnosis and solution to the problem.

Mixed and Integrated Approach

In their descriptions, some social workers expressed how they combine and integrate both the clinical as well as the problem-focused approach. This is illustrated in the following:

We [the social workers] go through some kind of process, and so do they [the self-neglectful older adults], at the end of which I can go to court and that is my obligation, and if not, then in fact, I am the one who will have to be answerable one day. There are times when it does help and there is some kind of change. Little things move. The goal is not to remove him from home right away, but to let him live in his own home with good service . . . I make an initial home visit and attempt to create that first connection and bonding and to get him to take care of himself. Sometimes it takes two meetings, not right away in the first meeting. When I see that it's not a success and I am afraid for his life, then I tell him that we have no choice but to involve the law. I explain the significance of my going to court and that I'm not the one to decide. He will be brought before a judge and will explain his position and the judge will decide whether we are right to be afraid for his life. Sometimes it helps and sometimes it doesn't.

(Tikvah, 20 years in the profession)

Tikvah tries to integrate the creation of a momentum in a clinically oriented way based on a change-based process ("little things move") with the problem-focused approach, which sometimes demands immediate intervention in life-threatening situations. For instance, an attempt is made to make room for the older person and to engage him in the treatment process. When the older person is not willing to cooperate, she turns to the court, in a more problem-focused manner.

Follow-Up

The final approach that arose in the interviews; is an approach of waiting for a change in the situation with continued follow-up, as illustrated by Ettie:

I have one woman who is caring for her husband alone and insists on not taking a foreign caregiver into the house. But she won't move him to a nursing home, either, and she is in a terrible state of self-neglect. I know that the first time anyone will be able to help will be when she has a fall. Those are the biggest dilemmas; when we sometimes know that nothing can be done with someone until they [*sic*] fall and something bad happens.

(Ettie, 17 years in the profession)

Ettie described the case of a self-neglectful couple who refused to receive help in the form of a foreign caregiver or by transferring the husband to an institution. Her approach is to remain on standby and to follow up on the situation in the knowledge that, one day, the reality will get worse because of aging and deterioration in the couple's functioning. A fall might bring about this change, potentially leading to an improvement in the situation of self-neglect.

In light of the older person's refusal to accept a wide variety of aids, the professionals do not give up, but move on to an alternative option of follow-up and control, as illustrated in the following quote:

[H]e used to cry bitterly, and at some stage, we used to stop listening because we saw that it wasn't leading anywhere. The man was completely clear-headed, and if that's how he wanted things to be, then so they would remain until the development of different circumstances that would allow . . . and it is never ending. We really tried to talk to him, we tried to persuade him to come out of this state of living, but he chooses to stay where he is . . . he says no . . . we presented him with all the possibilities, we tried to get him to talk and to convince him. He doesn't want to leave his home, so at least take a foreign caregiver to be with him around the clock because the man is bedridden, but he chose not . . . I think we went beyond the call of duty here. We stretched our capability to act to the limit here, and all we are doing today is a home visit from time to time. He is on our "red" list of people at high risk. The therapists . . . visit in the morning or in the afternoon and report if something isn't as it should be or if something has changed, or I don't know what; just to report.

(Vered, 26 years in the profession)

Vered described that the only help that this old man receives is home assistance in the form of two therapists who visit (morning and afternoon). The social worker has exhausted all the possibilities and intervention methods and the man's life is not in imminent danger, he is merely on the "red" list of people at high risk. The social workers chose to provide follow-up and control through therapists and other professionals who visit him at home. They are supposed to report any change for the worse in his situation.

Approaches to Intervention on the Societal Level

In the encounter with the self-neglect phenomenon, the social workers chose a variety of intervention approaches not only on the individual level but also on the more macro and societal levels. Specifically, these interventions included a multidisciplinary approach, awareness raising, and raising the issue of budgetary constraints.

Therapeutic Approach and Multidisciplinary Cooperation

On the system-wide level, within their intervention with self-neglecting older persons, the professionals attributed importance to multidisciplinary cooperation. This meant cooperation between the different welfare departments where they worked and the various other authorities and organizations in the community, including health funds (health maintenance organizations [HMOs]), hospitals, nongovernmental organizations, and so on. For example, Inbal raised the issue of the health systems' lack of cooperation, as follows:

> In the last case, I put pressure on the health fund [HMO]. I brought everyone there, the psychiatrists, the fund's social worker, the doctor. I forced them all to make home visits. I put pressure on the family doctor because you need special authorization for a psychiatrist to make a home visit. I was actually the one to manage this case. I think that the health care system is not aware enough of the need to inform us [the social welfare system]. You often have to pressurise the doctors, who are insufficiently aware of the issue of reporting harm and helpless people. The feeling is that the doctors don't cooperate enough with us in general because either they are very loyal to their patients or they are very scared that we will take extreme steps like removal from home. There isn't enough interest, in my opinion; I think there is not enough awareness about reporting and working in cooperation with us. We are working on this issue.
>
> (Inbal, 12 years in the profession)

Inbal describes an experience of helplessness and frustration derived from the need to push and to "force" the pertinent staff to make home visits. She describes the effort she had to make to lead the joint work of a multidisciplinary team. She explains why, in her opinion, cooperation is lacking: starting from a lack of awareness, through loyalty to the older person and fear that the welfare services will institutionalize the person, to a lack of social workers in the health system.

A contrasting experience of cooperation with authorities working in parallel is described in the following:

> In general, as social workers, we work with the health funds on a daily basis, with the Ministry of Housing, clubs, day centers, all sorts of community authorities; there is the Supportive Neighborhood. We work with them. We are in contact with these people almost every day. They know us, we know them. Everyone knows what can help so this cooperation is very profitable. We often hear about a self-neglectful person through one of these authorities and then the contact is made.
>
> (Sima, 19 years in the profession)

Sima described enlistment and cooperation of all the care authorities relevant to treating the self-neglect phenomenon. Her words reveal that all pertinent communication channels were open and interventions included input by each of the authorities, who had a joint aim—working toward providing assistance and treatment for the self-neglectful older adult.

Raising Awareness and Information Dissemination

In addition to the importance of cooperation, the social workers also mentioned the importance that they attributed to disseminating information and raising awareness of the phenomenon of self-neglect in the public in general, and among professionals in particular. This is illustrated in the following:

> I think that all the young women and young men who leave the school of social work to become social workers need to be made aware of this subject [self-neglect among older adults]. Until a year ago, we had an excellent project, which isn't continuing at present, that first-year medical students came to us with social workers throughout a semester to deal with cases and to see what's happening, what constitutes neglect, etc. I think that communication can really help here. I think that communication on the subject helps a lot . . . to raise awareness . . . in medical schools, among hospital doctors, sick-fund doctors, and schools of nursing. It seems to me that the teaching part and the educational part is [sic] currently one of the most important components.
>
> (Aliza, 23 years in the profession)

Aliza emphasized the importance of raising awareness in all the health professions, mainly among social work students, medical students, physicians, and nursing students. In her view, communication plays an important part in education and training, which in turn can lead to better and more effective treatment and can also contribute to changing attitudes about older adults engaged in self-neglectful behavior.

The next quote from one participant reinforces the need for information dissemination and raising awareness in the general public:

> The general public has very little awareness of self-neglect. It is not considered as abuse. This is a gray area at this time. People are not aware of older people's needs. It needs to be brought to people's notice that self-neglect is also abuse because people think that neglect isn't so terrible. It is better that he shouldn't eat at all than that he should eat too much, and all sorts of things . . . themselves, all sorts of stories that people tell themselves about neglect. But if self-neglect is included in the definition of abuse, like has already happened, then it only needs to be brought to other people's notice. Through the media, in films, even as a law.
>
> (Ettie, 17 years in the profession)

Public Policy Priorities and Budgeting

Another key issue raised by the social workers was the need to address the lack of appropriate budgeting and resource prioritizing in this field. This "neglecting the neglected" phenomenon is manifest in the lack of time, budget, staff, and intervention services. This is illustrated in the following:

> When there is no imminent risk to life, self-neglect is not on the priority list of the welfare agencies. It is not considered to be an important topic. . . . We forgot the values of social work, and in my opinion, self-neglect should be one of the top priorities, but it is not. Follow-up is almost impossible because we have 300 other clients. We do not honor our time schedule. Social

workers who work with older persons have a tremendous overload. . . . I believe that proper funding is needed.

(Odelia, 20 years in the profession)

Odelia described the lack of money needed to establish an appropriate intervention framework. According to her words, the social workers who are responsible for older clients are overloaded with work in general, but also with administrative duties, which do not leave them enough time for the actual care of the self-neglectful older adults. Moreover, the burden and overload harm the actual care provided to the older person, and, in this context, people who self-neglect do not receive the required attention. These issues are also echoed in the following:

I have a deep-rooted experience with a professional saying to me: "Don't bring us troubles." What does this mean? It means that the social welfare services are so overloaded that they do not want any extra work or responsibility. Moreover, why do we have to make an effort for people who do not want our assistance? At the moment, I don't believe that there are adequate services for self-neglectful older adults; it is convenient to leave them in such a reality and ignore them. These people can sometimes be in great distress but we don't have the resources to deal with them.

(Amalya, 6 years in the profession)

Persons who self-neglect are perceived as persons who refuse to receive assistance and treatment, and hence, in the context of overload, they are viewed as a waste of precious time. The overall "spirit" is then not to "raise" new issues when there is insufficient time and resources to deal with existing issues.

LIMITATIONS

This study was limited as it did not include significant viewpoints such as that of the self-neglecting elders themselves or their family members. Their voices and experiences are crucial for better understanding of the complete social picture regarding the meaning of the professional experience and impact on the realm of elder self-neglect. Future studies should focus on capturing these voices. In addition, the legal aspect of the self-neglect phenomenon should also be explored, through legal examination based on textual analysis of laws and court judgments. Furthermore, the sample was limiting because of the similar background and professional environment of the participants.

CONCLUSION

Professionals face difficulties in understanding and coping with older adults engaged in self-neglectful behavior. Nevertheless, they are expected to provide care and assistance, and to intervene for the prevention of harm. The complexity of the self-neglect phenomenon is experienced not only on the personal level, but also on the interpersonal, societal, and professional levels. As seen in the findings of this research, to provide appropriate intervention, the social workers developed intervention strategies based on the tension and the need for balance between preserving autonomy, protecting human rights, and respecting the older persons' wishes versus paternalism and client safety.

This attempt to find a "balanced" intervention approach was manifested in decision-making patterns based on different interventions, which attempted to try to answer not only the questions of when and how to intervene, but which approaches were appropriate to adopt. Each scenario related to the older person's level of risk and to the characteristics and severity of the neglect.

The different scenarios are a kind of "oral law" or practice wisdom (Chu & Tsui, 2008; Osmond, 2006). They were acquired through the social workers' years of work and experience. The nature of the self-neglect exposes the professionals to the use of accompanying knowledge and is expressed in attitudes, assumptions, and values and in their personal involvement regarding the phenomenon (Osmond, 2006; Rosen, 1994). In this context, the construction and choice of an intervention are the product of the use and the "infusion" of their existing knowledge regarding their accumulated experiences, which are a kind of practice wisdom. Practice wisdom made use of by social workers in the encounter with the self-neglect phenomenon is of great importance. It is used daily as a coping strategy, and it assists social workers in settling the constant tension between the personal and the professional.

However, it is important to note that these scenarios, which are the outcome of practice wisdom, are not based on empirical or evidence-based practice. In other words, it is not fully clear if, and to what extent, these scenarios actually provide the appropriate response to the needs of all self-neglecting older adults. Hence, there is need for future research to evaluate the success and/or failure of the different intervention scenarios described previously.

Moving from the intervention scenarios to a variety of approaches to address the phenomenon, it was found that, on the one hand, professionals have diverse instruments in their "tool box" for assessing older persons engaged in self-neglectful behavior. However, there is still a gap—in priorities, funding, and public awareness—between the capabilities of the social workers and their actual ability to execute and perform their duties. The actual outcome is that self-neglecting persons do not receive the appropriate and comprehensive treatment that they deserve and need.

IMPLICATIONS FOR RESEARCH AND PRACTICE

- Based on this research, it is apparent that each self-neglecting scenario warranted a different approach, as exemplified in this study.
- From a social policy perspective, the findings of this study point to the need to challenge the existing policy in the field of self-neglect among older adults.
- There is a need to address the phenomenon of self-neglect through a multidisciplinary approach, combining all relevant agencies and establishing integrated cooperation at the national and local levels.
- Funding needs to be allocated to address prevention, detection, intervention, and awareness.
- There is a need to change existing training programs by emphasizing a self-reflection process as an integral part of the professional intervention.
- Future research could focus on a more balanced professional perception between the genders by including more male social workers and comparing their meanings and experiences with those of the female social workers. The seniority variable could also be addressed, exploring the influence of seniority on burnout and stress issues in the context of treating elder self-neglect.

REFERENCES

Abrams, R. C., Lachs, M., McAvay, G., Keohane, D. J., & Bruce, M. L. (2002). Predictors of self-neglect in community-dwelling elders. *American Journal of Psychiatry, 159*(10), 1724–1730. doi:10.1176/appi.ajp.159.10.1724

Al-Haj, M. (1988). The changing Arab kinship structure: The effect of modernization in an urban community. *Economic Development and Cultural Change, 36*, 237–258. Retrieved from http://www.jstor.org/stable/1153766

Al-Haj, M. (2004). The political culture of the 1990s immigrants from the former Soviet Union in Israel and their views toward the indigenous Arab minority: A case of ethnocratic multiculturalism. *Journal of Ethnic and Migration Studies, 30*, 681–696. doi:10.1080/13691830410001699513

Alon, S., & Doron, I. (2009). Elder neglect: Theoretical, legal, and practical aspects [in Hebrew]. *Gerontology, 36*(1), 69–92.

Anetzberger, G. J. (2005). The reality of elder abuse. *Clinical Gerontologist, 28*(1–2), 1–25. doi:10.1300/J018v28n01_01

Band-Winterstein, T., & Alon, S. (2015). Theoretical knowledge and practice wisdom: Toward a comprehensive model for addressing elder abuse and neglect. In K. Jagielska, J. Malgorzata Lokasik, & N. G. Pikula (Eds.), *Violence against the elderly: Challenges—research—action.* Toronto, ON, Canada: Nova Printing.

Bar-Tur, L., & Hantman, S. (2010). Frontline therapists: Intervention methods to support elder-care therapists in times of war [in Hebrew]. *Gerontology, 37*(4), 43–58.

Bell, H. (2003). Strengths and secondary trauma in family violence work. *Social Work, 48*, 513–522. doi:10.1093/sw/48.4.513

Burnes, D., Pillemer, K., & Lachs, M. S. (2016). Elder abuse severity: A critical but understudied dimension of victimization for clinicians and researchers. *The Gerontologist*, 1–12. doi:10.1093/geront/gnv688

Burnett, J., Regev, T., Pickens, S., Prati, L. L., Aung, K., Moore, J., & Dyer, C. B. (2006). Social networks: A profile of the elderly who self-neglect. *Journal of Elder Abuse & Neglect, 18*(4), 35–49. doi:10.1300/J084v18n04_05

Campbell, R., & Wasco, S. M. (2005). Understanding rape and sexual assault: 20 years of progress and future directions. *Journal of Interpersonal Violence, 20*(1), 127–131. doi:10.1177/0886260504268604

Chu, W. C. K., & Tsui, M. (2008). The nature of practice wisdom in social work revisited. *International Social Work, 51*, 47–54. doi:10.1177/0020872807083915

Creswell, J. W. (2007). *Qualitative inquiry and research design: Choosing among five approaches* (2nd ed.). Thousand Oaks, CA: Sage.

Dekel, R., & Peled, E. (2000). Staff burnout in Israeli battered women's shelters. *Journal of Social Service Research, 26*(3), 65–76. doi:10.1300/J079v26n03_04

Doron, I., Alon, S., & Nissim, O. (2005). Time for Policy: Legislative response to elder abuse and neglect in Israel. *Journal of Elder Abuse & Neglect, 16*(4), 63–82.

Doron, I., Band-Winterstein, T., & Kornfield, M. (2016). Elder self-neglect: The Israeli legal response [in Hebrew]. *Alei-Mishpat, 13*, 219–259.

Doron, I., Band-Winterstein, T., & Naim, S. (2013). The meaning of self-neglect: Social workers' perspective. *International Journal of Aging and Human Development, 77*(1), 17–36. doi:10.1177/088626000015004004

Dutton, M. A. (1992). *Empowering and healing the battered women.* New York, NY: Springer Publishing.

Figley, C. R. (Ed.). (1995). *Compassion fatigue.* New York, NY: Brunner/Mazel.

Goldblatt, H. (2009). Caring for abused women: Impact on nurses' professional and personal life experiences. *Journal of Advanced Nursing, 65*, 1645–1654. doi:10.1111/j.1365-2648.2009.05019.x

Goldblatt, H., & Buchbinder, E. (2003). Challenging gender roles: The impact on female social work students of working with abused women. *Journal of Social Work Education, 39*(2), 255–275. doi:10.1080/10437797.2003.10779135

Goldblatt, H., Buchbinder, E., Eisikovits, Z., & Arizon-Messinger, I. (2009). Between the professional and private: The meaning of working with intimate partner violence in social workers' private lives. *Violence Against Women, 15*, 362–384. doi:10.1177/1077801208330436

Iliffe, G., & Steed, L. G. (2000). Exploring the counselor's experience of working with perpetrators and survivors of domestic violence. *Journal of Interpersonal Violence, 15*(4), 393–412. doi:10.1177/088626000015004004

Jenkins, S. R., & Baird, S. (2002). Secondary traumatic stress and vicarious trauma: A validational study. *Journal of Traumatic Stress, 15*(5), 423–432. doi:10.1023/A:1020193526843

Kvale, S. (1996). *Interviews*. Thousand Oaks, CA: Sage.

Lincoln, Y. S., & Guba, E. G. (1985). *Naturalistic inquiry*. Beverly Hills, CA: Sage.

Linley, P. A., & Joseph, S. (2006). The positive and negative effects of disaster work: A preliminary investigation. *Journal of Loss and Trauma, 11*, 229–245. doi:10.1080/15325020500494186

Lowenstein, A., & Doron, I. (2008). Times of transition: Elder abuse and neglect in Israel. *Journal of Elder Abuse & Neglect, 20*(2), 181–206. doi:10.1080/08946560801974695

Mautner, M. (1993). *The decline of formalism and the ascension of values in Israeli law* [in Hebrew]. Tel Aviv, Israel: Ma'agalei Da'at.

McCann, I. L., & Pearlman, L. A. (1990). *Psychological trauma and the adult survivor: Theory, therapy, and transformation*. New York, NY: Brunner/Mazel.

McDermott, S. (2010). Professional judgments of risk and capacity in situations of self neglect among older people. *Ageing & Society, 30*, 1055–1072. doi:10.1017/S0144686X10000139

Miller, I. (1998). Our own medicine: Traumatized psychotherapists and the stresses of doing therapy. *Psychotherapy, 35*, 137–146. doi:10.1037/h0087708

Morse, J. M. (2000). Determining sample size. *Qualitative Health Research, 10*(1), 3–5. doi:10.1177/104973200129118183

Moustakas, C. (1994). *Phenomenological research methods*. Newbury Park, CA: Sage.

Osmond, J. (2006). A quest for form: The tacit dimension of social work practice. *European Journal of Social Work, 9*(2), 159–181.

Patton, M. Q. (2002). *Qualitative research and evaluation methods*. Thousand Oaks, CA: Sage.

Payne, B. K., & Gainey, R. R. (2005). Differentiating self-neglect as a type of elder mistreatment: How do these cases compare to traditional types of elder mistreatment? *Journal of Elder Abuse & Neglect, 17*(1), 21–36. doi:10.1300/J084v17n01_02

Poythress, E. L., Burnett, J., Naik, A. D., Pickens, S., & Dyer, C. B. (2007). Severe self-neglect: An epidemiological and historical perspective. *Journal of Elder Abuse & Neglect, 18*(4), 5–12. doi:10.1300/J084v18n04_02

Rees, J., King, L., & Schmitz, K. (2009). Nurses' perceptions of ethical issues in the care of older people. *Nursing Ethics, 16*(4), 436–452. doi:10.1177/0969733009104608

Rosen, A. (1994). Knowledge use in direct practice. *Social Service Review, 68*(4), 561–577.

Slattery, S. M., & Goodman, L. A. (2009). Secondary traumatic stress among domestic violence advocates: Workplace risk and protective factors. *Violence Against Women, 15*(11), 1358–1379. doi:10.1177/1077801209347469

Strauss, A., & Corbin, J. (1997). *Grounded theory in practice*. London, UK: Sage.

Trevitt, C., & Gallagher, E. (1996). Elder abuse in Canada and Australia: Implications for nurses. *International Journal of Nursing Studies, 33*, 651–659. doi:10.1016/S00207489(96)00022-3

Trippany, R. L., White Kress, V. E., & Wilcoxon, S. A. (2004). Preventing vicarious trauma: What counselors should know when working with trauma survivors. *Journal of Counseling & Development, 82*, 31–37. doi:10.1002/j.1556-6678.2004.tb00283.x

Walker, M. (2004). Supervising practitioners working with survivors of childhood abuse: Counter transference, secondary traumatization and terror. *Psychodynamic Practice, 10*, 173–193. doi:10.10 80/14753630410001686753

Way, I., VanDeusen, K. M., Martin, G., Applegate, B., & Jandle, D. (2004). Vicarious trauma: A comparison of clinicians who treat survivors of sexual abuse and sexual offenders. *Journal of Interpersonal Violence, 19*(1), 49–71. doi:10.1177/0886260503259050

Weiss, I., & Welbourne, P. (Eds.). (2007). *Social work as a profession: A comparative cross-national perspective.* Birmingham, UK: Venture Press.

CHAPTER 16

HOW THE CITY OF CHICAGO ADDRESSES THE ISSUE OF SELF-NEGLECT AMONG SENIORS

Paul Dowling and Katharine Slover

The purpose of this chapter is to examine the extent to which helping professionals can facilitate positive change to the circumstances ("success") of self-neglecting older adults. We explore what it means to be successful in this context, and identify the areas where there is the most impact in improved functioning or stability. The Intensive Case Advocacy and Support program (ICAS) pioneered by the Chicago Department of Family & Support Services (DFSS)/Senior Services provides the backdrop against which these elements are explored. This chapter includes a history, program overview, client case studies to illustrate the reality of service provision, and a review of and update on quantitative research on program outcomes and provider agency survey responses.

Self-neglect remains an intractable, often hidden, and growing problem among older adults in Chicago. Chicago's DFSS/Senior Services and Area Agency on Aging have devised a method to address self-neglect among seniors in Chicago, through its innovative ICAS program.

HISTORY AND PROGRAM OVERVIEW

ICAS is one of the several programs hosted by DFSS, whose role is to support and coordinate services for city of Chicago residents:

> The Chicago Department of Family & Support Services (DFSS; 2016) is dedicated to supporting a continuum of coordinated services to enhance the lives of Chicago residents, particularly those most in need, from birth through the senior years. It works to promote the independence and well-being of individuals, support families and strengthen neighborhoods by providing direct assistance and administering resources to a network of community-based organizations, social service providers, and institutions.

The ICAS program is an offshoot of the city's long-running Senior Services Well-Being Task Force, an initiative that itself stemmed from concerns about seniors' ability for self-care in general, and in relation to summer heat emergencies in particular. The devastating 2003 heat wave across Europe, in which at least 35,000 people died—most of whom were elderly—brought to mind the July 1995 Chicago heatwave in which 700 died, 72% of whom were older than 65 years of age (Larsen, 2003). With these deadly events in mind, in 2003, the Well-Being Task Force began to develop best practices and collaboration of city and community organizations to foster safety and stability for older adults living in Chicago.

Since inception, the Well-Being Task Force has been composed of richly diverse sources. These include human services nonprofit organizations focused on older adult programming, city departments (buildings, streets and sanitation, water management, etc.), community mental health organizations, utility companies, hospitals and universities, faith-based councils, state of Illinois departments (Aging, Human Services), first responders (Chicago Police and Fire Departments), and many others.

This comprehensive, dynamic convergence of providers resulted in several significant accomplishments that brought substantive assistance to seniors in need. Over 30,000 field workers, including utility meter readers, cable company workers, garbage collectors, hospital emergency room personnel, and others, were trained to look for basic signs of neglect. Observations, such as newspapers or mail piling up on a front porch, an overgrown yard, or a senior outside dressed inappropriately for the weather, were shared with field workers as potential concerns. Field workers were strongly encouraged to be aware of such conditions and to simply call 3-1-1, Chicago's nonemergency information and assistance system, to report community issues. These calls generated a well-being check to determine whether the senior needed assistance.

During this same time period, the early- to mid-2000s, the state of Illinois (in which the city of Chicago is located) added language about self-neglect to the statute governing elder abuse. Although the Elder Abuse Act had been law in Illinois since 1988, self-neglect was not added until 2006; however, there was no funding attached to the self-neglect portion of this measure.

In order to provide funding so that self-neglect law could be enforced, DFSS/Senior Services leadership proposed using Community Development Block Grant (CDBG) money.

Enacted in 1974 as a means to "develop viable urban communities," CDBG is administered by the U.S. Department of Housing and Urban Development (HUD; 2016) (Figure 16.1). This is an entitlement program in which larger U.S. cities receive funds to delegate to organizations that successfully apply for program activities to aid the

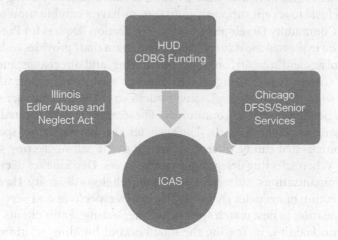

Figure 16.1 The ICAS structure.

CDBG, Community Development Block Grant; DFSS, Department of Family and Support Services; HUD, the U.S. Department of Housing and Urban Development; ICAS, Intensive Case Advocacy and Support.

enhancement of urban settings. CDBG allows for flexible and creative programs that can fit specific community needs. Chicago's DFSS/Senior Services leadership was successful in obtaining CDBG funds to address self-neglect among seniors in Chicago.

The result of this funding, which commenced in 2010, is known as Intensive Case Advocacy and Support (CAS) program. DFSS is responsible for the overall design and oversight of the ICAS program. It stipulates general policy and procedure for how the community agencies provide supportive services to self-neglectful seniors in the program.

Seniors are referred in one of two ways for participation in the ICAS program. As previously mentioned, hundreds of calls are received through 3-1-1, Chicago's nonemergency assistance line. The other avenue for referrals consists of calls that are made directly to the city's main senior services phone number.

If the CAS worker's assessment indicates the senior is not in imminent danger, but does appear to be self-neglectful and in need of further support, the CAS worker will report same to the city. That process is what leads to a senior's case being designated as ICAS (Intensive Case Advocacy and Support). Those cases are then assigned out by Chicago Department of Family and Support Services/Senior Services staff to one of the ten agencies that are contracted to provide case management and related services to self-neglectful seniors. The CAS team from an agency—also contracted with DFSS—makes the initial field assessment of the senior's condition. Should the senior be assessed as having an immediate, emergency situation or as in imminent danger, the CAS worker can intervene as deemed necessary to ensure the senior is safe. The CAS worker can call 9-1-1 (the city's emergency services phone number) for any police and/or fire department and emergency medical support required. On the other hand, if stabilization of the senior's situation appears to simply require in-home services, the CAS worker can make referrals for supportive care such as home-delivered meals. When the CAS assessment shows the senior to be appropriate for self-neglect intervention, the CAS worker alerts DFSS/Senior Services staff. The DFSS staff then refer to one of the 10 contracted agencies for this purpose.

Typically, a referral for ICAS is made when a senior is found to have a complex set of needs that require intensive, ongoing support in order to resolve and stabilize the senior's situation. Seniors who are referred for ICAS most frequently have either cognitive and/or mental health issues, unsafe/unsanitary living environments, as well as refusal to accept supportive services, or have a combination of these factors. As per the Community Development Grant Application Request for Proposals 2017–18, ICAS can be expressed most succinctly as a program that "provides in-home assessment, case advocacy and support, on-going monitoring, and direct assistance for at-risk seniors."

Currently, ICAS engages 10 Chicago nonprofit organizations to help stabilize the situations of self-neglecting seniors so that they can successfully remain living independently in the community. These agencies are located throughout the city in various neighborhoods. The agencies also have specific, specialized services and resources that can be offered as needed to the self-neglecting senior.

When selecting delegate/partner agencies, DFSS makes decisions in part based on the organizations' cultural, ethnic, and religious diversity. Having a comprehensive collection of agencies that offer distinct perspectives and services provides a strong foundation to best match specific self-neglecting senior clients with those who share commonalities, increasing the likelihood of building relationships and generating positive outcomes for the senior.

These unique factors are taken into account when the referral is made. For example, the Chicago Mitzvah Campaign (2016) is designed to, "assist individuals with information, social support and material aid, and avail them of spiritual counsel,

Jewish traditions and observances." Clearly, this would be relevant and a good fit for Jewish seniors who self-neglect. Housing Opportunities and Maintenance for the Elderly (H.O.M.E., 2016), another ICAS-delegated agency, offers a home-repair program. H.O.M.E. is, therefore, a good referral fit for self-neglecting senior home-owners who may need a new door lock or a toilet or bathtub repaired.

ICAS is designed to meet six predominant goals:

- Establish a trusting relationship with each senior.
- Make the senior aware of the issues that are causing problems for the senior, and the negative impacts of these issues.
- Educate the senior on available programs, services, and referrals that may be able to moderate or reverse the problematic situation or issue.
- Assist the senior in accepting necessary services, which can help improve and stabilize the senior's situation.
- Advocate for the senior in order to establish helpful services.
- Follow up to monitor the senior and the situation to ensure ongoing care.

Each goal builds upon the previous goals in the sequence. Taken as a whole, these goals serve to stabilize the senior's living situation.

MAJOR ICAS GOALS

Establish a Trusting Relationship

Isolation and lack of social interactions are almost always core elements of the self-neglecting senior's condition. Such seniors may have no remaining family, or family members may be estranged from, or living far from, the senior in need. Long-standing mental health issues or more recent dementia may leave the senior unable to interact appropriately with others. Such factors leave the self-neglecting senior without a so-cial network or resources to draw on when needs arise. One of the central tenets of the ICAS program, and a deeply held belief of the organizations that administer it, is that success in working with vulnerable, self-neglecting seniors often depends on the extent to which a meaningful rapport can be established with each senior client. This relationship, based on trust and mutual respect, can be leveraged to help the senior reach a point at which he or she has an increased understanding of the issues she or he is experiencing and is the basis of support to make positive changes. It is both revolutionary and foundational that previously isolated seniors, who lacked a social safety net, now have someone they trust. Creating such a relationship, however, can be quite challenging. Self-neglecting seniors are very often mistrustful and may have been taken advantage of by others in the past. Many self-neglecting seniors also seem to fear—not unreasonably—that allowing someone in to help, may in fact, bring about changes the senior does not want, even if objectively those changes would be positive.

Bring Awareness of Issues/Concerns

Self-neglecting seniors rarely can see or understand the issues they face that de-stabilize their living situations. An ICAS client may have a rodent infestation, for example, and see the rats as his "friends" rather than as a serious sanitation issue.

Living without a working toilet and using plastic bags and bottles to store human waste may result in a shrug. Water pipes that burst in winter as a result of no heat in the building may be accommodated by simply buying bottled water and eating less to avoid having to use a toilet that no longer has water in it. A hole in the roof that results in flooding on the second floor does not concern the senior, who no longer can walk upstairs anyway. Once a strong, trusting relationship is underway, the ICAS worker can begin to point out these issues and concerns and help the senior to recognize there are far better options.

Educate the Seniors

As isolation is a key underpinning of self-neglect, seniors may be unaware of community referrals, resources, programs, and services that can alleviate some of the issues they face. For example, ICAS agencies can refer their senior clients for assessments for home-delivered meals and homemaking services. The agencies can refer to the city for the Heavy Duty Chore (HDC) program, which consists of "extensive cleaning for those clients whose living conditions pose a threat to their health and safety" (City of Chicago, 2016). Other possibilities include adult day programs to reduce isolation, transportation for medical appointments, legal aid advice or representation, help with public benefit or energy assistance applications, home repairs, and moving help.

A self-neglecting senior may need one or more resources to help stabilize his or her living situation and to ensure the viability of safely aging in place. These same seniors may be unaware that such resources exist. The seniors also frequently do not acknowledge the need for this type of help. That is why developing a trusting relationship initially is crucial. Once that has been established, the senior is much more likely to have faith in the point of view and recommendations of the ICAS caseworker.

Help the Seniors Accept Necessary Services

Seniors can be reluctant to engage with support services for a variety of reasons. As mentioned earlier, many self-neglecting seniors do not have a great deal of insight into the issues they face and are often unwilling or unable to perceive their situation as problematic. When this is the case, merely educating the senior about the existence of community programs and supports that could be of assistance to them is unlikely to yield any significant positive changes. Even seniors who do understand the perils of their situations can refuse to engage with services because of anxiety, concerns around privacy, or shame. Having a self-neglecting senior agree to engage with support services can be a very lengthy process involving continued, consistent encouragement from the ICAS caseworker. The trusting relationship built between the ICAS caseworker and the senior must be leveraged to allay the senior's trepidations or bring the senior to a place where he or she has a better understanding of the prevalent issues.

Advocate for the Establishment of Services

Although convincing a senior to accept support services can be the most challenging part of making positive changes to the circumstances, it is only one part of the change process. Unfortunately, support services are often overburdened and susceptible to long wait times. A delay in the onset of services creates opportunities for seniors to change their minds. A senior who is still not entirely convinced of the want/need of support services will use even minor setbacks as a reason to refuse services. The caseworker must continue to nurture the senior's openness to services while simultaneously working to expedite the application and assessment process to ensure the initiation of services as quickly as possible. The ICAS worker will very often have to attend assessment meetings with service providers and facilitate the initiation of services.

Follow Up to Ensure Ongoing Care

Although ICAS is designed to be a short-term intervention, aftercare is an important element of the program. During the ICAS process, seniors are often asked to make significant changes that can initially be emotionally unsettling for them. The ICAS worker must try to guide seniors through the readjustment period. For a senior, the time following the initiation of support services can be fraught with challenges. The client must learn to interact with providers to schedule services. There can be personality clashes with providers as well as issues around disrupted services, whether on the part of the senior or the provider. A senior's desire to continue receiving services can be tenuous and the ICAS worker may need to provide follow-up support or to continue to act as a mediator between the senior and the service provider to protect the advances that have been made. The authors present two case studies (both worst and best case) of ICAS senior clients to illustrate and clarify the stages in this process.

DESIGNING FOR SUCCESS: KEY FEATURES OF THE ICAS PROGRAM

Understanding both the importance of building strong relationships with clients and the challenges involved in doing so, the DFSS set about crafting a program that would enhance the chances of developing such a connection. The broad parameters of the ICAS program allow caseworkers greater flexibility in how they interact with clients and the services they can provide. This increased scope greatly improves the chances that a meaningful relationship can be established with difficult-to-engage clients and that positive change can be facilitated.

The DFSS works with a variety of community-based agencies from an array of cultural and spiritual backgrounds. This allows clients to be "matched" with caseworks whom they view as being more relatable to them. This sense of affinity with a caseworker based on a perceived commonality can jumpstart the relationship-building process. This is not to say that all clients will invariably accept services from a caseworker from a similar background, nor does it suggest that caseworkers and clients from different backgrounds can't work very effectively together.

Duration of Contact

Despite the short-term nature of their services, ICAS agencies are encouraged to make repeated attempts to engage with clients. Clients often become more receptive to a caseworker if consistent attempts are made to engage them over a longer period of time. It is not uncommon for seniors to initially decline all services and refuse to engage with the ICAS caseworker. Despite this, the ICAS program allows caseworkers to be persistent in their efforts and continue to visit the senior. Often a senior will only be ready or willing to work with a caseworker when he or she has experienced a crisis such as a fall, utility shut-off, or eviction notice. Seniors who are socially isolated may have no one else they can or will call on for assistance. The senior remembers the persistent visits and offers of assistance from the ICAS caseworker and reaches out for help. Sometimes, it is months after a caseworker has tried to engage a senior that a call for assistance is made.

CASE STUDY 1: Ms. H

Establish a Trusting Relationship

Ms. H, a 66-year-old woman presenting with apparent mental health concerns, including paranoia, was referred to an ICAS provider because she was losing her home for failure to pay property taxes. Ms. H had refused to pay her taxes. She said since the house was paid for, she owned it, and therefore the government could not make her pay further. Our role was to help her accept this significant loss while finding appropriate alternate housing for her. Ms. H, however, refused to discuss her situation with the caseworker and stated she did not need help. The caseworker received the same response on each visit. Visits were frequent, given that eviction was looming and finding appropriate housing was urgent.

Make the Senior Aware of Issues Causing Problems

Despite ongoing negative responses from Ms. H, her caseworker tried several times to explain what had happened to Ms. H's house, and why. The senior's response, however, remained the same. She refused all efforts of help.

Educate the Senior

Ms. H's caseworker gave her many applications for housing and offered several times to escort her to see various housing options. Ms. H declined all such offers. Meanwhile, the eviction date grew nearer.

Assist the Senior to Accept Necessary Services

Despite prior refusals, the caseworker continued offering Ms. H help with housing applications and in going to see housing alternatives. Ms. H continued to refuse all offers of help and often refused to even meet with the caseworker.

Advocate for the Senior to Establish Helpful Services

The caseworker offered to alert Ms. H's adult daughter to this crisis, so the family could offer support as well. (Ms. H would not sign a release-of-information form, so the caseworker could not share this news, even with family.) Ms. H continued to refuse.

Follow Up to Monitor the Senior and the Situation to Ensure Ongoing Care

Despite all refusals from Ms. H to accept assistance, the caseworker was present when officials evicted her from the premises. The daughter was also present, having been called by Ms. H. The daughter stated that in her culture, respecting the parents' wishes comes before all else, and she therefore could not intercede against her mother's command. The caseworker was able to prevent Ms. H from being arrested for her behavior toward the police officers, but even at eviction, Ms. H would not accept housing help of any kind. Ms. H instead instructed her daughter to rent a moving truck, and she drove off with some of her belongings. The caseworker continued calling Ms. H to continue trying to help her find housing. Ms. H rarely answered or returned the caseworker's calls, and continued her resistance to any form of help. The caseworker later heard via voicemail that this senior was living in the basement of a former associate's house in suburban Chicago. Later, Ms. H temporarily moved out of the state to live with a family member. She occasionally calls the caseworker, but still does not agree to meet or accept any help to become stably housed.

CASE STUDY 2: Mr. O

Mr. O is a 92-year-old male immigrant from Eastern Europe. He walks with a cane but seems to get around well enough to spend most of his day out in the community. Mr. O has no family in the United States. Mr. O has a strong Catholic faith. He attends mass weekly and is part of a congregation originally from his country of origin.

Concerns were raised by Mr. O's bank. On several occasions, he had tried to withdraw considerable sums of money stating that he needed to give it to the people who had been calling him on the phone. Mr. O had given personal financial and identifying information to these callers and they had tried to make a large online transfer from his account. The bank blocked the transaction and had been refusing to give Mr. O the money he had been trying to withdraw. The bank made referrals to DFSS and the Office of the Public Guardian (OPG), which becomes the guardian of those who are deemed to lack the cognitive capacity to be their own agents.

Mr. O lived alone in a second-floor studio apartment. The home was very dirty, bug infested, and had a foul odor. Neighbors had complained about the smell coming from Mr. O's apartment. Although he always paid rent on time and has not caused any other trouble in the building, the condition of his apartment and his reluctance to work with the building exterminator have been enough for building management to threaten eviction.

Establish a Trusting Relationship With Each Senior

Initially, Mr. O interacted politely with the caseworker while insisting he had everything he needed. He concluded conversations as quickly as possible. Mr. O allowed the caseworker into his home on the second visit but again refused any services and very quickly ended the interaction. The caseworker visited Mr. O on a weekly basis and brought food from a nearby restaurant, which the client enjoyed. Mr. O gradually began to interact for longer periods of time and engage in conversation around the issues raised by his building manager and the bank. Although not from the same country, the caseworker was also an immigrant and Mr. O enjoyed finding out more about the caseworker's country of origin and opinions about life in the United States. Once a more solid relationship had been established, Mr. O was more comfortable speaking about his financial exploitation and the conditions of his home environment.

Make Senior Aware of Issues Causing Problems

After the trusting relationship was established, Mr. O was challenged to consider the complaints related to odors and the bug infestation. The client initially did not believe these were issues of concern and felt that insisting he address these problems was an invasion of his privacy and autonomy. The caseworker explained that the conditions in his home were now negatively impacting other tenants in the building. The caseworker also spoke with Mr. O about efforts to financially exploit him. He seemed to accept the true nature of the calls he had been receiving and was embarrassed that he had been duped. Mr. O was given materials on common scams and the caseworker talked him through the literature. The caseworker was able to identify a member of Mr. O's church who he was very close with; she agreed to attend meetings with the caseworker and Mr. O. Further convinced by his friend's opinions, Mr. O did come to understand that the condition of his home was problematic and needed to be addressed.

Educate the Senior

Mr. O was told about a DFSS program called Heavy Duty Chore (HDC), which provides deep cleaning, garbage removal, and/or organizing for seniors. The HDC program would benefit Mr. O and remedy the concerns about his home conditions. After completion of the HDC services, he would only need light, regular housekeeping. The caseworker also educated Mr. O about the OPG and why people were coming to his home to try to meet with him.

Assist Senior to Accept Necessary Services

At each visit with Mr. O, the caseworker would address the areas of concern and gauge any change that may have occurred with regard to his feelings on these issues or willingness to address them.

CASE STUDY 2: Mr. O (*continued*)

The caseworker also ensured that he understood the potential consequences of declining to deal with the problems he faced. Mr. O was also reassured that the caseworker would be available for support throughout the HDC process. Once the client understood the role and powers of the OPG, he was much more motivated to clean his home and to reassure the OPG that he was cognitively capable of managing his own affairs.

Advocate for Senior to Establish Helpful Services

Eventually, Mr. O agreed to the HDC program and the caseworker applied for this service. The caseworker mediated among the agency that provided the HDC program, the client, and the client's church friend, who also wanted to be a part of the process. The caseworker was present with Mr. O for the initial HDC assessment and checked in with him on HDC service days. The caseworker also advocated on Mr. O's behalf with the building's management to establish a timetable for insect extermination. This allayed his concerns about unscheduled visitors to his home. Furthermore, the caseworker supported Mr. O in having an official cognitive assessment performed by his own physician (with whom he felt very comfortable) in lieu of having the OPG bring a physician to his home to do so.

Follow Up to Monitor the Senior and the Situation to Ensure Ongoing Care

In Mr. O's case, the level of follow-up and monitoring was minimal as the caseworker had been successfully able to mobilize a support system for him in the form of his friend from the church. This friend was a very compassionate and trustworthy individual who cared very much for Mr. O's welfare. She was supported by the caseworker as she navigated the process of obtaining Mr. O's power of attorney. This created a mechanism to protect Mr. O should he one day be deemed cognitively incompetent. She also initiated an ongoing cleaning service for Mr. O.

Over the weeks following the HDC program, the caseworker did follow-up home visits with Mr. O and communicated with the building management and Mr. O's new power of attorney. Shortly afterward the case was officially closed.

Frequency of Contact

The ICAS program requires contact with clients at least every 2 weeks. However, the program allows for greater levels of service, if necessary. Meeting with clients often, particularly during the initial stages, can galvanize a relationship while providing an opportunity to address more pressing concerns, which may be time sensitive. Frequent visits allow a caseworker to garner the trust of clients incrementally and slowly establish a relationship with them.

Flexibility of Role

ICAS caseworkers can engage in a wide variety of activities with and on behalf of clients that extend beyond more circumscribed ideas of case management. Caseworkers can engage in such activities as counseling, transportation, money management, advocacy, accompanying clients to appointments, and cleaning and organization, as well as more traditional forms of case work such as making and making referrals for services. Essentially, caseworkers have the flexibility to provide an array of services to clients that can assist in developing a relationship with a client.

DETERMINING SUCCESS IN ICAS SELF-NEGLECT WORK

The primary purpose of the ICAS program is to stabilize the self-neglecting senior and make it possible to safely remain living in the community, whenever this is possible. When it is not possible for the senior's situation to be sufficiently stabilized to allow for safe continuation of community living, the next best alternative is to assist the senior with transitioning to a more structured setting (e.g., an assisted living facility or nursing home) that can provide necessary safety, sanitation, and overall care. When we can accomplish this purpose, the interactions and interventions with the senior are a success.

Success seems straightforward, and we all may believe we know it when we see it. Defining what *success* means in terms of helping self-neglecting seniors is more challenging. According to Merriam-Webster's (2016) online dictionary, perhaps the most fitting definition in this arena is "favorable or desired outcome." Although that definition offers some clarity, it still lacks clarification: Who will determine whether the outcome is favorable or desirable?

For example, from the self-neglecting senior's perspective, leaving his or her lifelong home of 83 years to move to an assisted living facility may seem to be quite unfavorable. From the caseworker's perspective, the senior leaving a structurally unsound, rodent-infested house with 80 years' worth of accumulated hoarded materials, broken toilets that are un-flushable, no electricity, and no means to store or prepare food to move to a safe, secure, sanitary assisted living building where a nurse, daily meals, medication assistance, laundry service, and socialization opportunities are readily available, is clearly a success.

Research to aid in gauging the success of the ICAS program utilizes a self-neglect assessment tool developed by Iris (Iris, Conrad, & Ridings, 2014); see Chapter 20 for more details on this tool.) The current version of this assessment tool includes a set of questions covering six principal domains associated with self-neglect concerns. (A previous version of this screening tool also included questions pertaining to financial issues.) The current domains include:

- Home environment
- Physical living conditions
- Social network
- Personal endangerment
- Physical health risk
- Mental health

The assessment is completed at the initial stages of engagement with self-neglect senior clients and again at case termination. Within the ICAS program, success is largely dictated by comparing responses from the initial and termination self-neglect assessments to determine the level of positive change within each domain.

The representative questions listed in the following from each domain illustrate the range of concerns being assessed.

- *Home environment:* Are the bathing facilities unsafe, unsanitary, or inoperable?
- *Physical living conditions:* Does the older adult's home lack at least one clear path for emergency evacuation?
- *Social network:* Does the older adult refuse to take advantage of socialization opportunities?

- *Personal endangerment:* Does the older adult lack sufficient care to meet his or her needs?
- *Physical health risk:* Has the older adult experienced recent, unplanned weight loss?
- *Mental health status:* Are the older adult's behaviors likely to cause imminent physical harm?

A DFSS/Senior Services intern performed a preliminary comparative analysis of initial versus termination self-neglect assessment responses in 2011, in which data from 98 ICAS senior clients were examined. As an indication of success in the ICAS program, the authors reviewed these findings and completed an updated analysis using similar 2015 assessment data. The 2015 analysis included 35 ICAS senior clients' data.

FINDINGS

The 2011 self-neglect assessment analysis showed that the most common areas of concern were personal endangerment and social network, with personal endangerment being the greatest area of concern. This finding was supported and echoed by the 2015 findings, in which 25 of the 35 seniors (71%) were evaluated as initially presenting with personal endangerment concerns. In the 2015 data, personal endangerment was more than twice as likely to be an initial concern than any other domain.

Areas of Greatest Improvement

The percentages of improvement from initial assessment to termination of services in 2011 are presented. As can be seen in Figure 16.2 the areas that improved are physical living conditions (38%), home environment (38%), social networks (36%), personal endangerment (34%), physical health risks (33%), and mental health (15%).

The percentages of improvement from initial assessment to termination of services in 2015 are presented in Figure 16.3. As can be seen in Figure 16.3 the areas that improved are physical living conditions (67%), home environment (64%), social networks (45%), personal endangerment (56%), physical health risks (50%), and mental health (80%).

Positive changes in physical health and home environment were highly rated in both 2011 and 2015. Positive changes in physical living conditions and home

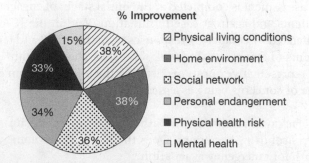

% Improvement

- ▨ Physical living conditions
- ■ Home environment
- ▨ Social network
- ▨ Personal endangerment
- ■ Physical health risk
- □ Mental health

Figure 16.2 Improvement from initial assessment, 2011.

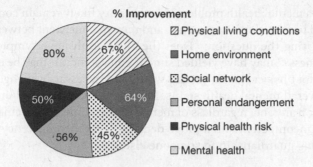

% Improvement

- ▨ Physical living conditions
- ■ Home environment
- ⊠ Social network
- ▤ Personal endangerment
- ■ Physical health risk
- ☐ Mental health

Figure16.3 Improvement from initial assessment, 2015.

environment were the highest rated in 2011, at 38% positive change in each category. Similarly, physical living conditions and home environment changes were closely and highly rated in 2015 (67% and 64% positive change, respectively).

These findings intuitively make sense. Deplorable living conditions and home environment are key indicators of self-neglect, as the senior is unable or unwilling to keep the surroundings clean and in good working order. It is relatively easy to affect a positive change in these areas, as they are external factors. Physical living conditions can be readily improved by upgrading lighting, getting utilities restored, fixing a toilet so it will flush, removing trash, and clearing a path for emergency evacuation (the indicator used in these studies). Safety in the home environment can be enhanced by installing working smoke detectors, clearing clutter, and repairing bathing facilities so that they are operable (the indicator used here). Making such changes makes a significant difference in the quality of a self-neglecting senior's life, without requiring much active participation from the senior.

Areas of Divergence in the Data Comparison

Although there are clearly significant differences between the two data sets, the reason(s) behind the differences remains unclear. One possible factor is the difference in sample size. The 2011 analysis was based on 98 senior ICAS clients, whereas the 2015 analysis was based on 35 seniors. Also, 19 agencies participated as ICAS providers in 2011, whereas 10 participated in 2015. A second potential factor was that ICAS agencies may have become more proficient in certain areas of assistance over time.

The radical difference in purported mental health improvement may be more a factor of the question asked. The authors believe that the change in results from 2011 (15% improvement in mental health—a reasonable figure) to 2015 (80% improvement in mental health) can be substantiated. In addition, just 10 of the 35 seniors in the 2015 analysis were assessed as having "behaviors likely to cause them imminent physical harm." For these reasons, the authors believe that most of the data from each year's analysis are accurate. The exception is the reported dramatic improvement in mental health in 2015. The other factors are fairly consistent and seem to make sense given that they are more about externals that can be more readily attained.

If one of the other questions in the mental health status section of the self-neglect assessment tool had been used both years, the result from each year may have been more consistent. For example, asking, "Do the older adult's behaviors appear to be related to a mental health problem?" would very likely remain consistent between the initial and termination assessments, and remain consistent between the 2 years being studied. Using the question: "Does the older adult have symptoms or a history of mental illness?" may have yielded similar consistency. It may be easier to address the potential for physical harm, yet this would not necessarily change the self-neglecting senior's overall mental health status. In Illinois, treatment and/or medication cannot be forced on anyone, regardless of mental illness, unless a psychiatrist agrees that the person is incompetent and a judge declares legal incompetency via signing a court order giving guardianship to someone else.

DISCUSSION: THINKING ABOUT SUCCESS

The survey administered to ICAS providers also solicited further qualitative feedback from caseworkers about how they conceptualize and measure "success," as well as what they believe to be the key challenges encountered in working with self-neglecting seniors.

How Do You Measure Success?

When asked: How do you define success for your ICAS clients? most respondents eschewed defining success in very specific terms. Overall, there was an emphasis on understanding that success tends to be both small and incremental. Only one responder equated success to something quantifiable when she reported that she defines success as "how many programs I get them (seniors) to participate in." Two other respondents referred to more vague conceptualizations of success when they cited "an improvement in their current situation" and "small progression toward minimal goals." One caseworker felt that success could be evaluated in relation to efforts to be caring and helpful, rather than the results of his attempts. This individual thought of success as being "process-focused" rather than "goal-focused." Of the remaining two respondents, one highlighted the building of relationships as a success in itself, whereas the other equated stabilization to success, and personal safety as a key consideration when evaluating success.

What Are the Key Successes, or Areas of Success, That You Have Seen With Regard to Your ICAS Seniors?

Two survey respondents specifically mentioned the building of a relationship as a key success. Moving a senior to a safer or more supportive living environment was highlighted by two caseworkers as a key element of success. One caseworker expressed the idea that the individuality of every client's situation required any evaluation of success to be equally unique; he further explained success as the ability to resolve the most pressing issues the senior was experiencing, whatever they might be. Both agencies providing home-repair services under their ICAS program indicated that having clients avail themselves of these services was a common success for them. Four agencies referenced making improvements to the home environment as a key success. Four of the six caseworkers surveyed mentioned the initiation of services such as home-delivered meals and benefits access.

What Are the Key Challenges You Have in Relation to Your ICAS Seniors?

Three of the six respondents expressly mentioned mental health explicitly as one of the key challenges when working with ICAS clients. Issues around building relationships with clients, such as overcoming initial suspicion and garnering trust, were highlighted by three agencies. On this theme, one caseworker felt that representing a department of the city of Chicago was viewed with suspicion by seniors and was something of an impediment to engagement. Three caseworkers felt convincing seniors to access support services that could be of assistance was a challenge.

It is interesting to note that only one agency specified housing as a key challenge to working with self-neglecting seniors. Equally surprising was that this was also the only agency to expressly identify a lack of financial assistance as a key challenge to working with self-neglecting seniors.

Two caseworkers thought that limited support services and resources were a key challenge to their work with self-neglecting seniors. One of these caseworkers felt that the number of support services to which she could refer seniors has been shrinking, whereas the other caseworker pointed to a lack of ongoing involvement from mental health services that would continually monitor and support seniors.

Is There Anything Else You'd Like to Add About Your ICAS Program or Your ICAS Seniors and Experiences?

Of the six agencies surveyed, four (two thirds) chose to add further thoughts on the program and their experiences in working with self-neglectful seniors. The common threads are representative of the issues one finds in attempting to build a relationship with such seniors:

- Caseworkers have to be willing to take time in developing the foundational relationships in order to effect positive change.
- Developing these relationships can lead to changes that enrich and secure the self-neglecting seniors' futures.
- Regardless of strong, longitudinal efforts, not all seniors will be ready and willing to make changes, despite the risks of not moving forward.
- Working over a long period of time on substantively challenging issues with seniors who mostly do not want the offered assistance can lead to burnout of the caseworkers.

CONCLUSION

This chapter examined specific datasets pertaining to a program that works with self-neglecting seniors as a means of contributing to a broader conversation around how we can conceptualize "success" with this group in a meaningful way. Our work with self-neglecting seniors brings us into contact with an especially troubled segment of an already vulnerable population. Their care needs are further complicated by mental illness, isolation, and an often impenetrable inability to fully understand the depths and dangers of their situations. Caseworkers are placed in the precarious position of balancing the duty of care and protecting the rights of the seniors to self-determination—the most venerated of all American entitlements. Despite the friction that can exist between these two ideals, it is important that both are somehow incorporated into any program assessment that claims to measure success.

In this chapter, we examined more concrete conceptualizations of success by reviewing the extent to which there were measurable improvements made to goals set from the perspective of the caseworkers/DFSS. Further thought needs to be given to incorporating the goals of seniors into the evaluation process, even when these are in opposition to what we as caseworkers deem appropriate. Interesting to note is that none of the ICAS caseworkers thought to frame their definition of success in terms of facilitating the goals of seniors. Although unquestioningly assisting a self-neglecting senior to meet his or her goals is without doubt often dangerous and inappropriate, it is important for us as social services professionals to constantly ask the big ideological and ethical questions that strike at the core of our profession and mandate thoughtful practice that balances the many conflicting values that guide us.

IMPLICATIONS FOR RESEARCH AND PRACTICE

- Communication is the key to success.
- The objective self-neglect assessment methods have been beneficial.
- Using caseworkers with the same experiences, ethnicity, and religious beliefs as the clients is appropriate.
- Individuals who self-neglect should be included in research involving multi-agency and multiprofessional interventions.

REFERENCES

Chicago Mitzvah Campaign. (2016). About us. Retrieved from http://chicagomitzvahcampaign.org/about_us

City of Chicago. (2016). Department of Family & Support Services page. Retrieved from http://www.cityofchicago.org/city/en/depts/fss.html

City of Chicago. (2016). Help in Your Home page. Retrieved from http://www.cityofchicago.org/city/en/depts/fss/supp_info/help_in_your_home.html

Housing Opportunities & Maintenance for the Elderly. Retrieved from http://www.homeseniors.org/services-in-the-community/upkeep-and-repair-services-program

Iris, M., Conrad, K. J., & Ridings, J. (2014). Observational measure of elder self-neglect. *Journal of Elder Abuse & Neglect, 26*, 365–397. doi:10.1080/08946566.2013.8011818

Larsen, J. (2003). Record heat wave in Europe takes 35,000 lives: Far greater losses may lie ahead. Retrieved from http://www.earth-policy.org/plan_b_updates/2003/update29

Success. (n.d.). In *Merriam-Webster online dictionary*. Retrieved from http://www.merriam-webster.com/dictionary/success

U.S. Department of Housing and Urban Development. Retrieved from https://portal.hud.gov/hudportal/documents/huddoc?id=DOC_16470.pdf CASE STUDY

RESEARCH EVIDENCE

CHAPTER 17

SELF-NEGLECT: A STATEWIDE ASSESSMENT IN VERMONT

Kelly Melekis

There is no unified, comprehensive definition for self-neglect in the United States. In an effort to enhance understanding and establish a coordinated community response to the issue of self-neglect in the state of Vermont, a statewide mixed-methods study was conducted. This study highlights the importance of definitional clarity to accurately assess the scope and severity of self-neglect, strategies for addressing the challenges to serving adults who are self-neglecting, such as refusal/lack of desire for services, inadequate access to and funding of services, cognitive and mental health issues, limited family and community connectivity, and lack of clarity on self-neglect/capacity determination. The study findings point to the need for innovative interprofessional and interagency collaboration to ensure a coordinated community response through a combination of expanding understanding of self-neglect, addressing systemic challenges, and implementing strategies to enhance the response to self-neglect.

Despite being the most commonly reported form of elder abuse and neglect in the United States, there is no unified, comprehensive definition for the concept of self-neglect. Medical and mental health practitioners have attempted to define self-neglect using specific diagnoses, including Diogenes syndrome and hoarding disorder, which is now included in the *Diagnostic and Statistical Manual of Mental Disorders* (5th ed., *DSM-5*; American Psychiatric Association, 2013), but ultimately have failed to achieve consensus or to incorporate the wide array of individual, social, and environmental factors often involved in self-neglect cases in their definition (Brandl et al., 2006; Kutame, 2007). Definitions are often laden with judgment-based principles and conceptualized solely through cultural and societal standards for self-care (Gibbons, Lauder, & Ludwick, 2006; Iris, Ridings, & Conrad, 2010). Gibbons et al. (2006) defined self-neglect as "the inability (intentional or nonintentional) to maintain a socially and culturally accepted standard of self-care with the potential for serious consequences to the health and well-being of the self-neglecter and perhaps even to their community" (p. 16). The definitions of self-neglect are typically characterized as the refusal or failure of an older adult to provide themselves with basic necessities such as food, water, shelter, medication, or basic hygiene. Self-neglect accounts for the largest percentage of reports to adult protective services (APS). Fulmer (2008) and O'Brien (2011) estimated that there are over 1 million cases per year in the United States.

Generally considered a geriatric phenomenon, the concept of self-neglect is rarely applied to individuals younger than the age of 60 in the United States. As a geriatric phenomenon, self-neglect is generally subsumed within the broad category of elder abuse and neglect. There are many arguments that self-neglect is not a form of abuse and "the immediate challenge with this classification is that with self-neglect there is no perpetrator and the classification does not fit the legal perpetrator/victim paradigm" (Vermont Department of Disabilities, Aging, and Independent Living [DAIL] Self-Neglect Task Force, 2012, p. 4).

Although there are no federal laws, rules, or regulations regarding the investigation and management of self-neglect reports, the 2006 amendments to the Older Americans Act (OAA) of 1965 provide the following definition of self-neglect:

> An adult's inability, due to physical or mental impairment or diminished capacity, to perform essential self-care tasks including (a) obtaining essential food, clothing, shelter, and medical care, (b) obtaining goods and services necessary to maintain physical health, mental health, or general safety, or (c) managing one's own financial affairs (p. 10).

In the United States, it is estimated that 13 states (including Vermont) do not explicitly include self-neglect within elder abuse and neglect statutes (Brandl et al., 2006). For those that do, definitions vary widely, including and excluding various clarifying elements such as the mental or physical capacity of the person considered to be self-neglecting, the presence and/or actions of a caregiver, and the severity of the impact of the self-neglect (Kutame, 2007; Rathborn-McCuan & Fabian, 1992). The use of these clarifiers not only speaks volumes to the complexity of defining self-neglect but also provides an important level of consistency for local service providers.

In Vermont, state statutes do not address the issue of self-neglect. Vermont State Statute, Title 33, Chapter 69, addresses reports of abuse, neglect, and exploitation of vulnerable adults, but does not include self-neglect. In 1996, a Memorandum from the Commissioner of Vermont's Department of Disabilities, Aging and Independent Living (DAIL) mandated that referrals for cases of suspected self-neglect among those older than 60 be directed to the Area Agencies on Aging (AAA) and those younger than 60 be directed to the APS (Flood, 1996). It was also directed that the APS would not provide case management, but would make referrals for such services. This position was restated in a 2005 communication from DAIL commissioner Patrick Flood to State Senator Richard Sears. It stated: "For persons over 60, that case management properly belonged to the AAA, which were already providing much of the case management. Unfortunately, there was no obvious party to provide those services for adults with physical disabilities younger than 60, so when those cases arise, APS is still directly involved" (as cited by DAIL Self-Neglect Task Force, 2012, p. 6). A review of state definitions and jurisdictions for self-neglect indicates that Vermont is one of only four states where self-neglect does not legally fall under the purview of the state's APS system.

In 2012, Vermont convened the Self-Neglect Task Force to address the problem of effectively helping people identified as self-neglecting. The task force expressed unanimous support for not recommending statutory requirements due to the sentiment that those engaging in self-neglect are in need of human services and support, not investigatory or legal approaches. Establishing an effective response to self-neglect requires an understanding of how the concept is defined. The Self-Neglect Task

Force (2012) adopted the OAA definition noted previously, with the addition of a clarifier: This definition excludes people who make a conscious and voluntary choice not to provide for certain basic needs as a matter of lifestyle, personal preference, or religious belief and who understand the consequences of their decision. In an effort to enhance understanding and establish a coordinated community response to the issue of self-neglect in Vermont, DAIL conducted a statewide mixed-methods study (Melekis, 2014a).

METHODS

The mixed-methods study of self-neglect reported in this chapter was part of a larger statewide assessment of the needs of and community resources for older adults and their caregivers in Vermont (Melekis, 2014b). Using a concurrent approach, a nonexperimental survey was used to investigate the service providers' perspectives, and key stakeholder interviews were utilized to gather in-depth information on the experiences of the respondents regarding existing resources and needs in disability and aging services.

Strategies for sampling and data collection were discussed in collaboration with the administrators and the staff from the DAIL Division of Disabilities and Aging Services (DDAS) and the five AAAs. Decisions were based on appropriateness, adequacy, and access, with particular attention paid to the costs and benefits of different strategies for various stakeholders. Both the survey instrument and key stakeholder interview protocols were designed by the researchers in conjunction with DAIL DDAS staff and AAA directors. In addition to the existing measures related to the community/state assessment of needs and resources among the older adults and self-neglect assessment, prior tools utilized by DAIL and the AAA were reviewed for item inclusion as appropriate.

Providers and key stakeholders were recruited via purposive and snowball sampling, with DAIL and each AAA recommending local providers and stakeholders for study inclusion. The survey was distributed via direct email that included a weblink to the survey for providers to complete and share with colleagues. A survey weblink was also included on several provider websites and social media tools, such as Facebook pages, and distributed via provider and partner lists at several agencies. For providers who were unable or did not wish to complete an online survey, there was an option to receive a paper version. The service provider survey was distributed for 1 month (mid-September to mid-October, 2013), with reminder emails sent weekly to encourage completion.

Descriptive statistics were utilized to summarize the data and analyze respondents' perspectives on the scope and severity of self-neglect cases, warning signs and symptoms, reporting processes, and recommendations for a community-based response.

The qualitative data analysis (QDA) software program Atlas.ti was utilized to assist with data management and analysis of the interviews. All interviews were transcribed verbatim by one transcriptionist. The researcher reviewed all transcriptions by simultaneously listening to the recording and reading the transcript. Errors in transcription or unclear words and passages were edited and clarified where necessary. One of the first steps in the analysis involved a close and careful reading of the transcripts "using filters and analytic axes to organize the process as it unfolds" (Padgett, 2008, p. 140). Repeated readings allowed for a search of meaning units that were descriptively labeled. Initially, the data were analyzed using an inductive approach, so that possible categories and themes could emerge from the data (Lincoln & Guba, 1985). The coding process occurred like a funnel, starting at a descriptive level and moving upward, reflecting greater selectivity and synthesis (Charmaz, 2006). The coding strategy utilized in this study followed Saldaña's first and second cycle coding, where the first cycle involved an open coding process and the second cycle was more focused, similar to the coding approach used in grounded theory (Charmaz, 2006). First-cycle coding methods included the use of descriptive, structural, and simultaneous coding (Saldaña, 2009). Descriptive coding was used to summarize the primary topic of excerpts. The descriptive codes and subcodes were helpful in categorizing and laying the groundwork for second-cycle coding and thematic analysis (Miles & Huberman, 1994; Saldaña, 2009). During the second cycle of coding, the goal was "to develop a sense of categorical, thematic, conceptual, and/or theoretical organization" from first-cycle codes (Saldaña, 2009, p. 149). Where appropriate, codes and subcodes were clarified and revised, similar codes were merged, and more advanced, detailed structural coding was applied. The primary method used during this time was focused coding to develop the major themes from the data (Saldaña, 2009). Coding and categorization are an iterative process used to identify patterns, themes, and interactions in the data (Patton, 2002). In order to reflect the voice of the participants, quotes are presented verbatim in the results and represented in *italics*.

FINDINGS

There were 137 survey respondents representing all areas of the state with a proportional distribution. For the stakeholder interviews, 10 to 15 individuals in each of the five areas were recruited for participation in a 1-hour interview in person or by phone. A total of 36 stakeholders throughout the state were interviewed, out of 68 who were invited to participate. Study participants represent entities conducting programs that receive assistance under the OAA, those conducting other federal programs for older individuals, as well as programs that serve a much broader community population, of which older adults and caregivers are included. Providers/programs represented include AAA, senior centers, health care and home health service providers, mental health practitioners, housing and residential services, community meals programs, and volunteer and employment programs.

Defining Self-Neglect

Although Vermont's definition of self-neglect includes adults of all ages, this study reveals provider experiences and perspectives that parallel the national distinction of self-neglect as a geriatric phenomenon. Indeed, survey and interview responses indicate that the term self-neglect is generally not utilized for those younger than 60, but that the same characteristics or behaviors are categorized under the realm of another descriptor. As one participant noted, "those people show up . . . they're not labeled as self-neglect, they're labeled as having developmental issues, or mental health issues . . . substance abuse issues." Further, when asked to distinguish between the needs of and resources for those older and younger than 60, there were fewer responses regarding those younger than 60. Some respondents indicated that they "don't have the experience with [the] younger-than-60 population to make an informed response," whereas others identified that there are "no specific services for [the] under 60 population, [they] fall into a crack."

It is important to note that several study participants noted the role of economics in our identification and categorization of self-neglect. As one respondent noted, "wealth can buy you a lot of leeway, so people who are self-neglecting who are really wealthy are just seen as eccentric." This raises some important questions about the role of poverty in self-neglect identification and intervention.

Scope and Severity

Although one of the study goals was to assess the scope of self-neglect in Vermont, it was extremely difficult to accurately estimate the number of individuals who could be described as self-neglecting, particularly those younger than the age of 60. Survey responses indicate that each year providers were involved in an average of 23 cases involving older adults (60+) and 10 cases involving adults younger than 60. However, estimates of the number of such cases ranged from 0 to 300, and there was no way of assessing how many of the cases are duplicative across sites and providers. Varying estimates and missing data make this data difficult to interpret.

Warning Signs and Symptoms

Respondents identified the common warning signs and symptoms in suspected cases of self-neglect for those younger than 60 and for those 60 and older. Warning signs and symptoms included inadequate nutrition, hygiene, home appliances and utilities, living conditions, management of financial affairs, utilization of necessary medical care, inadequate utilization of other services to maintain health and safety. In addition, inappropriate clothing, abuse, neglect, or exploitation by others were considered warning signs.

In addition, the majority of the respondents (59%) either strongly agreed (13%) or agreed (46%) that individuals identified as self-neglecting usually have underlying, untreated mental health problems, or cognitive impairment. Although it can be helpful to acknowledge the potential causes, common warning signs and symptoms, one participant clearly articulates the importance of individualized assessment and response: "Although most self-neglect cases have common denominators, each case is unique to the individual involved and there cannot be a blanket formula to address the needs of these unique folks who come to our attention."

Challenges in Responding to Self-Neglect

In addition to myriad challenges in their individual work with persons identified as self-neglecting, such as lack of desire for/refusal of services and cognitive/mental health issues, providers noted a number of systemic challenges, including (a) capacity determination and assessment, (b) reporting and referral process, and (c) the time-intensive nature of response to self-neglect in Vermont.

Capacity Determination and Assessment

The vast majority of the respondents (90%) strongly agreed (41%) or agreed (49%) self-neglect cases inherently present ethical challenges/dilemmas. These center mostly around the issue of capacity determination, with participants articulating a range of concerns on both ends of the spectrum such as "we too often use the right to self-determination to excuse our doing nothing" and "no one seems to remember the parts of that language that says 'due to diminished capacity.'" Indeed, the multilayered nature of capacity and the significant implications of capacity determination demand adequate resources for assessment.

Approximately 68% of respondents indicated that they (or someone else in their organization) conducted an assessment of self-neglect, which appeared to be happening in a myriad of ways, frequently on an informal, observational basis. Respondents included no references to formal or standardized measures and no standard measures were identified as being used across providers/sites in the state. It was repeatedly acknowledged that an essential part of the assessment was an opportunity to observe the individual in his or her home environment. One participant noted, "We do not have a formal system to assess self-neglect, however, I am in their homes on a regular basis and we can see [the warning signs]. I would not see it if they were coming to my office for appointments."

Although there were several indications of assessment of cognitive ability or decision-making capacity, it was unclear who was conducting the assessment of cognitive ability and decision-making capacity. While some respondents indicated they were comfortable conducting the assessment and consulting with mental health providers in questionable or challenging cases, others indicated that they felt this type of assessment was beyond the scope of their roles and responsibilities. Only one survey respondent noted the use of a specific tool for measuring cognitive status, the Mini-Mental State Examination (MMSE), which does not measure executive functioning.

Although the majority of the respondents (59%) either strongly agreed (13%) or agreed (46%) that individuals identified as self-neglecting usually have underlying, untreated mental health problems or cognitive impairment, there was widespread concern that "there is a serious lack of mental health services, and those we do have are not always easily accessible to the people who need them." Another fundamental concern was the role of dementia and cognitive impairment. One participant noted that the definition of self-neglect is "in a nutshell, what happens to somebody who has dementia . . . because it is by virtue of the disease process and trajectory going to happen if someone does not step in." Participants articulated a need for mental health professionals in terms of both determining capacity and helping to address issues underlying the presenting concern of self-neglect.

Reporting and Referral Process

Findings clearly indicate a lack of clarity regarding self-neglect reporting, with providers reporting cases of suspected self-neglect to a wide variety of organizations, programs, and providers (Figure 17.1). Providers most commonly reported to the APS (37%), with 15% of the respondents reporting to the AAA, and an equal number (15%) noting that they make reports to the APS *and/or* the AAA.

Respondent comments reflect the potential complexity of these situations, as well as confusion about where reports should be made. One clearly stated, "I don't know where to report this." The challenge in reporting cases of self-neglect for those younger than 60 was highlighted: "For people 60 or older, reports are made to the Area Agency on Aging providing services in the region where the person who is self-neglecting resides. For persons under 60 years old, referrals may vary. There is

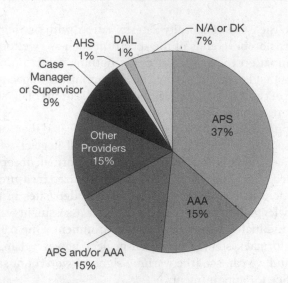

Figure 17.1 Where providers report suspected self-neglect.

AAA, Area Agencies on Aging; AHS, agencies of human services; APS, adult protective services; DAIL, Department of Disabilities, Aging and Independent Living; DK, don't know; N/A, not applicable.

no one place/source to make a referral for self-neglecting younger adults." To address this issue the following suggestion was made: "A single point of entry would help curb some of the community confusion and allow that agency to help clients while educating the community about the greater issues." However, it was acknowledged that regardless of age, it is a challenge that "there is no mandate to intervene in cases of self-neglect . . . so if someone refuses treatment no follow-up occurs."

Time-Intensive Nature of Self-Neglect Cases

As a result of the complex combination of contributing factors and challenges in assessment, service providers overwhelmingly reported that compared with the average workload, cases of self-neglect take more time. The important yet time-intensive nature of building rapport was evidenced in the following: "Building relationships that enable change takes time and repeat visits . . . often with little visible sign of success." The vast majority (85%) of the respondents reported that self-neglect cases take more time (33%) or much more time (52%) than their average cases/workload. This was often due to the emotional elements and common ethical dilemmas experienced. One participant commented, "Self-neglect is just that, a crisis waiting to happen most of the time and that's when change will happen or could happen" and several referred to the cyclical nature of such cases, in which a crisis is abated and there is a lull until the next anticipated crisis occurs. As one respondent stated, "even if this behavior is identified and addressed, it will most likely resurface."

Several provider respondents indicated that the concerns of community members can be difficult to manage. One participant said "a lot of time spent listening to community members' concerns . . . getting yelled at by community members that no one is helping the person [or] dealing with other agencies and individuals calling about the client [asking] why aren't you doing something . . . without understanding issues around working with someone who is self-neglecting." Those participants, particularly those on the frontlines of responding to self-neglect cases, expressed the difficulty of being on the receiving end of frequent frustrations and helping other service providers and community members understand the nature of confidentiality and the limits of intervention. The time and effort required on self-neglect cases points to the need for what one provider called *perseverance*, and another referred to as *consistent presence and compassion*. One participant articulately noted:

> Self-neglect is often very gray. Frequently, the person who is self-neglecting in our eyes, doesn't think there is a problem. Developing the necessary skills to meet the person on their own turf, and help them through the situation is essential. Approaching with respect, understanding what it is the person may want or need, is essential and often may not jive [be aligned] with what his/ her family or community find acceptable. There are no quick fixes, and it is not easy to know what the "right thing" is, or to avoid placing our own values on the person/the choices they've made. . . . Figuring out what can be done, should be done, what the individual wants or will accept, is not an easy task.

Responding to Self-Neglect

Participant responses offered a number of strategies and recommendations for enhancing the response to self-neglect. Common strategies included (a) training and education, (b) care management and collaboration, (c) and community involvement and support. Embedded throughout the recommendations was an acknowledgment of the need for financial resources and organizational leadership to ensure the effectiveness of a coordinated community response to self-neglect.

Training and Education

Participants expressed a strong need for specialized training and education about how to respond in cases of self-neglect. It was noted that this training was needed "across the continuum of health care providers." Participants articulated a need for trained providers to conduct assessments for self-neglect, particularly in terms of assessing decision-making capacity, mental health, and cognitive impairment. Furthermore, many frontline providers acknowledged that responding to cases of self-neglect requires unique expertise in establishing trust, building rapport, respecting self-determination, and assessing risk and capacity. Although many providers "really want to help," they often need training and resources to do so. Public awareness on self-neglect is also needed.

Care Management and Collaboration

Nearly 95% of the survey respondents reported the importance of engaging in interdisciplinary collaboration with colleagues and providers from other organizations. The following participant comment articulates the need for such collaboration: "Individuals respond uniquely to different types of intervention; someone might take the animal control officer's recommendation very differently than one with the same ends by the town health officer. For this reason, self-neglect needs to be approached in a customized way, which requires collaboration across a variety of sectors."

Many study participants articulated a desire for increased involvement from town health officers, animal control, and zoning authorities, as well as family members and community faith-based organizations. Many respondents identified a need for collaborative outreach and assessment, and specifically noted the prerequisite of adequate funding of mental health services and availability of geriatric mental health providers, in particular. Accessibility of mental health services was noted frequently, indicating that there was a need for "more accessible mental health services and supports, which are not only office based but community based" and "more access to mental health information, services, and support for self-neglect clients and the community partners who need guidance in how to help them." Although Vermont's Elder Care Clinician program was frequently highlighted as a valuable resource, significant variability in accessibility and utilization was noted throughout the state. Concerns were raised regarding inadequate funding of the program, inaccessibility to providers due to long wait lists, or inability to respond to crisis situations. Several respondents noted concerns that mental health providers were unwilling or unable to address cooccurring mental health issues and cognitive impairment, and that there is a serious need for mental health providers, particularly emergency/crisis responders, who can adequately conduct differential diagnostic assessments.

Community Involvement and Support

Generally, cases of suspected self-neglect come to the attention of service providers following a report or referral by the concerned family, community members, or providers. Although this often reflects a value of community and care for fellow community members, it also raises important questions and concerns reflecting the spectrum of perspectives regarding the role of personal choice and the balance of safety and risk. The majority of the survey respondents strongly agreed (12%) or agreed (43%) individuals of all ages should be able to do what they wish with their lives and their property. This result reflects the potential limits to personal choice perceived by some providers and community members. Comments illustrate the range of expectations regarding community involvement and impact from: "More community empathy for folks who may be different. . . . Less judgmental attitude to folks who are different" to "For many people it is a long-standing habit and lifestyle. . . . It should not be tolerated because it adversely affects the entire community."

Study participants offered several innovative strategies for a true community-based response to self-neglect, including community spaces, outreach, and the utilization of peer support networks consisting of volunteers and senior companions. It was suggested that we "need to have spaces in the community that are safe, community-centered spaces that are open cradle to grave." Local communities might "lead the community in frank discussions about the ethics and realities of those who might be self-neglecting and educate [about] available resources" and/or "establish strong volunteer networks for home visits and local companions." However, some respondents also noted a potential barrier in terms of "getting community partners or members to participate in helping the self-neglecting person."

Several participants indicated that since the nature of self-neglect cases is that people "don't want services" it is important to provide information and options via volunteers or a peer support network. However, some were clear that it would be important to utilize paid peers rather than unpaid volunteers, due to the nature of the work. Also, several expressed a significant concern that such a model would require extensive training, as well as ongoing support and supervision. It was noted that some individuals might be open to informal peer support—but perhaps only from a known neighbor or true peer (i.e., farmer to farmer), but might react negatively to perceived intervention via a network of community volunteers representing local teens, business people, or town leaders, for example.

Overall, many study participants reflected the sentiment that there was a significant need for providing family support and establishing a network of community volunteers to help when needed: "It is an issue that impacts not only the individual and their [sic] family but the community as a whole. If we can find ways to assist individuals with the underlying causes of self-neglect we will enhance the overall health and well-being of all."

DISCUSSION

The rapid aging of the U.S. population will likely exacerbate the problem of elder self-neglect (Dong, Simon, Fulmer, et al., 2010; Dong, Simon, Wilson, et al., 2010; Pavlou & Lachs, 2006). It is expected that by 2030, one in five Americans will be 65 years of age or older (U.S. Census Bureau, 2011). As a state with one of the oldest populations in the United States, Vermont must be prepared for a potential growth in self-neglect cases. The complex and challenging nature of self-neglect requires a locally informed strategy to ensure individuals and families receive support in a manner that maximizes safety, health, and well-being with respect to autonomy and individual/family decision making. A coordinated community response would involve collaboration among multiple systems and services at the local level. Based on the study findings presented in this chapter, a coordinated community response to self-neglect should involve a combination of (a) an expanded understanding self-neglect, (b) addressing systemic challenges, and (c) implementing strategies to enhance the response to self-neglect.

Understanding Self-Neglect

As demonstrated in the literature and illustrated in the study findings, the scope of self-neglect is particularly challenging to ascertain. Due to the aforementioned categorization of this issue as a geriatric syndrome, self-neglect estimates are generally embedded within estimates of the incidence and prevalence of elder abuse and neglect overall, which are considered to be underreported nationally and internationally. Furthermore, states and localities have varying definitions of self-neglect and reporting processes, adding to the difficulty of obtaining clear numbers of confirmed cases and accurate estimates (Teaster, 2003). Vermont faces perhaps a unique challenge given the structure of self-neglect reporting (younger-than-age 60 cases to the APS and older-than-age 60 cases to the AAA) and the lack of inclusion of self-neglect in state statutes. Although the aging service network (most notably the AAA) provides essential care and response in cases of self-neglect and has a fundamental role in supporting the overall health and well-being of the older adults and caregivers, the definition of self-neglect indicates that systems of care involved in addressing the physical or mental impairment, or diminished capacity, should be active collaborative partners, not peripheral responders. The apparent difficulty in defining self-neglect stems from both the ambiguous nature of the concept itself, the limited research on the topic, and a lack of consensus among national, state, and local service providers. It is also important that we enhance the understanding of self-neglect from the clients' perspective (Band-Winterstein, Doron, & Naim, 2012). Furthermore, although often vital for the provision of services, the connection of self-neglect to elder abuse and neglect may exacerbate the difficulty of defining and conceptualizing both the term and its response (Rathborn-McCuan & Fabian, 1992). The need for definitional clarity, more accurate reporting of self-neglect, and consistent documentation is not only important for the development and provision of services but also vital to the health and well-being of those involved.

Though many studies have shed light on the potential risk factors and causes for self-neglect, it is still unclear exactly how these aspects inform, influence, and compound one another to cause and perpetuate self-neglect. Mental health issues and cognitive impairment are among the most commonly cited causes or risk factors for self-neglect and weigh heavily on discussions of capacity and competence. Those who self-neglect are likely to have some form of mental illness or cognitive impairment (Dong, Simon, Wilson, et al., 2010; Dong, Wilson, Mendes de Leon, & Evans, 2010), with dementia and depressive symptoms being the most common (Abrams, Lachs, & McAvay, 2002; Bartley, Knight, O'Neill, & O'Brien, 2011; Burnett et al., 2006; Dyer, Pavlik, & Murphy, 2000). Likewise, cognitive impairment and declines in executive functioning are often found in conjunction with self-neglect (Abrams et al., 2002; Dong, Simon, Fulmer, et al., 2010). Study findings are aligned with the existing literature, with the vast majority of the respondents reporting underlying, untreated mental health problems, or cognitive impairment among individuals identified as self-neglecting. It is important to recall that Vermont's definition of self-neglect includes a clarifier that "excludes people who make a conscious and voluntary choice not to provide for certain basic needs as a matter of lifestyle, personal preference, or religious belief and who understand the consequences of their decision." Perhaps inherent in this definition is an assumption that anyone identified as self-neglecting has some mental health problem or cognitive impairment that results in a lack of understanding of consequences of their decisions. Regardless, there is a clear call for effective assessments of decisional capacity, access to mental health services, and interprofessional collaboration.

Addressing Systemic Challenges

As illustrated in the study findings, frontline responders are often in the center of the inherent conflict between society's desire to protect vulnerable adults from harm and respect for individual autonomy. An essential element of cases in which services are refused is deciding whether someone has the capacity to make that decision. Determining capacity and competence are extremely difficult tasks, and often prove to be a gray area for most practitioners, who have very few specific guidelines for such determinations. As White (2014) stated, "the tension between an adult person's right to make [his or her] own decisions and the responsibility of society to protect the individual from harm has made defining, researching, and addressing self-neglect an arduous and often debated process" (p. 134). One of the biggest difficulties for practitioners is that they often lack the tools or resources to determine capacity (Braye, Orr, & Preston-Shoot, 2011). Usually, capacity determinations can only officially be made by a geriatrician or psychiatrist (Day, 2010), which often requires an office visit. For individuals who are homebound or wary of office visits, obtaining an official determination can prove difficult.

In addition to the challenge of obtaining a capacity determination, there are few accurate or official measurements for the assessment of self-neglect. This is due in part to the lack of a universal definition and the limited research on effective self-neglect assessment tools (Brandl et al., 2006; Kelly, Dyer, Pavlik, Doody, & Jogerst, 2008).

As illustrated in the study findings, there is no standardized measure or even common/shared assessment method being used throughout Vermont. Most often, individual judgments of APS field workers, AAA case managers, or health professionals are used to initially determine cases of self-neglect. There are an increasing number of measures for determining capacity (Naik, Lai, Kunik, & Dyer, 2008; Parmar, Bremault-Phillips, & Charles, 2015; Skelton, Kunik, Regev, & Naik, 2010) and assessing for self-neglect (Day & McCarthy, 2016; Kelly et al., 2008; Pickens et al., 2013), which could inform a more universal and coordinated process for assessment. "Building therapeutic relationship with self-neglecting clients and sensitive comprehensive assessment are key to evaluating situations" (Day, Mulcahy, Leahy-Warren, & Downey, 2015, p. 114).

Given that one of the defining features of self-neglect is the failure to obtain goods and services necessary to maintain health and safety, those considered to be self-neglecting rarely present for services. This points to the need for an efficient reporting and referral process. Study findings indicate notable confusion about this process in Vermont and point to the need for clarity among both providers and the public. Research indicates significant gaps between expert and public views of elder abuse in that "many experts and organizations that deal with elder abuse treat self-neglect as a form of elder abuse, yet the public excludes self-neglect from the concept and assumes that the term 'elder abuse' refers only to cases in which one person abuses another" (Volmert & Lindland, 2016, p. 5). In order to put self-neglect on the map and/or raise public awareness, "strategies are needed to bring self-neglect into the conversation, under the heading of 'elder abuse' or as a twin concept" (Volmert & Lindland, 2016, p. 7). Furthermore, in Vermont, there is a need to raise public awareness and provider understanding about where to report suspected cases of self-neglect.

Findings indicate that self-neglect cases are among the most time-consuming of provider caseloads. Given that one of the defining features of self-neglect is the failure to obtain goods and services necessary to maintain health and safety, those considered to be self-neglecting rarely present for services. Those on the frontlines of response face a challenging situation in engaging individuals who frequently do not desire involvement with formal service providers, and in working on high-risk, high-demand cases with diminishing resources. Outreach and engagement are essential for assessment and service provision, however, they are frequently time-consuming and demanding. Although this may require resources at the front end, it could help to distinguish between those cases that qualify as self-neglect or not, so that services can be referred, utilized, and coordinated most appropriately and efficiently. This could help to avoid allocation of provider time and resources to inaccurately categorized cases/situations, potentially reducing costs in the long term. Through outreach efforts and adequate time invested in establishing trust, service providers can assess for self-neglect and either provide or connect individuals to essential case management and health/mental health services as appropriate.

Implementing Strategies

Clarification of the reporting and referral process, and the establishment of this process via formal policy is fundamental to an effective response to self-neglect. Study findings point to a vital need for clarity around the reporting and referral process for suspected cases of self-neglect. The reporting process in Vermont may benefit from review and modification to establish a single point of entry and reflect the most appropriate location for coordinating the response to cases of self-neglect. Service providers across the continuum of health and social services are in need of training to enhance the recognition of and response to self-neglect. Nearly 75% of respondents reported that training on self-neglect was an extremely important component of responding to it. Not only did providers express a need for more training and education for themselves, but for their families and community members as well. Given the role of community concern and involvement in reporting/referring suspected cases of self-neglect, public education is essential in terms of raising awareness about warning signs, resources, and referral options. Of particular concern is raising public awareness regarding self-determination and the limits to intervention.

Study findings point to the need for specialized training and/or access to expertise via consultation when responding to cases of self-neglect. Several respondents indicated a desire for the designated staff to respond to self-neglect cases. Although some indicated a preference for a specially trained and/or experienced staff to be hired/assigned to address self-neglect cases, given the high need and expectations for engagement and unique characteristics of these cases, others suggested having all staff trained and/or having a specialist available for consultation so that all staff are able to respond accordingly. Another option is teaming case managers and mental health providers together for a response. Ultimately, there is a significant need for expertise in this area and resources to support the provision of specialized services for complex self-neglect cases.

Study findings illustrate that care management services are an essential component of the response to cases of suspected self-neglect. Case managers play a crucial role in coordinating care and facilitating interdisciplinary collaboration. Unfortunately, in a time of financial constraints and increasingly limited resources, service agencies and providers face challenges to collaboration, including time and competition. Findings indicate that although collaboration is perceived as key to an effective response to self-neglect, there is limited time for additional team meetings. Local areas may prefer to utilize existing interagency meetings or collaborate on a one-on-one, case-by-case basis. It was also noted that although agencies need to work together, and often have a long history of doing so, they are simultaneously vying for limited resources, creating a competitive rather than collaborative environment. Whether through existing teams and collaborative meetings, the development of new partnerships, or individual provider relationships, it is clear that interprofessional, interagency collaboration is essential to accessing expertise, maximizing resources, and providing a comprehensive response to self-neglect.

Given the role of concerned community members in bringing suspected cases of self-neglect to the attention of providers, there are several ways that community support and involvement could enhance the response to self-neglect. It is of primary importance that the public is informed regarding the nature of self-neglect and process for report, referrals, and response. Related to the recommendation provided under training and education, a public awareness campaign may be useful in providing information and education about elder self-neglect to the concerned community members and families. There is a clear need for additional support for families and caregivers, specifically for individuals suspected to be self-neglecting. Of particular concern and worthy of further investigation is the issue of caregivers who may be neglecting to address their own needs in the process of caring for a loved one. As long-term care services are increasingly home and community based, family caregivers will likely need additional supports to help reduce cases of self-neglect as well as potential abuse and neglect resulting from caregiver stress. Ultimately, the movement toward a coordinated community response to self-neglect could be strengthened by an effort to involve community members through an organized volunteer/peer/companion network. As community members are generally the concerned party who brings self-neglect to the attention to others, they may be well positioned to be an active part of the response. Providers can partner with communities to engage in both prevention and intervention efforts, however, it is clear that significant attention to and resources for training and support will be essential to success.

CONCLUSION

Findings from this study and related recommendations should be considered in light of several limitations. First, this study represents the perspectives of service providers and stakeholders in Vermont. The purpose of this study was a statewide assessment, and although results may be applicable to other areas, there is no guarantee that findings would be replicated across other state, national, and/or international regions. In addition, use of alternative methods, such as the inclusion of elders and caregivers, could have resulted in different findings and recommendations to inform a community response. That said, study findings point to several implications for research and practice.

IMPLICATIONS FOR RESEARCH AND PRACTICE

- Further research is needed to better understand the relationship between self-neglect mental health/cognitive impairment, and the utilization and impact of different capacity-determination and self-neglect assessment measures.
- There is a paucity of research on the outcomes of various self-neglect interventions, indicating a need for comparative, longitudinal studies.
- There is a need for practitioners trained in capacity determination and assessment of self-neglect.
- Care management and coordination services are essential to a coordinated community response. Interprofessional and interagency collaboration will require practitioner education and systemic support for interprofessional practice.
- Increasingly, innovative peer, family, and community support models may serve as a valuable resource in a coordinated community response to self-neglect.

REFERENCES

Abrams, R.C., Lachs, M., & McAvay, G. (2002). Predictors of self-neglect in community-dwelling elders. *American Journal of Psychiatry, 159*(10), 1724–1730. doi:10.1176.appi.ajp.159.10.1724

American Psychiatric Association. (2013). *Diagnostic and statistical manual of mental disorders* (5th ed.). Arlington, VA: American Psychiatric Publishing.

Band-Winterstein, T., Doron, I., & Naim, S. (2012). Elder self-neglect: A geriatric syndrome or a life course story? *Journal of Aging Studies, 26*, 109–118.

Bartley, M., Knight, P.V., O'Neill, D., & O'Brien, J. G. (2011). Self-neglect and elder abuse: Related phenomena? *Journal of the American Geriatrics Society, 59*(11), 2163–2168. doi:10.1111/j.1532-5415.2011.03653.x

Brandl, B., Dyer, C. B., Heisler, C.J., Otto, J. M., Stiegel, L. A., & Thomas, R. W. (2006). *Elder abuse detection and intervention: A collaborative approach*. New York, NY: Springer Publishing.

Braye, S., Orr, D., & Preston-Shoot, M. (2011). *Self-neglect and adult safeguarding: Findings from research* (SCIE Report 46). London, UK: Social Care Institute for Excellence. Retrieved from http://bit.ly/1IGGyOf

Burnett, J., Regev, T., Pickens, S., Prati, L. L., Aung, K., Moore, J., & Dyer, C. B. (2006). Social networks: A profile of the elderly who self-neglect. *Journal of Elder Abuse & Neglect, 18*(4), 35–49. doi:10.1300/J084v18n04_05

Charmaz, K. (2006). *Constructing grounded theory: A practical guide through qualitative analysis*. London, UK: Sage.

DAIL Self-Neglect Task Force. (2012). *Report and recommendations on self-neglect in Vermont*. Report submitted to the Vermont Department of Disabilities Aging and Independent Living (DAIL). Retrieved from http://dail.vermont.gov/dail-whats-new/whats-new-documents/report-and-recommendations-on-self-neglect-in-vt

Day, M.R. (2010). Self-neglect: A challenge and a dilemma. *Archives of Psychiatric Nursing, 24*(2), 73–75.

Day, M. R., & McCarthy, G. (2016). Self-neglect: Development and evaluation of a self-neglect (SN-37) measurement instrument. *Archives of Psychiatric Nursing, 30*(4), 480–485. doi:10.1016/j.apnu.2016.02.004

Day, M. R., Mulcahy, H., Leahy-Warren, P., & Downey, J. (2015). Self-neglect: A case study and implications for clinical practice. *British Journal of Community Nursing, 20*(3), 110–115.

Dong, X., Simon, M., Fulmer, T., Mendes de Leon, C. F., Rajan, B., & Evans, D. A. (2010). Physical function decline and the risk of elder self-neglect in a community-dwelling population. *The Gerontologist, 50*(3), 316–326. doi:10.1093/geront/gnp164

Dong, X., Simon, M. A., Wilson, R. S., Mendes de Leon, C. F., Rajan, K. B., & Evans, D. A. (2010). Decline in cognitive function and risk of elder self-neglect: Finding from the Chicago Health Aging Project. *Journal of the American Geriatrics Society, 58*(12), 2292–2299.

Dong, X., Wilson, R. S., Mendes de Leon, C. F., & Evans, D. A. (2010). Self-neglect and cognitive function among community-dwelling older persons. *International Journal of Geriatric Psychiatry, 25*(8), 798–806.

Dyer, C. B., Pavlik, V. N., & Murphy, K. P. (2000). The high prevalence of depression and dementia in elder abuse or neglect. *Journal of the American Geriatrics Society, 48*(2), 205–208. doi:10.1111/j.1532-5415.2000.tb03913.x

Flood, P. (1996, December 13). *Self-neglect reporting*. Memorandum to Vermont HHA Executive Directors.

Fulmer, T. (2008). Barriers to neglect and self-neglect research. *Journal of the American Geriatrics Society, 56*, S241–S243.

Gibbons, S., Lauder, W., & Ludwick, R. (2006). Self-neglect: A proposed new NANDA diagnosis. *International Journal of Nursing Terminologies & Classifications, 17*(1), 10–18. doi:10.1111/j.1744-618X.2006.00018.x

Iris, M., Ridings, J. W., & Conrad, K. J. (2010). The development of a conceptual model for understanding elder self-neglect. *The Gerontologist, 50*(3), 303–315. doi:10.1093/geront/gnp125

Kelly, P. A., Dyer, C. B., Pavlik, V. N., Doody, R. S., & Jogerst, G. (2008). Exploring self-neglect in older adults: Preliminary findings of the Self-neglect Severity Scale and next steps. *Journal of the American Geriatrics Society, 56*(Suppl. 2), S253–S260. doi:10.1111/j.1532-5415.2008.01977.x

Kutame, M. M. (2007). *Understanding self-neglect from the older person's perspective* (Unpublished doctoral dissertation). Ohio State University, Columbus, OH.

Lincoln, Y. S., & Guba, E. G. (1985). *Naturalistic inquiry*. Beverly Hills, CA: Sage.

Melekis, K. (2014a). *Responding to self-neglect*. Prepared for the Vermont Department of Disabilities, Aging, and Independent Living.

Melekis, K. (2014b). *Vermont statewide assessment of needs and resources for older adults and caregivers*. Prepared for the Vermont Department of Disabilities, Aging, and Independent Living.

Miles, M. B., & Huberman, A. M. (1994). *Qualitative data analysis*. Thousand Oaks, CA: Sage.

Naik, A. D., Lai, J. M., Kunik, M. E., & Dyer, C. B. (2008). Assessing capacity in suspected cases of self-neglect. *Geriatrics, 63*(2), 24–31.

O'Brien, J. G. (2011). Self-neglect in old age. *Aging Health, 7*(4), 573–581.

Padgett, D. K. (2008). *Qualitative methods in social work research* (2nd ed.). Thousand Oaks, CA: Sage.

Parmar, J., Bremault-Phillips, S., & Charles, L. (2015). The development and implementation of a decision-making capacity assessment model. *Canadian Geriatrics Journal, 18*(1), 15–28.

Patton, M. Q. (2002). *Qualitative research and evaluation methods* (3rd ed.). Thousand Oaks, CA: Sage.

Pavlou, M., & Lachs, M. (2006). Could self-neglect in older adults be a geriatric syndrome? *Journal of the American Geriatrics Society, 54*, 831–842.

Pickens, S., Ostwald, S. K., Pace, K. M., Diamond, P., Burnett, J., & Dyer, C. B. (2013). Assessing dimensions of executive function in community-dwelling older adults with self-neglect. *Clinical Nursing Studies, 2*(1), 17–29.

Rathborn-McCuan, E., & Fabian, D. R. (Eds.). (1992). *Self-neglecting elders: A clinical dilemma*. New York, NY: Auburn House.

Saldaña, J. (2009). *The coding manual for qualitative researchers*. London, UK: Sage.

Skelton, F., Kunik, M. E., Regev, T., & Naik, A. D. (2010). Determining if an older adult can make and execute decisions to live safely at home: A capacity assessment and intervention model. *Archives of Gerontology and Geriatrics, 50*(3), 300–305. doi:10.1016/j.archger

Teaster, P. (2003). *A response to the abuse of vulnerable adults: The 2000 survey of state adult protective services*. Washington, DC: National Committee for the Prevention of Elder Abuse/National Association of Adult Protective Services Administrators/National Association of State Units on Aging and National Center on Elder Abuse.

Teaster, P. B., Dugar, T. A., Mendiondo, M. S., Abner, E. L., & Cecil, K. A. (2006). *The 2004 survey of state adult protective services: Abuse of adults 60 years of age and older*. Washington, DC: The National Center on Elder Abuse. Retrieved from http://www.napsa-now.org/wp-content/uploads/2012/09/2-14-06-FINAL-60+REPORT.pdf

U.S. Census Bureau. (2011). *Age and sex composition: 2010*. Washington, DC: U.S. Department of Commerce.

Volmert, A., & Lindland, E. (2016). *You only pray that somebody would step in: Mapping the gaps between expert and public understandings of elder abuse in America*. Washington, DC: Frame Works Institute.

White, W. (2014). Elder self-neglect and adult protective services: Ohio needs to do more. *Journal of Law and Health, 27*, 130–162.

CHAPTER 18

MEDICATION USE AND POLYPHARMACY IN OLDER ADULTS WITH SUBSTANTIATED SELF-NEGLECT: A CASE STUDY

Jason Burnett, Leslie E. Clark, Sharon Abada, Kimberlee Parker, Renee J. Flores, and Kathleen Pace-Murphy

Self-neglect is defined as the inability or unwillingness to provide oneself with necessary resources to maintain safety and health. Self-neglecting elders tend to experience increased functional and cognitive decline as well as increased morbidity and mortality. Adherence to chronic disease medications is low in this population, whereas polypharmacy (more than five prescribed medications) is high (73%). Medication usage patterns and polypharmacy may underlie some of the negative social and physical conditions and outcomes of self-neglect. An interprofessional team (IPT) approach is imperative to the development of a comprehensive plan of care for older adults with substantiated self-neglect and polypharmacy. This chapter presents a case study of substantiated self-neglect and discusses medication use and polypharmacy.

This chapter begins with a case study of substantiated self-neglect that highlights polypharmacy in an older adult. Negative social and physical conditions and outcomes of self-neglect may be associated with medication usage patterns and polypharmacy. An IPT approach is imperative for a comprehensive plan of care in older adults with substantiated self-neglect and polypharmacy.

SELF-NEGLECT

Mr. R's situation is not unusual or rare but quietly remains a hidden epidemic across the United States. In fact, self-neglect is the most common cause for referral to adult protective services (APS) across the United States despite only 20% being brought to the attention of social services (Teaster, Dugar, Mendiondo, Abner, & Cecil, 2006). Self-neglect prevalence has been estimated to be 38% to 56% of all APS cases nationwide. The National Center on Elder Abuse defines self-neglect as:

> The inability, due to physical or mental impairments or reduced capacity, to provide oneself with the necessary resources (e.g., food, medical services,

shelter) to maintain physical health, mental health and overall well-being (The National Center on Elder Abuse, 2016).

In addition, self-neglect can be described as intentional or unintentional behaviors that threaten older adults' health, safety, and/or the ability to live independently (Dyer, Pickens, & Burnett, 2007).

Older adults with substantiated self-neglect often present to the health care community with one or more of the following conditions:

- Untreated or undertreated acute and chronic medical conditions, including asthma, heart failure, diabetes mellitus, or hypertension (medical neglect) (Burnett, Coverdale, Pickens, & Dyer, 2006)
- Nonadherence to medical plans of care, including not filling prescriptions or taking medications as prescribed, missing multiple medical appointments, frequent emergency department visits (medical neglect; Turner, Hochschild, Burnett, Zulfiqar, & Dyer, 2012)
- Isolated and unsanitary living conditions, including squalor, hoarding, lack of utilities (environmental neglect; Dyer, Pickens, et al., 2007)
- Poor or unkempt appearance, overgrown nails and hair, pressure ulcers, excoriated perineal areas, body odor (physical and medical neglect; Abrams, Lachs, McAvay, Keohane, & Bruce, 2002; Dyer, Pickens, et al., 2007)
- Poorly managed depression and other psychiatric conditions (i.e., mental health neglect; Burnett et al., 2006; Dyer, Pavlik, Murphy, & Hyman, 2000)

CASE STUDY 1: MR. R

Mr. R is a 75-year-old bilingual Hispanic man. He is living in a low-income, one-bedroom apartment with his wife and autistic son in a high-crime neighborhood in a large metropolitan city. With substantiated elder self-neglect, Mr. R was a client of APS. He was referred by the APS to an interventional outreach health program. The health program's registered nurse contacted Mr. R. She described the aim of the year-long program, which was to help older adults with APS-substantiated self-neglect become healthier through improved medical self-management. Mr. R was interested and consented to participate.

Upon arrival for his initial assessment, the RN walked into Mr. R's home through the front door, and entered the living room, which is used as Mr. R's bedroom. It was musky and dark, with one bedside lamp cramped next to a king-sized mattress. A dresser was squeezed in on either side of the bed and there was no visible wall space due to clutter. A walker and a motorized chair sat at the foot of the bed, just out of the way of the television, leaving little to no walking space. Mr. R was sitting, propped up on his bed with several pillows, wearing only shorts. His respiratory distress was visibly apparent with the use of accessory muscles, and he was self-administering his nebulizer. Next to him, hidden underneath the soiled sheets, was his emaciated, late-stage HIV-positive wife. Across the room, seen through a crack in the door was a television-illuminated dining and kitchen area currently serving as a bedroom for multiple disheveled people who trafficked in and out during the visit. These people were later determined to be transients/homeless persons, drug users, and prostitutes who occupied the room for little to no money. As part of the comprehensive assessment, Mr. R's medication knowledge was assessed to determine his health literacy. It was clear that he had scarce comprehension into the medical indications or side effects of his medications. He was also not aware of how to take his medications to prevent poor outcomes. In fact, he stated that he could not discern which medications were prescribed to take once, twice, or three times per day, so he stated that he would take all his medications ($N = 17$) at the same time so that he would not miss a dose. This approach required Mr. R to take 22 pills all at once.

Dyer, Pickens, et al. (2007) described an etiological model of elder self-neglect based on over 500 cases evaluated and treated by an interprofessional clinical team. This model describes cognitive, nutritional, and mental health deficits as precipitating factors that lead to executive function and activities of daily living impairments. When these impairments are met with the absence of adequate support services, conditions of self-neglect result (Dyer, Goodwin, Pickens-Pace, Burnett, & Kelly, 2007). Moreover, recent research has identified four clusters/types of self-neglect: (1) financial, (2) environmental (e.g., clutter, poor living conditions), (3) global, and (4) physical and medical self-neglect (Kelly, Dyer, Pavlik, Doody, & Jogerst, 2008). These clusters are differentiated by unique sets of conditions and associated risk factors, indicating the possibility for various etiologies (Burnett et al., 2014). For example, cognition and mental health are considered to be primary risk factors for self-neglect in older adults, yet, mental health problems are only prominent in the global self-neglect cluster.

Consistent among the studies of elder self-neglect are associations with poor outcomes. Elder self-neglecters have significantly higher rates of emergency department visits, hospitalizations, functional decline, subsequent elder abuse, institutionalization, and two- to threefold increases in all-cause mortality compared to non-neglecting older adults (Dong, Mendes de Leon, & Evans, 2009; Dong, Simon, et al., 2009; Dong, Simon, & Evans, 2012a, 2012b, 2013; Lachs, Williams, O'Brien, & Pillemer, 2002; Lachs, Williams, O'Brien, Pillemer, & Charlson, 1998). Many of these risks are independent of measured cognitive, functional, medical, and social conditions.

Mr. R's Conditions of Self-Neglect

Table 18.1 provides an overview of Mr. R's initial assessment findings. Conditions specific to self-neglect are included to paint a picture of his self-neglect status at the time of the initial assessment.

As reviewed in Table 18.1, Mr. R presented with several conditions commonly identified in older adults with substantiated self-neglect. Medically, Mr. R was determined to be dehydrated based on physical examination and self-report. Mr. R was prescribed multiple diuretics and upon examination he had dry mucous membranes, dry skin, and expressed complaints of increased thirst, decreased urine output, muscle fatigue, and explained that he did not want to increase his fluid intake due to concerns about multiple trips to the bathroom and fear of falling. Mr. R did not appear to be malnourished but did explain that he eats only one meal a day and shares most of his food with his wife, son, and "friends" who visit their apartment. Although Mr. R reports seeing physicians to manage his chronic disease diagnosis he reports several conditions that he does not believe he is being treated for, which include chronic back and neck pain, multiple caries and chronic oral infections and pain, worsening bilateral hand tremors, and pain in the right hand. Mr. R appears to have the medical aids he needs at home, which include blood pressure cuff, nebulizer, oxygen concentrator, manual and electric wheelchairs, and a walker. Despite Mr. R's functional limitations and chronic debilitating pain, his physical appearance was well kept. This may reflect his prior military training.

Unlike the majority of the self-neglecters, Mr. R did not live in isolation, but he did have poor social networks consisting of transients and sex workers. These

TABLE 18.1   Mr. R's Initial Assessment Findings and Conditions of Self-Neglect

Evidence-Supported Indicators	Clinical Assessment	Condition Observed Yes or No
Social		
Isolation	Lives with wife and cognitively impaired son	No
Poor social networks	Multiple vagrants, drug abusers, and sex workers in and out of home daily	Yes
Environment		
Unsanitary living conditions	Very dirty, trash present, odors, multiple mattresses and bedding in common living area, and bug infestation	Yes
Insects and rodents	Bedbug and cockroach infestation	Yes
No utilities	All working appropriately	No
Hoarding	Unremarkable	No
Physical		
Poor hygiene	No odors or dirty skin	No
Inadequate clothing	Appropriate and clean clothing	No
Unkempt appearance	Unremarkable	No
• Dry mucous membranes, increased thirst, decreased urine output, fatigue • Oral mucosa and tongue fissured and coated with dried mucus	Dehydration secondary to multiple prescribed diuretics	Yes
BMI within normal limits, no serum evaluation, limited food present in home	Malnutrition suspected secondary to nutritional deficiency; need to assess nutritional serum parameters	No
• Back, neck, and right hand pain • Multiple dental caries with acute chronic oral infections and dental pain • Bilateral hand tremors	• Multiple undertreated or untreated medical conditions • Multiple health care providers, no coordinated medical plan of care, unable to articulate when health care provider appointments are scheduled • Transportation issues	Yes

(continued)

TABLE 18.1 Mr. R's Initial Assessment Findings and Conditions of Self-Neglect (*continued*)

Evidence-Supported Indicators	Clinical Assessment	Condition Observed Yes or No
Mental Health		
Depression	Severe depression as measured by the Geriatric Depression Scale	Yes
Psychosis	No indication of psychosis or altered mental status	No
Anxiety	Severe anxiety and depression	Yes
Executive dysfunction	• Normal Trail Making Test: Parts A and B • Normal CLOX I and II	No
Medical		
Lack of medical aids	Had a medical scooter	No
Polypharmacy—currently taking 17 different medications all at one time per day	• Prescriptions are written by multiple health care providers, received from multiple pharmacies. • Medications do not appear to be current. • Two medications are "borrowed" from a friend who "thought they would help."	Yes
Medication adherence	Concerns regarding his daily routine of taking all medications and doses at once to avoid missed doses	Yes

Note: This table compares the literature and evidence-based indicators of self-neglect to the clinical assessment findings of Mr. R to identify his present areas of self-neglect.
BMI, body mass index; CLOX, an executive clock-drawing task.

poor relationships may have contributed to his self-neglect. Mr. R stated that he made poor decisions when making his apartment available to vagrants and drug users because they would commonly use his limited resources for their benefit. Consistent with many self-neglect situations, Mr. R's environment was extremely unkempt as evidenced by dirty, stained, damp floors and bedding, severe bedbug and cockroach infestation, trash and mildew odors combined with the malodorous evidence of multiple unsanitary people living in his home. He was not lacking basic utilities and explained that the utilities were covered under his rent so all utilities are paid. There was no evidence of hoarding, however, multiple mattresses, bedding and various belongings on the floor promote a hoarder-like situation with unsafe mobility and health hazards.

Mr. R did express feelings of extreme anxiety and depression and when he was administered the Geriatric Depression Scale (GDS) he scored 14 out of 15, indicating severe depression. Mr. R verbalized his sadness over making poor decisions and "paying the consequences" for those decisions. He felt helpless to change his situation.

Review of Mr. R's medications indicated excessive polypharmacy and medication nonadherence. Mr. R described the desire to take his medications as prescribed but felt overwhelmed with the dosing instructions. In fact, he described taking all 17 medications at the same time each morning. Even if the medication was scheduled to be taken multiple times a day, he took all of the doses at the same time. However, before we assess and discuss Mr. R's medication list, we briefly review the definitions of polypharmacy and the interactions between pharmacology and aging.

DEFINING POLYPHARMACY

Polypharmacy is a significant concern among older adults living with chronic diseases, yet health care professionals have struggled to reach a consensus on its definition. The two most common definitions are the concomitant use of five or more medications or the use of potentially inappropriate medications (Mion & Sandhu, 2016). Research by Gnjidic et al. (2012) found that the use of four or more medications concomitantly provided the best prediction for adverse outcomes in a population of 1,705 community-dwelling men, aged 70 years and older (Gnjidic et al., 2012). A national survey of adults 65 and older, residing in the United States, found that 57% of women took five or more concurrent prescription medications, whereas 12% took 10 or more concurrent prescription medications. Therefore, the concept of excessive polypharmacy, which is defined as the concomitant use of 10 or more medications, may be especially relevant when describing general medication trends in the older adult community-dwelling population. Although pharmacologic management has many benefits, such as alleviation of clinical signs and symptoms, enhanced quality of life, and perhaps life extension, there are also risks associated with this intervention (Liu, 2016; Steinman & Hanlon, 2010). Both polypharmacy (5–9 medications) and excessive polypharmacy (≥10 medications) are predictors of adverse drug events, hospitalization, nursing home placement, functional decline, falls, delirium, and death (Charlesworth, Smit, Lee, Alramadhan, & Odden, 2015; Frazier, 2005; Mion & Sandhu, 2016). Older adults prescribed seven or more medications have up to an 82% risk of adverse drug events (Scott, Gray, Martin, & Mitchell, 2016).

AGING AND PHARMACOLOGY

Increased drug consumption may be harmful to the aging population due to altered physiology. The geriatric literature has cited that older adults are more susceptible to anticholinergic adverse effects, orthostatic hypotension, cognitive impairment, increased fall risk, and difficulty with adherence to medication plans. Some of these risks are increased as a result of age-related changes affecting medication absorption, distribution, metabolism, and elimination. Absorption is the only process not affected by age in the gastrointestinal (GI) system. As one ages, the distribution of medications may change as a result of (1) increase in body fat, which causes lipophilic medications to have a significantly longer half-life, increasing the risk for side effects related to high medication levels; (2) decrease in total body water, which causes a decrease in the volume of distribution of water-soluble medication, resulting in higher concentration of hydrophilic medications; (3) decrease in albumin, an important plasma protein associated with malnutrition, leading to decrease in the effectiveness of some medications not being bound to target proteins; (4) increased permeability of the blood–brain barrier, causing a higher potential for central nervous system adverse effects; and (5) changes in subcutaneous fat, which may alter the absorption of transdermal medication, influencing the distribution of the medication prescribed. Demographics, such as gender, lifestyle choices (e.g., smoking), and chronic comorbidities (e.g., heart failure), can all influence liver function, causing either decreases or elevations of medication metabolism. Associated with aging are decreases in renal clearance and reductions in the elimination of medications. These changes, along with the use of multiple and potentially harmful medications, may have a synergistic effect on the function and well-being of the older adult.

MEDICATION USE AND SELF-NEGLECT

The intersection of medication use and self-neglect is vastly understudied but is emerging as an important area of research. The majority of APS self-neglect cases occur in adults 65 years and older living with multiple chronic health conditions. Complex and sometimes potentially harmful therapeutic regimens increase these individuals' risk for adverse events. In 2011, Culberson et al. reported that individuals determined by APS to be suffering elder self-neglect are more likely to be taking benzodiazepines compared with older adults without substantiated self-neglect. This class of medications could play an important role in self-neglect given its sedative properties and its association with falls and depression. In a separate self-neglect study, Turner et al. (2012) reported that approximately 90% of a community-based sample of APS-substantiated self-neglecting individuals were nonadherent to their chronic disease medication regimens and 59% were nonadherent to three or more chronic disease medications. More recent data support a link between medication regimen complexity and medication nonadherence behaviors in older adults who self-neglect, independent of memory and executive dysfunction (Burnett et al., 2016). This study found that the mean medication complexity score for elder self-neglecters was as high as the medication complexity scores of hospitalized and institutionalized older adults. Moreover, new unpublished data indicate that 73% of elder self-neglecters exhibit polypharmacy. This number increases to 90% if over-the-counter (OTC) medications are included in the count. Given the age-related changes, and inappropriate medication use and polypharmacy in self-neglecters, a review of Mr. R's medical history and prescribed medication regimen for problems and concerns that may have increased his propensity for self-neglect is appropriate.

Mr. R's Medical History and Medication Regimen

During the first home visit, Mr. R self-reported a medical history consisting of myocardial infarction (MI), cerebrovascular accident (CVA), hepatitis (A, B, and

C) and chronic diseases: congestive heart failure (CHF), peripheral vascular disease (PVD), osteoarthritis (OA), chronic obstructive pulmonary disease (COPD), pulmonary hypertension, and hypertension. Mr. R's prescribed medication regimen is presented in Table 18.2.

One does not need to be a seasoned nurse or a pharmacologist to be concerned at the number of medications ($N = 17$) Mr. R was taking on a daily basis. Moreover, the total pill-count was actually 22. This number becomes even more alarming when one remembers that Mr. R stated that he took *ALL* his medications at one time because he could not keep up with the regimen and was afraid to miss a dose. If we did not know his method of medication administration and we simply counted his medications to assess adherence, Mr. R would appear to be adherent. However, a more complete picture of his medication and chronic disease management informed the team of the many problems and potential feedback effects that

TABLE 18.2 Mr. R's Medication List, Doses, Diagnoses, and Pills Taken per Day

Medication	Instructions	Diagnosis	Pills Daily
Levothyroxine 0.05 mg	1 tablet daily	Hypothyroidism	1
Xarelto 10 mg	1 tablet daily	Atrial fibrillation	1
Gabapentin 100 mg	1 cap 3× daily	Neuropathic	3
Metoprolol Tartrate 25 mg	1 tablet 2× daily	CHF	2
Spironolactone 25 mg	1 capsule 2× daily	CHF	2
Torsemide 20 mg	1 tablet daily	CHF, ascites	1
Pantoprazole 40 mg	1 tablet daily	GERD	1
Isosorbide Mononitrate ER 30 mg	1 tablet daily	CHF	1
Ranexa 500 mg	1 capsule 2× daily	Angina	2
Furosemide 40 mg	1 tablet daily	CHF	1
Bumetanide 1 mg	1 tablet daily	CHF	1
Aspirin 81 mg	1 tablet daily	CAD antianginal	1
Montelukast 10 mg	1 tablet every PM	Asthma, bronchospasm prophylaxis	1
Valsartan/HCTZ 320/12.5 mg	1 tablet daily	CHF/CAD	1
Levofloxacin 500 mg	1 tablet daily for 14 days	Oral infection	1
Tramadol ER 200 mg	1 tablet daily	Oral pain, neuropathic pain	1
Sertraline 50 mg	1 tablet daily	Depression	1

CAD, coronary artery disease; CHF, congestive heart failure; ER, extended release; GERD, gastroesophageal reflux disease; HCTZ, hydrochlorothiazide.

may be leading to exacerbated conditions, new onset of symptoms and conditions, as well as increased risks for self-neglect. For instance, Mr. R had multiple health care professionals who prescribed medication while caring for him and he never brought his medications with him to his doctors/office/outpatient visits for review. This increases the potential for medication interactions or duplication of medications as in Mr. R's regimen. He was prescribed five diuretics, which could result in dehydration, hypotension, dizziness, and falls; all of which could negatively impact his function and ability to engage in activities of daily living. In addition, Mr. R had multiple people going to different pharmacies to help him get his medications so pharmacists were unaware of the potentially harmful combinations of medications that he was taking. This is a perfect example of what not to do when managing chronic multiple illnesses and provides an insight into the importance of performing in-depth assessments of the patient's medications and usage patterns. There are several steps that should be implemented to help prevent these and other kinds of problems.

MEDICATION RECONCILIATION

Medication Review

The medication safety assessment can begin with a complete detailed inventory and review of the prescribed medications. The health care team needed to visually inspect Mr. R's medications at every visit. Medication review in the older adult with self-neglect begins with an accurate listing of all medications that are being taken, including prescription medications, OTC medications, and herbal and alternative therapies. Identifying the full list of medications for review in the elder self-neglecting population can prove to be difficult given that they often store their medications in many different areas of the home and combine new prescriptions with old prescriptions (Turner et al., 2012). Moreover, older adults who self-neglect often have limited health literacy and are poor historians (Burnett, Cully, Achenbaum, Dyer, & Naik, 2011).

Mr. R is a perfect example of how a medical history and medication regimen may tell two different stories and why taking a conservative approach, by performing a comprehensive medication safety assessment, is a best practice for this population. After review of Mr. R's medications and chronic disease history it was apparent he was taking medications for conditions that were not included in his self-report. For example, Mr. R was prescribed gabapentin, which is typically prescribed as an anticonvulsant or for pain associated with neuropathic pain. Mr. R did not report a diagnosis that would warrant the gabapentin medication. Another example would be his prescription for levothyroxine, which is prescribed for thyroid insufficiency, which he denied. It is common for underserved populations, similar to those who self-neglect, to have limited health literacy and provide incomplete medical histories (Ciechanowski, Wagner, & Schmaling, 2004).

Medication Safety Assessment

The next step for the health care team is to perform a series of assessments to ensure that each medication is appropriately prescribed and is the best option for the older adult given his or her medical conditions. What does this mean? It means that the health care team needs to ensure that the prescribed medication, dose, frequency, and route of administration are appropriate given the older adults' health conditions and characteristics. Inappropriate prescribing can lead to poor health outcomes, including cognitive impairments, falls, and increased mortality. Mr. R is taking 17 different medications, which adds up to 22 pills taken all at once, one time per day. It was immediately noted that the timing was not appropriate (i.e., nonadherent) and he was not experiencing the desired effects of his medications. Taking all of these medications at once places him at a high risk for adverse drug–drug interactions. As part of the reconciliation process, the question must be asked whether he really needs all these medications. Were there any medications that were not appropriate or no longer necessary that could arguably be removed from his regimen? Mr. R is taking five diuretic medications. Could this number potentially be reduced to decrease his reported side effects of dizziness and dehydration? In addition to the diuretics, a health care professional would likely want to investigate what additional chronic diseases or diagnosis he might have to align or account for the medication regimen. For example, he did not report a diagnosis that would support his prescription for gabapentin and sertraline. As his medications could potentially lead to drug–drug and drug–disease interactions, it is important to check the safety of these medications prior to contacting his prescribing physicians(s). There are many tools that can be used to review the safety and appropriateness of Mr. R's medication regimen, which include the Beers Criteria for Potentially Inappropriate Medication Use, the multi-drug interaction tool (Micromedex), Medication Appropriateness Index (MAI), and STOPP/START (screening tool of older people's prescriptions/screening tool to alert to right treatment) criteria (Hanlon & Schmader, 2013; O'Mahony et al., 2014; The American Geriatrics Society, 2015; Truven Health Analytics, 2016).

Beers Criteria for Potentially Inappropriate Medications

We now know that aging can change the effect of medications, making some potentially inappropriate for the older population. The Beers Criteria for Potentially Inappropriate Medications in older adults was first created in 1991 and last updated in 2015 (The American Geriatrics Society, 2015). The Beers Criteria provides evidence-based recom-mendations on medications to be used with caution, drug interactions to avoid, drugs to be avoided in renal impairment, and medications with highly anticholinergic properties. If the patient is on medications that are contraindicated on the Beers list and assessed as inappropriate for the older adult, it could potentially be the cause or may increase the incidence of poor health outcomes and cognitive decline. In the case of Mr. R, of his 17 prescribed medications, four (24%) had alerts that indicated a contraindication with patients who are diagnosed with renal insufficiency. Although he did not report a diagnosis of renal insufficiency his other multiple diagnoses of chronic disease and polypharmacy would promote the need to use these medications with caution.

Multidrug Interaction Tool

Another important consideration when performing the medication reconciliation is checking for drug-to-drug and drug-to-disease interactions. We used Micromedex to assess for possible drug-to-drug and drug-to-disease interactions. Upon reviewing Mr. R's medications and the possible drug-to-drug interactions, we found 10 of the 17 (59%) prescribed medications had a possibility of causing a drug-to-drug reaction or adverse event. The tool we used gave a severity scale rating of "contraindicated: major, moderate, or minor" with supporting evidence that was excellent, good or fair. For example, Mr. R was prescribed both aspirin and sertraline. On the severity scale, the contraindication was major and the evidence to support the severity scale was good. Summary of the contraindication of these two medications stated that the concurrent use of sertraline and antiplatelet agents may result in an increased risk of bleeding. Given this kind of possible adverse effect, the health care team would evaluate the medications to determine whether these were the best options for Mr. R given his chronic conditions.

The MAI and STOPP/START Criteria

The MAI and the STOPP/START criteria may also be used to review an older adult's medications. The MAI uses 10 criteria to assess the appropriateness of each prescribed and OTC medication (Spinewine, Dumont, Mallet, & Swine, 2006). Some examples of the specific MAI criteria include whether the medication is indicated, the dosage is correct, the medication is effective for the condition, and the directions are practical (Hanlon & Schmader, 2013). In addition, the STOPP/START criteria is a set of inappropriate combinations of medicines and disease systems (the STOPP component), as well as a list of recommended medications for a given disease (Gallagher, O'Connor, & O'Mahony, 2011). Geriatricians and older adult health care professionals may use a combination of the three methods described to elicit medication appropriateness during the medication reconciliation process.

Utilizing the findings from the Beers and Micromedex tools, the health care team could then complete the 10-question MAI tool. Of the 17 medications Mr. R was prescribed, six (35%) were scored as inappropriate for him based on the MAI. For instance, as stated previously he was prescribed gabapentin and, according to his self-reported medical history, there was no indication the medication was necessary. Because there was no indication, the health care team was unable to determine whether the medication was effective, whether the correct dose was prescribed, or whether the duration of therapy was acceptable. Gabapentin was scored as an inappropriate medication for Mr. R. The other five inappropriate medications were levothyroxine, Xarelto, pantoprazole, furosemide, and bumetanide. Until discussed with his prescribing physician, it is a good practice not to target these medications using evidence-based adherence strategies because doing so may inadvertently increase the likelihood of poor health outcomes.

Anticholinergic Cognitive Burden Scale

There are other available tools that provide information regarding medication effects on an older adult's heath and mortality burden. One popular scale is the Anticholinergic Cognitive Burden Scale (ACB; Indiana University Center for Aging Research, 2012). The ACB is a tool that can be utilized to identify medications in an older adult's regimen that may affect cognition due to anticholinergic properties. If applied to Mr. R, each medication in his regimen would be given a score of 0, 1, 2, or 3, depending on the strength of its anticholinergic effects, with higher scores indicating worse effects. The cumulative score represents the overall anticholinergic burden of Mr. R's medication regimen. For example, of the 17 medications prescribed to Mr. R, only three (18%; i.e., furosemide, isosorbide, and metoprolol) were on the ACB scale. Each received a score of 1, resulting in a cumulative score of 3. Notably, for each 1-point increase in the ACB total score, there is a 26% increase in the risk of death. Moreover, cognitive burden related to the use of anticholinergics by older adults significantly increased the 6-year risk for cognitive impairment and a 2-year increased risk for lowered Mini-Mental State Examination scores.

For Mr. R, some of his self-neglect behaviors, such as the inability to coordinate his medication regimen or make better decisions regarding his social and environmental situations, could possibly be attributed to the negative cognitive burden caused by his medication regimen. Moreover, his anticholinergic medication regimen has the possibility of creating an increased decline in cognitive function, self-neglect, and mortality (Fox et al., 2011). To date, anticholinergic use and other medication use practices within the self-neglecting population have not been included as risk factors or important moderators of self-neglect conditions and health outcomes.

In summary, Mr. R exhibited excessive polypharmacy ($N = 17$ medications), nonadherence to his prescribed medication regimen (taking all medications and doses at once), demonstrated poor health literacy and a complete inability to articulate his medical plan of care. After review of his medications, four (24%) were found to be potentially inappropriate based on the Beers Criteria, 10 (59%) were identified for potential drug–drug interactions, six (35%) were suggested to be inappropriate based on the MAI, and three (18%) contributed to cognitive burden that may decrease cognitive functioning and increase mortality risks.

THE INTERPROFESSIONAL TEAM

The case of Mr. R highlights the complexity that can and often does accompany self-neglect cases encountered by health care and social service professionals. Intervening in self-neglect, especially medically, is likely to be more efficient and long-lasting when multiple intervention perspectives are implemented. Such interventions are best led by the IPTs working together to ensure that a comprehensive and individualized plan is in place for the older adult. The IPT is one of the fundamental cornerstones of geriatric medicine and provides services (comprehensive geriatric assessment and screenings) to identify pertinent risk factors and assess vulnerabilities that may account for the current conditions and impact the future health and well-being of the older adult leading to negative outcomes such as self-neglect. A multitude of studies provide evidence-based data supporting the superiority of the IPT model for reducing clinical error and improving patient outcomes and safety in complex cases (Oandasan & Reeves, 2005a, 2005b; West, Guthrie, Dawson, Borrill, & Carter, 2006). This approach has been tested in older adults with substantiated elder self-neglect and has demonstrated improved health outcomes compared to a non-IPT intervention (Burnett, Pickens, Aung, Reilley, & Dyer, 2010).

The central strengths of the IPT are expertise, flexibility, and efficiency. In an elder self-neglect case, the core IPT members would at the very least consist of a geriatrician, nurse (i.e., nurse practitioner or RN), and a geriatric social worker. Based on the evaluation, other professionals, including, but not limited to neurologists, psychologists, physician assistants, physical and occupational therapists, and pharmacists would be consulted to participate in the review of the case and develop the optimal plan of care. For instance, in the case of Mr. R, the best IPT would likely consist of the core team plus a pharmacist and a cardiologist. This team could have worked together to perhaps reduce the number of medications Mr. R was taking, worked to combine his medication taking in ways that posed less of a risk for drug–drug interaction, making his regimen less complicated and safer. Another important function would be to ensure that his medication regimen was optimized to promote control of chronic conditions while preserving functional status, which appears to be an important limitation for Mr. R. Moreover, the IPT may have been able to propose an educational plan with environmental supports to increase his health literacy and remind him of when his medications were to be taken throughout the day.

IPT Steps for Evaluating Mr. R's Polypharmacy and Medication Use

Principles for caring for older adults with multiple comorbidities have been developed by the American Geriatric Society (Burke et al., 2013). These guidelines may be used by the IPT as a guide to work with Mr. R in formulating a plan of care, including medication management. Informed by patient values and preferences, decisions are based on the impact on Mr. R's overall health condition. Functional and cognitive status, degree of comorbidity, frailty, and overall life expectancy frame the likelihood of attaining Mr. R's desired outcomes (Smith, Williams, & Lo, 2011). The guiding principles and parameters, which were important for IPT members when evaluating Mr. R for polypharmacy and proposing an individualized plan of care, are shown in Table 18.3, which provides a list of proposed questions that could be addressed to ensure that the plan of care, specifically medication management, is individualized, comprehensive, and sustainable given Mr. R's characteristics and circumstances.

Comprehensive Geriatric Assessment and Screening

Performing a comprehensive geriatric assessment (CGA) is a widely supported evidence-based approach to gathering functional, cognitive, social, medical, and environmental information necessary for developing an effective comprehensive plan of care for older adults (Stuck, Siu, Wieland, Rubenstein, & Adams, 2016). The CGA includes a thorough medical and social history, physical examination, and medication review and may include several of the following exams:

- The MMSE
- The St. Louis University Mental Status Exam (SLUMS)
- The GDS
- The CLOX: An executive clock-drawing task
- The Trail Making Test (TMT): Parts A and B

For medication purposes, the medication review could consist of several or all of the aforementioned assessments of medication appropriateness. Moreover, assessing functional, cognitive, and psychosocial well-being provides the IPT with a more complete profile of Mr. R's conditions and appropriateness of his prescribed medications. This information could be used by the IPT to discuss concerns about his medication regimen and to recommend ways in which polypharmacy and risks can be reduced for medication-related adverse events.

One approach to reducing polypharmacy and the potential risks for medication-related adverse events is to consider deprescribing some of his medications. Deprescribing is the process of tapering, withdrawing, discontinuing, or stopping medications when

TABLE 18.3   Guiding Principles for Evaluating Polypharmacy for Mr. R

Guiding Principle	Factors to Consider	IPT Members Who Can Take Ownership
Elicit patient preferences	What is the clinical situation?	MD, NP, PA, PharmD
	What is the home situation?	RN, SW, OT, PT
	What are Mr. R's objectives?	IPT
	What are Mr. R's personal values? What are Mr. R's cultural values?	IPT IPT
Interpret evidence	Is there evidence-based literature available regarding polypharmacy and the older adult?	MD, NP, PA, PharmD
	Does the evidence translate into Mr. R's particular situation?	MD, NP, PA, PharmD
	Does the treatment plan of care exacerbate other physical, psychological, or social conditions?	IPT
Estimate prognosis	What are the risks, burdens, and benefits to changing the current pharmacologic plan of care?	MD, NP, PA, PharmD
	What is Mr. R's life expectancy?	MD, NP, PA, PharmD, IPT
	What is Mr. R's functional status?	IPT
	What is Mr. R's quality of life?	IPT
Determine clinical feasibility	What is the anticipated burden of this change in the pharmacologic plan of care?	IPT
	How will these changes impact multiple comorbidities?	IPT
	How will these changes impact his cognitive and functional status?	IPT
Prioritize the pharmacologic plan of care	Is the polypharmacy intervention a priority? How can changing the pharmacologic plan of care optimize benefit, minimize harm, and enhance quality of life?	IPT

IPT, interprofessional team; MD, geriatrician or other medically trained physician; NP, nurse practitioner; OT, occupational therapist; PA, physician assistant; PharmD, pharmacist; PT, physical therapist; RN, registered nurse; SW, social worker.

they are found to be no longer necessary or if the risk of the medication outweighs the benefit. Deprescribing is most effective when a stepwise approach is taken. The IPT would first ensure that Mr. R has a condition indicating the need for each medication. Team members would then evaluate how effective the medication has been for Mr. R, discuss observation/findings with Mr. R, evaluate whether the medication is of benefit or high risk, and then determine whether or not the medication should be discontinued. Scott et al. developed an evidence-based 10-step discontinuation guide that can be used to decrease medication use and reduce the number of inappropriate medications prescribed (Scott, Gray, Martin, Pillans, & Mitchell, 2013). Of course, this process may lead to replacing more harmful medications with less harmful medications and, thus, may not always reduce polypharmacy.

Regardless of whether polypharmacy can be reduced, the CGA can also be used to identify ways for improving adherence. Recent evidence by Turner et al. (2012), suggest that adherence in self-neglecting older adults is correlated with functional status. Determining which cognitive, functional, and environmental barriers may be affecting adherence levels could lead to modifications in daily life to overcome some of these barriers to medication adherence. In the case of Mr. R, the establishment of a specific location where all of his medications could be stored and the use of other environmental supports were important to increasing adherence. In his care plan, medications were organized in pill boxes indicating the days and times taken for each medication along with a medication alarm set to remind him to take his medications at specific times throughout the day. This program appeared to improve Mr. R's self-reported adherence levels, as measured by the Morisky Adherence Scale, from a score of 2 at the initial assessment to a score of 5 at the final assessment (Morisky, Ang, & Krousel-Wood, 2008). His Geriatric Depression Scale-15 scores decreased from a 14 (i.e., clinical depression) at the initial assessment to a 2 (i.e., little or no depression) at the final assessment (Burke, Roccaforte, & Wengel, 1991). His functional status remained constant throughout the program, as measured by the Short Form Health Survey (SF-36), and his level of social interaction and satisfaction with those interactions remained low as measured by the Duke Social Support Inventory (Parkerson, Broadhead, & Tse, 1991; Ware & Sherbourne, 1992). These findings suggest that the program component targeting Mr. R's medication adherence may have had a positive effect on his medication adherence as well as his depression levels.

CONCLUSION

Elder self-neglect is a prevalent condition among older adults and increases their risks for hospitalization, emergency room visits, nursing home placement, and mortality. Like Mr. R, older adults who neglect themselves often present with multiple comorbidities and other circumstances requiring multifaceted interventions to promote positive health and quality-of-life outcomes. Hazardous medication-use patterns share many of the same potentially harmful outcomes as self-neglect, yet it has been a widely understudied and overlooked component of self-neglect. New evidence highlights its importance among self-neglecters; health care professionals should consider polypharmacy, medication nonadherence, drug–drug interactions and the use of potentially harmful medications as possible contributors to self-neglect.

Increasing screening for risk factors consistent with self-neglect, through the use of CGAs, is important for identifying the most likely contributors. Likewise, the CGA would inform the need for specific IPT members when developing an effective and individualized intervention or prevention program for an older adult with self-neglect. In the case of Mr. R and likely that of other older adults with substantiated self-neglect, a comprehensive review of medications and the development of a medication-related interventional plan are important steps for improving the quality-of-life outcomes such as depression. More studies are needed to better understand the association between medication use and self-neglect as well as to inform educational programs on how best to train health care professionals to prevent and intervene in community-dwelling older adults with substantiated self-neglect.

IMPLICATIONS FOR PRACTICE AND EDUCATION

- It is critical to educate physicians, nurses, and all health care professionals regarding the clinical risk factors and manifestations of elder self-neglect. Given the complexities of self-neglect, often brought on by multiple comorbid conditions, prescribing physicians, prescribing health care professionals, and environmental influences, a strong foundation in geriatric principles of care and IPT approaches are important in responding to self-neglect cases. Thus, both undergraduate and graduate health care education should include aging as a focus, especially regarding the interaction between age-related physiologic changes and medication use.
- Health care professionals must understand the physiology of aging and how specific medications may play a role in diminishing cognitive and functional status, negatively impacting the inability of a person to live safe and independently.
- Strategies to detect and reduce polypharmacy and increase appropriate medication taking behaviors in older adults are imperative.
- There is a drastic need for health education and literacy among older adults to help them understand the prescribed plan of care and the importance of adherence to this plan. This may require targeting knowledge of medications, self efficacy, and skills to adequately adhere to the medication regimen and the recognition of expected and dangerous side effects.
- Education of the patient and family, especially related to OTC medications is necessary. Older adults are the largest consumers of OTC medications (Qato et al., 2008). Older adults often self-medicate and may place themselves at additional risk by thinking OTC medications are safe to take without physician supervision. Chui, Stone, Martin, Croes, and Thorpe (2014) report that on average, older adults take nearly four OTC medications, regularly. These medications can interact with the prescribed medications and medication complexity increases with each new medication added to an older adult's plan of care; therefore, education of the older adult and family regarding ways to reduce or manage this complexity is critical to chronic disease self-management at home.

IMPLICATIONS FOR RESEARCH

- Elder self-neglect is a complex biopsychosocial phenomenon with a myriad of risk factors and potential causal pathways. Despite the many studies identifying associated risk and protective factors, medication use has been widely overlooked as a potential contributor to the etiology or exacerbation of self-neglect in older adults. Given the adverse effects of polypharmacy and inappropriate medication use among older adults and the similarities in outcomes that these factors share with self-neglect (i.e., cognitive impairment, hospitalization, mortality), at the very least, future studies should include measures of both polypharmacy and inappropriate medication use (i.e., medication adherence, Beers Criteria) as contributing factors. Polypharmacy and inappropriate medication use may be more readily modifiable compared to changing someone's social network or living environment. This may be enough to restore one's energy level, cognition, function, or mood and, thus, stymie the negative effects on self-management and independent living.

(continued)

- Like other risk factors for self-neglect, there is a need for well-developed, retrospective and prospective longitudinal studies to help establish the temporality of polypharmacy and inappropriate medication use in this population. If these factors fall within the causal pathways, early intervention and prevention studies may target these to reduce the risks for subsequent self-neglect within certain settings and contexts. This is especially important for older adults who are living alone with multiple chronic conditions and concomitant medication use. Medication reconciliation studies and medication monitoring studies would be highly beneficial in reducing risks for declines in function or cognition that result in the need for a stronger social support network where none may be available. Both functional and cognitive decline have been linked to higher odds of self-neglect (Dong et al., 2010; Dong, Mendes de Leon, et al., 2009).

REFERENCES

Abrams, R. C., Lachs, M., McAvay, G., Keohane, D. J., & Bruce, M. L. (2002). Predictors of self-neglect in community-dwelling elders. *American Journal of Psychiatry, 159*(10), 1724–1730. doi:10.1176/appi.ajp.159.10.1724

American Geriatrics Society. (2015). American Geriatrics Society 2015 updated Beers Criteria for potentially inappropriate medication use in older adults. *Journal of the American Geriatrics Society, 63*(11), 2227–2246. doi:10.1111/jgs.13702

Burke, W. J., Roccaforte, W. H., & Wengel, S. P. (1991). The short form of the Geriatric Depression Scale: A comparison with the 30-item form. *Journal of Geriatric Psychiatry and Neurology, 4*(3), 173–178. doi:10.1177/089198879100400310

Burke, W. J., Roccaforte, W. H., Wengel, S. P., Chui, M. A., Stone, J. A., Martin, B. A., . . . Carter, M. (2013). Patient-centered care for older adults with multiple chronic conditions: A stepwise approach from the American Geriatrics Society. *Journal of the American Geriatrics Society, 300*(8878), 173–178. doi:10.1001/jama.2008.892

Burnett, J., Coverdale, J. H., Pickens, S., & Dyer, C. B. (2006). What is the association between self-neglect, depressive symptoms, and untreated medical conditions? *Journal of Elder Abuse & Neglect, 18*(4), 25–34. doi:10.1300/J084v18n04_04

Burnett, J., Cully, J. A., Achenbaum, W. A., Dyer, C. B., & Naik, A. D. (2011). Assessing self-efficacy for safe and independent living: A cross-sectional study in vulnerable older adults. *Journal of Applied Gerontology, 30*(3), 390–402. doi:10.1177/0733464810362898

Burnett, J., Dyer, C. B., Halphen, J. M., Achenbaum, W. A., Green, C. E., Booker, J. G., & Diamond, P. M. (2014). Four subtypes of self-neglect in older adults: Results of a latent class analysis. *Journal of the American Geriatrics Society, 62*(6), 1127–1132. doi:10.1111/jgs.12832

Burnett, J., Jackson, S. L., Sinha, A. K., Aschenbrenner, A. R., Murphy, K. P., Xia, R., & Diamond, P. M. (2016). Five-year all-cause mortality rates across five categories of substantiated elder abuse occurring in the community. *Journal of Elder Abuse & Neglect, 28*(2), 59–75. doi:10.1080/08946566.2016.1142920

Burnett, J., Pickens, S., Aung, K., Reilley, B., & Dyer, C. B. (2010, May). *Caring for vulnerable elders reported to Adult Protective Services for self-neglect: A multidimensional approach.* Poster presented at the American Geriatrics Society 63rd Scientific Meeting, Orlando, FL.

Charlesworth, C. J., Smit, E., Lee, D. S. H., Alramadhan, F., & Odden, M. C. (2015). Polypharmacy among adults aged 65 years and older in the United States: 1988–2010. *Journals of Gerontology, Series A: Biological Sciences and Medical Sciences, 70*(8), 989–995. doi:10.1093/gerona/glv013

Chui, M. A., Stone, J. A., Martin, B. A., Croes, K. D., & Thorpe, J. M. (2014). Safeguarding older adults from inappropriate over-the-counter medications: The role of community pharmacists. *The Gerontologist, 54*(6), 989–1000. doi:10.1093/geront/gnt130

Ciechanowski, P., Wagner, E., & Schmaling, K. (2004). Community-integrated home-based depression treatment in older adults: A randomized controlled trial. *The Journal of the American Medical Association, 291*(13), 1569–1577. doi:10.1001/jama.291.13.1569

Culberson, J. W., Ticker, R. L., Burnett, J., Marcus, M. T., Pickens, S. L., & Dyer, C. B. (2011). Prescription medication use among self neglecting elderly. *Journal of Addictions Nursing, 22*(1–2), 63–68. doi:10.3109/10884602.2010.545089

Dong, X., Mendes de Leon, C. F., & Evans, D. A. (2009). Is greater self-neglect severity associated with lower levels of physical function? *Journal of Aging and Health, 21*(4), 596–610. doi:10.1177/0898264309333323

Dong, X., Simon, M. A., & Evans, D. (2012a). Elder self-neglect and hospitalization: Findings from the Chicago Health and Aging Project. *Journal of the American Geriatrics Society, 60*(2), 202–209. doi:10.1111/j.1532-5415.2011.03821.x

Dong, X., Simon, M. A., & Evans, D. (2012b). Prospective study of the elder self-neglect and emergency department use in a community population. *American Journal of Emergency Medicine, 30*(4), 553–561. doi:10.1016/j.ajem.2011.02.008

Dong, X., Simon, M., & Evans, D. (2013). Elder self-neglect is associated with increased risk for elder abuse in a community-dwelling population: Findings From the Chicago Health and Aging Project. *Journal of Aging and Health, 25*(1), 80–96. doi:10.1177/0898264312467373

Dong, X., Simon, M., Mendes de Leon, C., Fulmer, T., Beck, T., Hebert, L., . . . Evans, D. (2009). Elder self-neglect and abuse and mortality risk in a community-dwelling population. *Journal of the American Medical Association, 302*(5), 517–526. doi:10.1001/jama.2009.1109

Dong, X., Simon, M. A., Wilson, R. S., Mendes de Leon, C. F., Rajan, K. B., & Evans, D. A. (2010). Decline in cognitive function and risk of elder self-neglect: Finding from the Chicago Health Aging Project. *Journal of the American Geriatrics Society, 58*(12), 2292–2299. doi:10.1111/j.1532-5415.2010.03156.x

Dyer, C., Pickens, S., & Burnett, J. (2007). Vulnerable elders: When it is no longer safe to live alone. *Journal of the American Medical Association, 298*(12), 1448–1450. doi:10.1001/jama.298.12.1448

Dyer, C. B., Goodwin, J. S., Pickens-Pace, S., Burnett, J., & Kelly, P. A. (2007). Self-neglect among the elderly: A model based on more than 500 patients seen by a geriatric medicine team. *American Journal of Public Health, 97*(9), 1671–1676. doi:10.2105/AJPH.2006.097113

Dyer, C. B., Pavlik, V. N., Murphy, K. P., & Hyman, D. J. (2000). The high prevalence of depression and dementia in elder abuse or neglect. *Journal of the American Geriatrics Society, 48*(2), 205–208. doi:10.1111/j.1532-5415.2000.tb03913.x

Fox, C., Richardson, K., Maidment, I. D., Savva, G. M., Matthews, F. E., Smithard, D., . . . Brayne, C. (2011). Anticholinergic medication use and cognitive impairment in the older population: The Medical Research Council Cognitive Function and Ageing Study. *Journal of the American Geriatrics Society, 59*(8), 1477–1483. doi:10.1111/j.1532-5415.2011.03491.x

Frazier, S. C. (2005). Health outcomes and polypharmacy in elderly individuals: An integrated literature review. *Journal of Gerontological Nursing, 31*(9), 4–11.

Gallagher, P. F., O'Connor, M. N., & O'Mahony, D. (2011). Prevention of potentially inappropriate prescribing for elderly patients: A randomized controlled trial using STOPP/START criteria. *Clinical Pharmacology & Therapeutics, 89*(6), 845–854. doi:10.1038/clpt.2011.44

Gnjidic, D., Hilmer, S. N., Blyth, F. M., Naganathan, V., Waite, L., Seibel, M. J., . . . Le Couteur, D. G. (2012). Polypharmacy cutoff and outcomes: Five or more medicines were used to identify community-dwelling older men at risk of different adverse outcomes. *Journal of Clinical Epidemiology, 65*(9), 989–995. doi:10.1016/j.jclinepi.2012.02.018

Hanlon, J. T., & Schmader, K. E. (2013). The Medication Appropriateness Index at 20: Where it started, where it has been, and where it may be going. *Drugs & Aging, 30*(11), 893–900. doi:10.1007/s40266-013-0118-4

Indian a University Center for Aging Research. (2012). *Anticholinergic Cognitive Burden Scale*. Retrieved from http://www.agingbraincare.org/uploads/products/ACB_scale_-_legal_size.pdf

Kelly, P. A., Dyer, C. B., Pavlik, V., Doody, R., & Jogerst, G. (2008). Exploring self-neglect in older adults: Preliminary findings of the Self-neglect Severity Scale and next steps. *Journal of the American Geriatrics Society, 56*, S253–S260. doi:10.1111/j.1532-5415.2008.01977.x

Lachs, M. S., Williams, C. S., O'Brien, S., & Pillemer, K. A. (2002). Adult protective service use and nursing home placement. *The Gerontologist, 42*(6), 734–739. doi:10.1093/geront/42.6.734

Lachs, M. S., Williams, C. S., O'Brien, S., Pillemer, K. A., & Charlson, M. E. (1998). The mortality of elder mistreatment. *Journal of the American Medical Association, 280*(5), 428–432. doi:10.1001/jama.280.5.428

Liu, L. M. (2016). Deprescribing: An approach to reducing polypharmacy in nursing home residents. *Journal for Nurse Practitioners, 10*(2), 136–139. doi:10.1016/j.nurpra.2013.09.010

Mion, L. C., & Sandhu, S. K. (2016). Adverse drug events in older hospitalized adults: Implications for nursing practice. *Geriatric Nursing, 37*(2), 153–155. doi:10.1016/j.gerinurse.2016.02.006

Morisky, D. E., Ang, A., & Krousel-Wood, M. (2008). Predictive validity of a medication adherence measure in an outpatient setting. *Journal of Clinical Hypertension, 10*(5), 348–354.

National Center on Elder Abuse. (n.d.). What is elder abuse? Retrieved from https://ncea.acl.gov/faq/index.html#faq1

Oandasan, I., & Reeves, S. (2005a). Key elements for interprofessional education. Part 1: The learner, the educator and the learning context. *Journal of Interprofessional Care, 19*(Suppl. 1), 21–38. doi:10.1080/13561820500083550

Oandasan, I., & Reeves, S. (2005b). Key elements of interprofessional education. Part 2: Factors, processes and outcomes. *Journal of Interprofessional Care, 19*(Suppl. 1), 39–48. doi:10.1080/13561820500081703

O'Mahony, D., O'Sullivan, D., Byrne, S., O'Connor, M. N., Ryan, C., & Gallagher, P. (2014). STOPP/START criteria for potentially inappropriate prescribing in older people: Version 2. *Age and Ageing, 44*(2), 213–218. doi:10.1093/ageing/afu145

Parkerson, G. R., Broadhead, W. E., & Tse, C. K. (1991). Validation of the Duke Social Support and Stress Scale. *Family Medicine, 23*(5), 357–360.

Qato, D. M., Alexander, G. C., Conti, R. M., Johnson, M., Schumm, P., & Lindau, S. T. (2008). Use of prescription and over-the-counter medications and dietary supplements among older adults in the United States. *Journal of the American Medical Association, 300*(24), 2867–2878. doi:10.1001/jama.2008.892

Scott, I. A., Gray, L. C., Martin, J. H., & Mitchell, C. A. (2016). Minimizing inappropriate medications in older populations: A 10-step conceptual framework. *American Journal of Medicine, 125*(6), 529–537. doi:10.1016/j.amjmed.2011.09.021

Scott, I. A., Gray, L. C., Martin, J. H., Pillans, P. I., & Mitchell, C. A. (2013). Deciding when to stop: Towards evidence-based deprescribing of drugs in older populations. *Evidence Based Medicine, 18*(4), 121–124. doi:10.1136/eb-2012-100930

Smith, A. K., Williams, B. A., & Lo, B. (2011). Discussing overall prognosis with the very elderly. *New England Journal of Medicine, 365*(23), 2149–2151. doi:10.1056/NEJMp1109990

Spinewine, A., Dumont, C., Mallet, L., & Swine, C. (2006). Medication Appropriateness Index: Reliability and recommendations for future use. *Journal of the American Geriatrics Society, 54*(4), 720–722. doi:10.1111/j.1532-5415.2006.00668_8.x

Steinman, M. A., & Hanlon, J. T. (2010). Managing medications in clinically complex elders: "There's got to be a happy medium." *Journal of the American Medical Association, 304*(14), 1592–1601. doi:10.1001/jama.2010.1482

Stuck, A. E., Siu, A. L., Wieland, G. D., Rubenstein, L. Z., & Adams, J. (2016). Comprehensive geriatric assessment: A meta-analysis of controlled trials. *Lancet, 342*(8878), 1032–1036. doi:10.1016/0140-6736(93)92884-V

Teaster, P. B., Dugar, T. A., Mendiondo, M. S., Abner, E. L., & Cecil, K. A. (2006). *The 2004 Survey of State Adult Protective Services: Abuse of adults 60 years of age and older.* Washington, DC: The National

Center on Elder Abuse. Retrieved from http://www.napsa-now.org/wp-content/uploads/2012/09/2-14-06-FINAL-60+REPORT.pdf

Truven Health Analytics Inc. (n.d.). Micromedex medication, disease and toxicology management. Retrieved from https://www.micromedexsolution.com/home/dispatch/ssl/true

Turner, A., Hochschild, A., Burnett, J., Zulfiqar, A., & Dyer, C. B. (2012). High prevalence of medication nonadherence in a sample of community-dwelling older adults with adult protective services-validated self-neglect. *Drugs & Aging, 29*(9), 741–749. doi:10.1007/s40266-012-0007-2

Ware, J., & Sherbourne, C. D. (1992). The MOS 36-Item Short-Form Health Survey (SF-36). I. Conceptual framework and item selection. *Medical Care, 30*(6), 473–483.

West, M. A., Guthrie, J. P., Dawson, J. F., Borrill, C. S., & Carter, M. (2006). Reducing patient mortality in hospitals: The role of human resource management. *Journal of Organizational Behavior, 27*(7), 983–1002. doi:10.1002/job.396

CHAPTER 19

SELF-NEGLECT IN IRELAND: A PILOT STUDY

David McCann

Self-neglect is a hidden and undeniably complex problem that presents a serious public health issue. It is associated with multiple issues, including serious adverse health outcomes, hospitalization, institutionalization, and ill health. Health and social care professionals are often faced with a multiplicity of ethical challenges related to refusal of services, mental capacity, and whether to intervene. The research presented in this chapter was inspired by my experiences as a student on a social care work placement at a community organization for older people. The aim of the pilot study was to explore the perspectives of a public health nurse (n = 1) and a senior caseworker (n = 1) on self-neglect. A qualitative methodology that used semi structured interviews was employed. Data were analyzed using content analysis. The findings of the study identified four themes: prevalence and contributing factors, current referral pathways and service interventions, professional challenges, and outcomes in cases of self-neglect. Despite the small sample size, the study highlights the significance of self-neglect for health and social care professionals.

Although the needs of older people can be varied and complex, self-neglect, as a serious public health issue, presents multifaceted problems for family members, communities, as well as health and social care professionals. As part of my undergraduate bachelor degree program, I spent 12 weeks in a work placement at a multidisciplinary agency and research center in Ireland. This research center is dedicated to improving the lives of older people and is funded by a number of agencies. During this work placement, I encountered several instances of self-neglect for the first time and saw firsthand the multiplicity of issues that encompass self-neglect work. I attended several multidisciplinary case conferences and witnessed discussions on processes and approaches used by team members to work with people engaging in self-neglecting behavior. After my 12-week placement, I remained as a volunteer on a day-visiting program. These experiences motivated me to pursue research on self-neglect, the aim of which was to investigate the perspectives of a public health nurse and a senior caseworker on self-neglect. This chapter describes the results of that research.

BACKGROUND LITERATURE

Defining Self-Neglect

As a starting point, a clear definition of self-neglect is paramount. Given the Irish context of this research, the following definition by Day (2010, p. 74) is perhaps the most pertinent:

> Self-neglect can present along a continuum of severity ranging from failure to attend to self-care, leaving bills unattended, noncompliance with treatment regimens, not eating or drinking, service refusal with evidence of self-neglect; to dilapidated homes and environments, faulty electrics, hoarding of rubbish, squalor, and hoarding of animals.

This definition illustrates and describes a whole range of diverse behaviors, which can manifest among individuals who self-neglect, from personal idiosyncrasies to severe environmental hazards. Much of the literature offers similar definitions, as well as outlines myriad consequences such behaviors have on the health and well-being of older persons. Although Dong and Simon (2013) assert that there are some significant gaps in current knowledge regarding the exact consequences of self-neglect, they concur that the available evidence identified an increased rate of mortality (Dong & Simon, 2015), high rate of health care utilization (Franzini & Dyer, 2008), increased risk for nursing home placement (Lachs, Williams, O'Brien, & Pillemer, 2002), all-cause mortality (Lachs, Williams, O'Brien, Pillemer, & Charlson, 1998), a 15-fold increase in cancer, and a tenfold increase in nutritional- and endocrine-related mortality (Dong, 2005). Self-neglect is also associated with a high rate of hospitalization, in addition to longer stays in hospitals (Dong, Simon, & Evans, 2012a). Furthermore, in instances of extreme self-neglect and squalor, where hygiene and environmental conditions are very poor, such circumstances pose not only a threat to the health and safety of the individual but also to those surrounding them, such as neighbors and community members (Dong, Simon, Mosqueda, & Evans, 2012).

Although it can vary in its presentation and degree of severity, self-neglect is predominantly characterized by extensive environmental neglect and aggregate diverse behaviors and deficits, which can have devastating consequences for the person's health, safety, and well-being (Day, Leahy-Warren, & McCarthy, 2016). Self-neglect is often associated with other conditions, sometimes labeled "risk factors," such as depression, dementia, cognitive and/or physical impairments, poor social networks, living alone, economic decline, old age, and alcohol or substance abuse (Gibbons, 2009; Pickens, Ostwald, & Pace, 2013). Although self-neglect behaviors can occur among the young and old, research has primarily focused on older people (Lauder, Roxburgh, Harris, & Law, 2009). This is largely due to the overwhelming absence of age-related morbidities among younger people, suggesting that it may be a somewhat different phenomenon in this particular age group (Iris, Ridings, & Conrad, 2010).

Prevalence and Policy Context

Although self-neglect behaviors are more often associated with older people, in particular older men (Dong et al., 2012), determining its prevalence has been very difficult given that it is often hidden and under-reported (Day, Mulcahy, Leahy-Warren, &

Downey, 2015). Moreover, there is a divergence of self-neglect classifications across the literature, as some countries, particularly Canada and the Unites States, and even different states/provinces within those countries, choose to include self-neglect under the definition of elder abuse (Day, 2010). This is not the case in Ireland, where self-neglect is excluded from the definition of elder abuse because it does not occur within a relationship (Health Service Executive [HSE], 2014). Some argue that inclusion is necessary (O'Brien, 2011), yet others maintain that exclusion is appropriate to avoid ambiguity and confusion (Doron, Band-Winterstein, & Naim, 2013). This does not rule out the possibility that in some instances self-neglect can occur simultaneously with elder abuse (Bartley, O'Brien, & O'Neill, 2010; HSE, 2014). Arguably, these divergent definitions have contributed to the underdeveloped epidemiology of self-neglect (Day et al., 2015).

In Ireland, cases of self-neglect account for approximately 21% (or 631) of the referrals received by senior caseworkers who specifically deal with cases concerning elder abuse (HSE, 2014). However, current policy dictates that senior caseworkers may only take on a referral if the criterion of *extreme* self-neglect is present, a concept not very well defined. Of the 21% of individuals referred to senior caseworkers, 53% have come from public health nurses, with 15% comprising hospital staff and 13% family members (HSE, 2014). In a recent study, Day and McCarthy (2015) revealed that 89% of public health nurses and other health and social care professionals had come into contact with cases of self-neglect in the previous 12-month period. Nevertheless, these statistics may only be the tip of the iceberg, as individuals who self-neglect are difficult to profile, with under-reporting and nonengagement issues obscuring the true scope of the phenomenon (Day, Mulcahy, & Leahy-Warren, 2016).

At present, older persons (65 and older) represent less than 10% of Ireland's population based on the 2011 census (Central Statistics Office [CSO], 2012). But population predictions by the CSO suggest that by the year 2036 older people could account for 20% to 23% of the country's total population (Gallagher, 2013). The implication, then, is that the prevalence of self-neglect will increase and create myriad challenges for health and social care professionals and for society in general (Day, Leahy-Warren, & McCarthy, 2013). Consider that in 94% of the cases referred to senior caseworkers the older person lived alone. This elucidates how the behavior can potentially go unnoticed, and possibly become deep-seated for a long period of time before ever coming to the attention of health and social care professionals (HSE, 2014).

Self-Neglect: Geriatric Syndrome or Sociocultural Phenomenon?

Numerous theories have been postulated as to why self-neglect typically occurs from biological causes, such as cognitive or physical impairments, to more social and environmental factors, like poverty and social isolation brought about by bereavement or dwindling social networks (Braye, Orr, & Preston-Shoot, 2011). However, although some correlations have been uncovered, there is no one absolute explanatory model for self-neglect, and a complex interaction of these factors is said to be the best interpretation for why the behavior takes place. Diogenes syndrome, also known as senile squalor syndrome, is described as a behavioral disorder of the elderly, typically associated with frontotemporal dementia, characterized by an extremely neglected physical and environmental state, social isolation, lack of shame, and a tendency to hoard excessively (Capriani, Lucetti, Vedovello, & Nuti, 2012). Similar theories have been described, which emphasize the role that dementia, depression, or other cognitive changes in the frontal lobe area of the brain may play in bringing about a functional decline that can lead to self-neglect behaviors (Dong et al., 2010). This type of cognitive impairment, coupled with physical dysfunction and exacerbated further by a lack of financial or social support, could easily aggravate the overall condition, resulting in a plethora of self-neglecting behaviors (Dong, Simon, & Evans, 2012b). In contrast, others maintain that poor self-care could be the result of society's failure to ensure adequate quality care for the elderly in general (Choi, Kim, & Asseff, 2009; Gill, 2009). Another theoretical model attempts to distinguish between older people who self-neglect by choice and those struggling to cope due to cognitive, functional, and financial constraints (Iris et al., 2010).

The belief that self-neglect is solely attributable to biological dysfunction is quite pervasive, despite limited empirical evidence for this claim, with literature being self-referential and comprising reviews and case studies opposed to actual original research (Lauder et al., 2009). McDermott (2010) uses critical theory to highlight how the prominence of biomedical explanations in the literature can obscure the influence of professional judgments in shaping understandings of and responses to self-neglect among older people. There is a gray area between what is considered living a "nonconformist" lifestyle and a pathological state (Lauder et al., 2009). Perception of self-neglect, then, becomes an identifiable theme and the literature reveals that cultural attitudes toward the elderly and perceptions of self-neglecting behaviors play a role in the detection of the phenomenon. For instance, San Filippo, Reiboldt, White, and Hails (2007) found that self-neglect is viewed differently by various cultures and cohorts, which can inhibit the ability of professionals to intervene in a timely manner. However, Snowdon, Shah, and Halliday (2007, p. 48) argue that "some people live in conditions so filthy and unhygienic that almost all observers, in whatever culture, would consider them unacceptable." And yet, one only has to consider that throughout history human beings have managed to live in all sorts of diverse environmental conditions that would be in stark contrast to contemporary standards of domestic living.

One caveat to consider in light of these findings is that people who self-neglect, especially those who live in squalor, may differ from the "nonconformists" in that they can recognize what others should do in instances when their health is at risk because of self-neglecting behaviors but not actually do it themselves (Naik, Pickens, Burnett, Lai, & Dyer, 2006). This corresponds with further research, which reveals that older people living in environmentally hazardous conditions who possess emotional processing can recognize pictures of other filthy homes but also exhibit executive dysfunction (or lack of capacity), which might explain why they do not consider their own homes to be filthy (Gregory, Halliday, Hodges, & Snowdon, 2011). Hildebrand, Taylor, and Bradway (2013) suggest that proper self-care may require the person's recognition of both societal expectations of hygiene as well as having the capacity and problem-solving ability to execute these particular standards. In a study with individuals who self-neglect, Kutame (2007) found that participants did not interpret their behavior as self-neglect and, instead, portrayed the problems as being outside of their control. Band-Winterstein et al. (2012) report similar self-perceptions among self-neglecting individuals, who largely disassociate themselves from any responsibility or agency.

Identification of self-neglect by health and social care professionals is a highly subjective matter, hindered more so by the lack of any validated self-neglect instruments, suggesting that professional judgments are not standardized but rather susceptible to individual interpretation (Day, McCarthy, & Leahy-Warren, 2012). Although severe cases of self-neglect more often than not are referred to specialist services such as senior caseworkers, other instances that present challenges and ethical dilemmas may not be classified as extreme and could subsequently lose service intervention prioritization because of demanding caseloads among professionals (O'Donnell et al., 2012).

Capacity and Ethical Considerations

Throughout the literature, one major theme emerges concerning how cases of self-neglect can present challenges and ethical dilemmas for professionals mandated with responsibility for safeguarding the older person (Blagodatny, Skudlarska, & Tocchi, 2007). Such challenges include legal frameworks for intervention and the nature of the older person's decision-making capacity and autonomy (Braye et al., 2011). Torke and Sachs (2008) state that trying to establish a safe living environment for the older person who is self-neglecting can be extremely difficult if they are at risk and simultaneously resist any kind of help. The ideal of respecting self-determination and achieving a person-centered approach in many cases of extreme self-neglect poses a considerable challenge to practitioners, especially for senior caseworkers and public health nurses (Day, 2010; Day, Leahy-Warren, et al., 2016).

Hurley, Scallan, Johnson, and De La Harpe (2000) describe those who self-neglect as "service refusers," highlighting the general unwillingness to accept treatment or services as being one of the defining features of the phenomenon. Naturally, such an inclination of service refusal can become a key issue and impede service providers from building a therapeutic relationship of trust, as the older person either outright rejects or merely tolerates myriad interventions, which they deem as unnecessary and intrusive (Lauder, Anderson, & Barclay, 2005). Perhaps the most difficult issue for professionals working with older persons who self-neglect is recognizing the kind of extreme situations that merit overriding the person's wishes to be left alone and the ramifications of such actions. In many instances, it is the lack of capacity as a result of physical illness, mental illness, or cognitive impairment that is the primary characteristic that health professionals cite as the justification for making such judgments (McDermott, 2010). *Capacity* is defined as the ability to understand the consequences of decisions as well as being able to execute decisions (Dyer, Goodwin, Pickens-Pace, Burnett, & Kelly, 2007). Yet, capacity is not always completely present or totally absent, but rather, it appears on a gradient or sliding scale (Dong & Simon, 2013).

In Ireland, when a person is deemed mentally incapacitated to the extent that he or she is unable to manage his or her person and/or property, an application to have the individual legally deemed a ward of court can be made (O'Neill, 2006). This specific action substitutes the legal decision-making capacity of the person, who is brought into state wardship concerning his or her property and person, with the court appointing a substitute decision maker. This entire process can involve the forced removal of the person to an institutional facility (i.e., a nursing home), which although intended to safeguard the person, may cause psychological harm rather than physical good (Mauk, 2011). In essence, appropriate consideration is needed and community health teams and other social care professionals should be well trained in self-neglect and risk assessments (Day, Leahy-Warren, et al., 2016).

Conversely, the wardship system is currently being phased out, soon to be supplanted by the Assisted Decision-Making (Capacity) Act 2015, which will repeal the Lunacy Regulation (Ireland) Act 1871. Thus, adults with diminished mental capacity can no longer become a ward of court and, instead, they will have an assistant decision maker, codecision-maker, or attorney appointed based on the extent of his or her capacity (Griffen, 2015). However, at the time of writing, the legislation is not fully operational. It is difficult to predict how it will impact the practice of health and social care professionals.

Day, Mulcahy, et al. (2016), along with Braye, Orr, and Preston-Shoot (2014), draw particular attention to the more complex and challenging cases of self-neglect in which people choose to self-neglect and have capacity while, at the same, remain steadfast in their refusal of services. Bergeron (2006) implies that accepting service refusal could be construed as client abandonment. Yet, trespassing without permission can infringe the property rights of owners and home surveillance visits without any clear purpose can have the effect of stigmatizing individuals who self-neglect (Ballard, 2010). As such, the most frequent dilemma raised by professionals appears to be not whether to intervene in cases of self-neglect, but how to intervene (McDermott, 2010).

Effective Practice in Responding to Self-Neglect

The primary role for all health and social care professionals is to take a coordinated interagency approach to cases of self-neglect and establish a holistic assessment to inform what, if any, intervention should take place (Braye et al., 2011). Good governance structures and procedural guidelines are recommended (Braye, Orr, & Preston-Shoot, 2015). Dong and Gorbien (2006) state that a comprehensive geriatric assessment should take place. Murray and Upshall (2009) underscore the benefits of global assessments in determining how best to proceed. Understandably, the early detection of self-neglect is identified as being of paramount importance as, in doing so, it can prevent the behavior from becoming too entrenched and, thus, it is much easier to put early intervention supports in place (Day & Leahy-Warren, 2008; Snowdon & Halliday, 2009).

Maintaining positive relationships and regular contact with older people who self-neglect is, perhaps, the greatest responsibility health care professionals have and Lauder et al. (2005) recommend that any ongoing monitoring plans should be shared across various agencies to be sustainable and effective. This is because outcomes of self-neglect are generally poor and associated with high rates of relapse and mortality (Dong, Simon, et al., 2009). A key area for intervention is assistance with activities of daily living (ADL), which is provided for by various agencies (i.e., home help services) as self-neglect is often linked to disability and poor functioning (Dong, Mendes de Leon, & Evans, 2009; Naik, Pickens, Burnett, & Dyer, 2007; Pickens et al., 2007; Poythress, Burnett, Naik, Pickens, & Dyer, 2007). Focusing on ADL can yield substantial improvements in cases of self-neglect (Griebling, 2010).

In summary, the literature encompasses the broad scope of self-neglect behaviors and manifestations, from its prevalence and diverse contributory factors to the means in which health and social care professionals can be multifarious in their attempts to address the behavior. What should be apparent is that self-neglect is far from being a straightforward phenomenon with simplistic solutions, and, as the population grows policy makers and other stakeholders will need to pay greater attention to this public health issue.

METHODS

Participants and Sample

A qualitative research approach was chosen to provide a detailed perspective on how cases of self-neglect can be identified and how they are managed by health and social care professionals. Two professionals from the HSE were selected to comprise the research sample: a public health nurse ($n = 1$) and a senior caseworker ($n = 1$). The justification for choosing these particular individuals was made on the grounds of purpose-based, nonprobability sampling, given that both possessed, by virtue of their job descriptions, extensive knowledge and firsthand experience of encountering self-neglect in their line of work.

Data Collection

Semistructured interviews were conducted using open questions to elicit a series of in-depth responses. The interview questions were informed by the myriad themes uncovered in the literature review, representing a more deductively orientated strategy intended to answer focused questions in relation to professionals' experience of self-neglect. The interviews began with basic questions that were relatively easy to answer before progressing toward a more detailed line of inquiry designed to illicit more intricate responses, as recommended by Berg and Lune (2012). Furthermore, each question was centered on a single topic or concept. Although the degree of control over interview proceedings may vary, there is, nevertheless, a tacit agreement embedded within the whole process of being interviewed that the agenda for discussion will be at the sole discretion of the researcher (Denscombe, 2010). Notwithstanding, both participants were given the opportunity at the end of their respective interviews to add anything further that they deemed relevant to the topic of research that had *not* been covered in the preceding set of questions put to them. In doing so, the researcher was satisfied that the participants' freedom to openly discuss the topic of self-neglect had not disproportionately limited.

Both participants were provided with an information sheet and consent form on the day of their respective interviews and the consent forms were signed. Participants were also advised that they were under no obligation to answer all or any of the questions and that they could "pass" on any given question if they so wished. Upon completion of the interviews, the audio data was transcribed and stored as two password-protected text files. All personal data and identifying locations were made private, shielded under the protection of anonymity with each of the participants being assigned a pseudonym and any references made to their geographical location of work removed to uphold the participants' sense of privacy (Christians, 2000).

Data Analysis

The interviews were processed using content analysis, which is a systematic examination and interpretation of the raw data by the researcher to identify any patterns, themes, biases, or meanings (Berg & Lune, 2012). Familiarization with the interview transcripts was the first step undertaken through a process of immersion in the data by reading it over several times, taking memos of anything deemed noteworthy, and employing theoretical sensitivity, a specific type of researcher insight and self-awareness (Corbin & Strauss, 2008). The second stage involved minutely coding the data in order to help identify any concepts and themes. At this early stage, the *open code* names were rough and involved labeling chunks of data with either a word or a phrase that described said data sufficiently (Rivas, 2012). This was then followed by *axial coding*, in which the researcher searched for relationships among the codes, establishing links and associations that allowed certain codes to be incorporated into larger headings or categories, as well as particular codes being perceived as more frequent or crucial than others in relation to the research questions (Denscombe, 2010).

Finally, having identified a number of salient themes in the data, the concluding stage of analysis involved integrating the particular findings into the research document through a mixture of summarization and verbatim quotes, for the sake of clarity. Four prominent themes emerged.

FINDINGS

Prevalence and Contributing Factors

Both the public health nurse (Jane) and the senior caseworker (Aoife) stated that their workloads included cases of self-neglect. Jane reported that these particular cases accounted for 10% of her total caseload, whereas Aoife stated that it comprised 20% but added that elder abuse services only dealt with cases of extreme self-neglect. The major contributing factors to self-neglect were identified as dementia, cognitive deterioration or delirium, in addition to mental health behavioral issues or addiction.

Current Referral Pathways and Service Interventions

Instances of self-neglect often come to the attention of public health nurses through a general practitioner (GP), a personal carer, or a neighbor, whereas the senior caseworker was usually contacted by a public health nurse who had made a referral for a case of extreme self-neglect. Jane stated that usually something public had happened with the older person when public health nurses were notified. Similarly, Aoife explained that there would be a crisis in the older person's medical presentation by the time elder abuse services became involved. However, there was a lack of a formal self-neglect assessment procedure among public health nurses for determining the degree of self-neglect. When asked whether there was a comprehensive assessment tool used by her agency Jane stated that:

> There isn't, no. We'd be just using our own nursing assessments and making our own determinations. I suppose it would be a classification of the type of neglect rather than the degree of it because we don't have a tool that determines degree.

Aoife explained that the closest thing to a comprehensive assessment tool utilized by the elder abuse services was a referral form, which identified the self-neglect behaviors involving environmental and individual characteristics (dirty, matted hair, etc.). These details would inform the referral process for the senior caseworker to make a determination of extreme self-neglect. Service interventions included providing specific services such as home supports. For example, a caregiver who can assist the older person with keeping himself or herself and/or the environment clean and tidy. Financial services could also be provided, particularly in instances in which a clean-up of the home environment was deemed necessary. Other interventions included admission for assessment to acute hospitals, or to long-term-care beds in nursing homes. More complex interventions necessitated a GP medical assessment and referral to the psycho-geriatrician.

Professional Challenges

Based on the interviews, a number of distinct challenges were identified. Aoife elucidated some of the main barriers such as gaining access to the older person (i.e., engagement) and the understanding of the older person and his or her perception of the situation, especially when there are other contributing factors. She said:

> There could be issues in terms of capacity or there could be issues in terms of mental health or addiction. So, you could have somebody who lacks the insight as to what's happening. So, they're very vulnerable and could be living in total squalor.

Similarly, Jane stated that if the person has dementia or a behavioral problem it can be very difficult because they will not see self-neglect as a problem. She also asserted that family is a problem encountered by public health nurses and not the older person. On the topic of service refusal, Jane went on to say:

> Service refusal is often the refusal of the family more than the refusal of the client. The refusal of the client would be from maybe somebody who has dementia or a mental health issue . . . but if they're deeper issues, sometimes it can be the family who doesn't want somebody going into the home. That can be it, more than anything else.

When asked to elaborate upon this point she added:

> Well, if it's somebody with dementia the family just haven't come to the point of acceptance. If it's behavioral, then maybe some of the family members have similar behavioral issues and they don't see it as someone else does. Sometimes, they just probably don't want the intrusion and you can have a bit of house politics going on and often the client can be neglected in the middle of it all because there's family dynamics going on.

In terms of service refusal, Aoife highlighted how senior caseworkers ought to try to engage with the older person to build up a level of trust and make incremental changes, but added that any attempts to make considerable progress in a short time are ill-advised:

> I don't think you can go into a very squalid situation and completely remove everything because I think that can be quite traumatic, particularly if you're looking at the whole aspect of hoarding.

Another significant professional challenge identified was the area of accessing the necessary medical assessments in a timely fashion to confirm whether the older person lacks capacity. Such instances typically come about when professionals have identified the risks as being too high to respect the older person's autonomy. Jane described the current system as being archaic, referring to the laws under which it's governed as being outdated. She also highlighted how public health nurses have no direct referral pathways to old-age psychiatry services. The referral must come from the GP, who may not be aware that the older person is self-neglecting. Indeed, instances of self-neglect, which require a medical determination of capacity, can become very complex, by way of the sheer number of persons involved, as illuminated by Jane in this quote:

> There are too many people involved in the decision. We can't do it ourselves so we have to refer to a GP or a social worker or somewhere and then you have to get solicitors on board, you have to get family agreement . . . it's a very complex process, which takes months and months and in the meantime the patient is still refusing care or the patient is getting deeper into a complicated scenario.

From Aoife's perspective, a determination of capacity and any decision to override the older person's autonomy are quite individual and depend on the context of the case.

> Hopefully, now with our new assisted decision-making legislation, whilst it's not operational yet, we would hope that would assist us in this because it will give us more focus in trying to ascertain the views of the individual to the very best we can. I think it is very important that we try and do that.

However, she expanded on a number of challenges that still lie ahead in trying to address some of the more progressive concepts given the current state of service provision:

> I think there's a lot of discussion around person-centered care and positive risk taking. I think it's wonderful to have such discussions ongoing. I don't actually think, however, that we have been able to marry the discussions around the concepts to what is available on the ground. I think we're talking, and I think the talking is good, but it's not being replicated on the ground because we don't have the options available to us.

Outcomes in Cases of Self-Neglect

Outcomes in cases of self-neglect can include both positive and negative aspects, with instances of negative outcomes serving to illustrate the role played by the aforementioned professional challenges. As summarized by Jane:

> Good ones are just a matter of getting the appropriate services in place. If somebody has lost the will to keep themselves [sic] clean or tidy and you get in a good carer with a good relationship, good communication skills, I mean it can completely turn the situation around. You get somebody then who accepts social connections and it brings them [sic] into other services because

of that. If it doesn't work out, then it's very difficult. You're hitting off a brick wall all the time and you're going nowhere and that's when you end up then having to go through the legal process because nothing is changing and the neglect persists and the danger persists. And you have to keep reminding yourself, once you're aware of it you have to make sure you close the loop somehow. Pass it on. Keep it and do nothing, you're in trouble.

This quotation underscores the responsibility and difficulties around engagement with cases of self-neglect as stated by Aoife:

Well, hopefully, we have, in all cases of extreme self-neglect, what you're trying to achieve is, maintaining the person's independence whilst minimizing risk. We can't eliminate the risk and we can't eliminate behaviors that may lead to the hoarding. But we can minimize it in terms of trying to engage positively.

CONCLUSION

The research described investigated the perspective of two experienced professionals who have firsthand experience of self-neglect. The study findings have deepened the recognition of the multifaceted nature of self-neglect, from manifestations of the behavior and contributing factors, to the potential role played by family members and the myriad challenges faced by health and social care professionals in trying to deal with cases, which can involve both service refusal as well as multidisciplinary impediments.

The prevalence of self-neglect based on both participants' estimations of their caseloads is corroborated by the literature. Jane approximated that 10% of her public health nursing work involved cases of self-neglect. In a recent study, Day and Mc-Carthy (2015) revealed that 89% of public health nurses, including other health and social care professionals, had come into contact with cases of self-neglect in the previous 12-month period. Aoife stated that cases of self-neglect made up 20% of her workload as a senior caseworker. Cases of self-neglect account for roughly 21% of the referrals received by senior caseworkers for elder abuse (HSE, 2014). However, one must remember that these are just cases that come to the attention of professionals and may not be representative of the true extent of self-neglect within the population.

The absence of a formal self-neglect assessment tool for use by public health nurses and social workers identified in this research means the assessment of self-neglect is subjective and not standardized, a fact recognized by Day et al. (2012). Jane and Aoife indicated that in the absence of such a comprehensive tool they were using their own assessments and making their own determinations. This is a concern given that these health and social care professionals have a key role to play in the identification of vulnerable older people at risk of self-neglect. The results revealed that until a medical determination of capacity is made, health and social care professionals cannot intervene against the older person's wishes, even when there is a huge risk and they are a clear danger to themselves.

Service intervention for self-neglect clearly presented a number of issues causing significant impediments. These included greater access to multidisciplinary services to speed up the process of assessment and intervention and access to a nursing home placement or supervised home support or sheltered accommodation (Mauk, 2011).

The research findings state that putting in the right supports can completely turn the situation around. Going the legal route should be the last resort and acknowledging that the process takes considerable time is paramount. The research findings reveal that professionals are tasked with having to monitor ongoing situations involving deep-seated self-neglecting behaviors while trying to maintain the older person's independence and also minimizing the risk. This approach has been described as "positively engaging" with the older person and, thus, keeping the lines of communication open. According to Day et al. (2015), gradually building up a therapeutic relationship with the older person and including him or her in any decision-making and negotiation processes can be one of the key factors in achieving more positive outcomes. Lauder et al. (2005) recommended that any ongoing monitoring plans should be shared across various agencies to be sustainable and effective.

What may be one of the most significant implications of this pilot study is that self-neglect has no easy solutions. This phenomenon continues to remain a hidden and undeniably complex problem, presenting a serious public health issue. Given the association between self-neglect and dementia or other forms of cognitive deterioration, the numbers of people at risk for self-neglect is expected to increase significantly. Good governance structures, self-neglect policy and legislation, and training and support are required for effective practice. Self-neglect is a burgeoning area of study, that should continue to be researched to add to the existing body of knowledge. This way, policy makers and other stakeholders can be fully informed of its prevalence and how society can try to best minimize its impact for the benefit of both the individuals and communities affected.

IMPLICATIONS FOR RESEARCH AND PRACTICE

- A comprehensive self-neglect assessment tool will support health and social care professionals in identifying and responding to self-neglect cases in a more objective and standardized way.
- Assessment and intervention in self-neglect cases requires an interdisciplinary team approach as manifestations of self-neglect can present along a diverse spectrum and usually require diverse skill sets and resources to address self-neglect phenomena.
- Research on self-neglect will need to focus on specific interventions and associated outcomes.

REFERENCES

Ballard, J. (2010). Legal implications regarding self-neglecting community-dwelling adults: Practical approach for the community nurse in Ireland. *Public Health Nursing, 27*(2), 181–187. doi:10.1111/j.1525-1446.2010.00840.x

Bartley, M., O'Brien, J. G., & O'Neill, D. (2010). Elder abuse and self-neglect: Reading between the lines. *Irish College of General Practitioners Hot Topics 2010.* Retrieved from https://www.icgp.ie/assets/47/14BA7FA8-19B9-E185-83D899492F60F95A_document/elderabuse18-19.pdf

Berg, B. L., & Lune, H. (2012). *Qualitative research methods for the social sciences* (8th ed.). Boston, MA: Pearson.

Bergeron, L. (2006). Self-determination and elder abuse: Do we know enough? *Journal of Gerontological Social Work, 46*(3/4), 82–102. doi:10.1300/J083v46n03_05

Blagodatny, M. L., Skudlarska, B., & Tocchi, C. (2007). Management of Diogenes Syndrome: Behavioral disorder of self-neglect. *Journal of the American Geriatrics Society, 55*(4), 41.

Braye, S., Orr, D., & Preston-Shoot, M. (2011). *Self-neglect and adult safeguarding: Findings from research.* London, UK: Social Care Institute for Excellence.

Braye, S., Orr, D., & Preston-Shoot, M. (2014). *Self-neglect policy and practice: Building an evidence base for adult social care.* London, UK: Social Care Institute for Excellence.

Braye, S., Orr, D., & Preston-Shoot, M. (2015). Learning lessons about self-neglect? An analysis of serious case reviews. *Journal of Adult Protection, 17*(1), 3–18. doi:10.1108/JAP-05-2014-0014

Capriani, G., Lucetti, C., Vedovello, M., & Nuti, A. (2012). Diogenes syndrome in patients suffering from dementia. *Dialogues in Clinical Neuroscience, 14*(4), 455–460.

Central Statistics Office. (2012). *Highlights from the census 2011, part 1.* Retrieved from http://www.cso .ie/en/media/csoie/census/documents/census2011pdr/Census,2011,Highlights,Part,1,web,72dpi.pdf

Choi, N. G., Kim, J., & Asseff, J. (2009). Self-neglect and neglect of vulnerable older adults: Reexamination of etiology. *Journal of Gerontological Social Work, 52*(2), 171–187. doi:10.1080/01634370802609239

Christians, C. G. (2000). Ethics and politics in qualitative research. In N. K. Denzin & Y. S. Lincoln (Eds.), *Handbook of qualitative research* (2nd ed.). London, UK: Sage.

Corbin, J., & Strauss, A. (2008). *Basics of qualitative research* (3rd ed.). London, UK: Sage.

Day, M. R. (2010). Self-neglect: A challenge and a dilemma. *Archives of Psychiatric Nursing, 24*(2), 73–75. doi:10.1016/j.apnu.2010.02.002

Day, M. R., & Leahy-Warren, P. (2008). Self-neglect 1: Recognizing features and risk factors. *Nursing Times Research, 104*(24), 26–27.

Day, M. R., Leahy-Warren, P., & McCarthy, G. (2013). Perceptions and views of self-neglect: A client-centered perspective. *Journal of Elder Abuse & Neglect, 25*(1), 76–94. doi:10.1080/08946566.2012.712864

Day, M. R., Leahy-Warren, P., & McCarthy, G. (2016). Self-neglect: Ethical considerations. *Annual Review of Nursing Research, 34*(1), 89–107. doi:10.1891/0739-6686.34.89

Day, M. R., & McCarthy, G. (2015). A national cross-sectional study of community nurses' and social workers' knowledge of self-neglect. *Age and Ageing, 44*(4), 717–720. doi:10.1093/ageing/afv025

Day, M. R., McCarthy, G., & Leahy-Warren, P. (2012). Professional social workers' views on self-neglect: An exploratory study. *British Journal of Social Work, 42*(4), 725–743. doi:10.1093/bjsw/bcr082

Day, M. R., Mulcahy, H., & Leahy-Warren, P. (2016). Prevalence of self-neglect in the caseloads of public health nurses. *British Journal of Community Nursing, 21*(1), 31–35.

Day, M. R., Mulcahy, H., Leahy-Warren, P., & Downey, J. (2015). Self-neglect: A case study and implications for clinical practice. *British Journal of Community Nursing, 20*(3), 110–115. doi:10.12968/bjcn.2015.20.3.110

Denscombe, M. (2010). *The good research guide* (4th ed.). Berkshire, UK: McGraw-Hill.

Dong, X. (2005). Medical implications of elder abuse and neglect. *Clinics in Geriatric Medicine, 21*(2), 293–313. doi:10.1016/j.cger.2004.10.006

Dong, X., & Gorbien, M. (2006). Decision-making capacity: The core of self-neglect. *Journal of Elder Abuse & Neglect, 17*(3), 19–36. doi:10.1300/J084v17n03_02

Dong, X., Mendes de Leon, C. F., & Evans, D. A. (2009). Is greater self-neglect severity associated with lower levels of physical function? *Journal of Aging and Health, 21*(4), 596–610. doi:10.1177/0898264309333323

Dong, X., & Simon, M. A. (2013). Elder self-neglect: Implications for health care professionals. *Canadian Geriatrics Society Journal of Continuing Medical Education, 3*(1), 25–28.

Dong, X., & Simon, M. A. (2015). Elder self-neglect is associated with an increased rate of 30-day hospital readmission: Findings from the Chicago Health and Aging Project. *Gerontology, 61*(1), 41–50. doi:10.1159/000360698

Dong, X., Simon, M. A., & Evans, D. (2012a). Elder self-neglect and hospitalization: Findings from the Chicago Health and Aging Project. *Journal of the American Geriatrics Society, 60*(2), 202–209. doi:10.1111/j.1532-5415.2011.03821.x

Dong, X., Simon, M. A., & Evans, D. (2012b). Prevalence of self-neglect across gender, race, and socio-economic status: Findings from the Chicago Health and Aging Project. *Gerontology, 58*, 258–268. doi:10.1159/000334256

Dong, X., Simon, M., Fulmer, T., Mendes de Leon, C. F., Rajan, M., & Evans, D. (2010). Physical function decline and the risk of elder self-neglect in a community-dwelling population. *The Gerontologist, 50*(3), 316–326. doi:10.1093/geront/gnp164

Dong, X., Simon, M. A., Mendes de Leon, C. F., Fulmer, T., Beck, T., Hebert, L., . . . Evans, D. (2009). Elder self-neglect and abuse and mortality risk in a community-dwelling population. *Journal of the American Medical Association, 302*(5), 517–526. doi:10.1001/jama.2009.1109

Dong, X., Simon, M., Mosqueda, L., & Evans, D. A. (2012). The prevalence of elder self-neglect in a community-dwelling population: Hoarding, hygiene, and environmental hazards. *Journal of Aging and Health, 24*(3), 507–524. doi:10.1177/0898264311425597

Doron, I., Band-Winterstein, T., &Naim, S. (2013). The meaning of elder self-neglect: Social workers' perspective. *International Journal of Aging and Human Development, 77*(1), 17–36. doi:10.2190/AG.77.1.b

Dyer, C. B., Goodwin, J. S., Pickens-Pace, S., Burnett, J., & Kelly, P. A. (2007). Self-neglect among the elderly: A model based on more than 500 patients seen by a geriatric medicine team. *American Journal of Public Health, 97*(9), 1671–1676. doi:10.2105/AJPH.2006.097113

Franzini, L., & Dyer, C. B. (2008). Healthcare costs and utilization of vulnerable elderly people reported to Adult Protective Services. *Journal of the American Geriatrics Society, 56*(4), 667–676. doi:10.1111/j.1532-5415.2007.01629.x

Gallagher, C. (2013). Social care and the older person. In K. Lalor & P. Share (Eds.), *Applied social care: An introduction for students in Ireland* (3rd ed., pp. 259–272). Dublin, Ireland: Gill & Macmillan.

Gibbons, S. W. (2009). Theory synthesis for self-neglect: A health and social phenomenon. *Nursing Research, 58*(3), 194–200.doi:10.1097/NNR.0b013e3181a3092c

Gill, T. M. (2009). Elder self-neglect: Medical emergency or marker of extreme vulnerability? *Journal of American Medical Association, 302*(5), 570–571. doi:10.1001/jama.2009.1136

Gregory, C., Halliday, G., Hodges, J., & Snowdon, J. (2011). Living in squalor: Neuropsychological functioning, emotional processing, and squalor perception in patients found living in squalor. *International Psychogeriatrics, 23*(5), 724–731. doi:10.1017/S1041610210002103

Griebling, T. L. (2010). Is greater self-neglect severity associated with lower levels of physical function? Editorial comment. *Journal of Urology, 183*(1), 288.

Griffen, D. (2015, June 17). Assisted Decision-Making Bill reaches committee stage. *The Irish Times*. Retrieved from http://www.irishtimes.com/news/social-affairs/assisted-decision-making-bill-reaches-committee-stage-1.2253229

Health Service Executive. (2014). Open your eyes: HSE elder abuse services 2014. Retrieved from http://www.hse.ie/eng/services/publications/olderpeople/elderabusereport14.pdf

Hildebrand, C., Taylor, M., & Bradway, C. (2013). Elder self-neglect: The failure of coping because of cognitive and functional impairments. *Journal of the American Association of Nurse Practitioners, 26*(8), 452–462. doi:10.1002/2327-6924.12045

Hurley, M., Scallan, E., Johnson, H., & De La Harpe, D. (2000). Adult service refusers in the greater Dublin area. *Irish Medical Journal, 93*, 207–211.

Iris, M., Ridings, J. W., & Conrad, K. J. (2010). The development of a conceptual model for understanding elder self-neglect. *The Gerontologist, 50*, 303–315. doi:10.1093/geront/gnp125

Kutame, M. M. (2007). *Understanding self-neglect from the older person's perspective* (Doctoral dissertation, Ohio State University). Retrieved from https://etd.ohiolink.edu/rws_etd/document/get/osu1186597966/inline

Lachs, M. S., Williams, C. S., O'Brien, S., & Pillemer, K. A. (2002). Adult protective service use and nursing home placement. *The Gerontologist, 42*(6), 734–739. doi:10.1093/geront/42.6.734

Lachs, M. S., Williams, C. S., O'Brien, S., Pillemer, K. A., & Charlson, M. E. (1998). The mortality of elder mistreatment. *Journal of the American Medical Association, 280*(5), 428–432. doi:10.1001/jama.280.5.428

Lauder, W., Anderson, I., & Barclay, A. (2005). A framework for good practice in interagency interventions with cases of self-neglect. *Journal of Psychiatric and Mental Health Nursing, 12*(2), 192–198. doi:10.1111/j.1365-2850.2004.00817.x

Lauder, W., Roxburgh, M., Harris, J., & Law, J. (2009). Developing self-neglect theory: Analysis of related and atypical cases of people identified as self-neglecting. *Journal of Psychiatric and Mental Health Nursing, 16*, 447–454. doi:10.1111/j.1365-2850.2009.01397.x

Mauk, K. L. (2011). Ethical perspective on self-neglect among older adults. *Rehabilitation Nursing, 36*(2), 60–65. doi:10.1002/j.2048-7940.2011.tb00067.x

McDermott, S. (2010). Professional judgements of risk and capacity in situations of self-neglect among older people. *Ageing and Society, 30*, 1055–1072. doi:10.1017/S0144686X10000139

Murray, B. L., & Upshall, E. (2009). Risk to self. In A. M. Kettles (Ed.), *Risk assessment and management in mental health nursing* (pp. 143–197). Oxford, UK: Wiley Blackwell.

Naik, A. D., Pickens, S., Burnett, J., & Dyer, C. B. (2007). The association between elder self-neglect and functional impairment in community-living older adults. *Journal of the American Geriatrics Society, 55*(4), 17.

Naik, A. D., Pickens, S., Burnett, J., Lai, J., & Dyer, C. B. (2006). Assessing capacity in the setting of self-neglect: Development of a novel screening tool for decision-making capacity. *Journal of Elder Abuse & Neglect, 18*(4), 79–91. doi:10.1300/J084v18n04_08

O'Brien, J. G. (2011). Self-neglect in old age. *Aging Health, 7*(4), 573–581. doi:10.2217/ahe.11.47

Pickens, S., Naik, A. D., Burnett, J., Kelly, P. A., Gleason, M., & Dyer, C. B. (2007). The utility of the Kohlman Evaluation of Living Skills test is associated with substantiated cases of elder self-neglect. *Journal of the American Academy of Nurse Practitioners, 19*(3), 137–142. doi:10.1111/j.1745-7599.2007.00205.x

Pickens, S., Ostwald, S., & Pace, K. (2013). Assessing dimensions of executive function in community-dwelling older adults with self-neglect. *Clinical Nursing Studies, 2*(1), 17–29. doi:10.5430/cns.v2n1p17

Poythress, E. L., Burnett, J., Naik, A., Pickens, S., & Dyer, C. B. (2007). Severe self-neglect: An epidemiological and historical perspective. *Journal of Elder Abuse & Neglect, 18*(4), 5–12. doi:10.1300/J084v18n04_02

Rivas, C. (2012). Coding and analyzing qualitative data. In C. Seale (Ed.), *Researching society and culture* (3rd ed., pp. 366–392). London, UK: Sage.

San Filippo, S. M., Reiboldt, W., White, B., & Hails, J. (2007). Perceptions of elderly self-neglect: A look at culture and cohort. *Family and Consumer Sciences Research Journal, 35*, 215–231. doi:10.1177/1077727X06296624

Snowdon, J., & Halliday, G. (2009). How and when to intervene in cases of severe domestic squalor. *International Psychogeriatrics, 21*(6), 996–1002. doi:10.1017/S1041610209990597

Snowdon, J., Shah, A., & Halliday, G. (2007). Severe domestic squalor: A review. *International Psychogeriatrics, 19*(1), 37–51. doi:10.1017/S1041610206004236

Torke, A. M., & Sachs, G. A. (2008). Self-neglect and resistance to intervention: Ethical challenges for clinicians. *Journal of General Internal Medicine, 23*(11), 1926–1927. doi:10.1007/s11606-008-0807-6

ASSESSMENT AND MEASUREMENT OF SELF-NEGLECT

CHAPTER 20

SHORT-FORM ELDER SELF-NEGLECT ASSESSMENT

Madelyn A. Iris

This chapter describes the development of the Short-Form Elder Self-Neglect Assessment (SF-ESNA) and presents findings from its use by practitioners in the field of self-neglect assessment and intervention. Developed and tested as a 73-item measure, the full ESNA was reduced to a 25-item version to encourage its practical application. The SF-ESNA includes 12 indicators of self-neglect relating to physical and psychosocial aspects of self-neglect, and 13 indicators related to environmental and personal living conditions. Data from 50 SF-ESNA assessments were used to compare findings from data on the same items, using the database derived from the 73-item version. Results confirmed that elder self-neglect stemming from personal behaviors and psychosocial characteristics is more common, as compared to self-neglect involving inadequate or deplorable environmental and personal living conditions. This suggests that self-neglect conditions may progress over time, from self-care deficits to more severe housing conditions. In addition, investigators noted cognitive impairments and mental health problems in over half of the 50 older adults suffering from self-neglect. Those scoring high on the SF-ESNA were more likely to have some type of cognitive impairment or mental illness as compared to those with lower scores. Implications for research and practice are discussed.

Elder self-neglect (ESN) has long been described as a complex, multifaceted, and controversial condition (Connolly, 2008; Iris, Ridings, & Conrad, 2010; Lauder, Anderson, & Barclay, 2005; Rathbone-McCuan & Fabian, 1992). It is the most common form of elder mistreatment reported to adult protective services (APS) (Dyer, Goodwin, Pickens-Pace, Burnett, & Kelly, 2007), with rates exceeding those of all other forms of elder abuse combined (Dong, 2014).

In very general terms, ESN represents "the inability (intentional or nonintentional) to maintain a socially and culturally accepted standard of self-care with the potential for serious consequences to the health and well-being of the self-neglecter and perhaps even to their community" (Gibbons, Lauder, & Ludwick, 2006, p. 16). Per this definition, ESN includes lack of accommodation to normative standards of self-care and culturally specific practices and behaviors, and individual tolerance for divergent views regarding health and well-being.

In their review of the characterization of ESN over time, Rathbone-McCuan and Fabian (1992) cite conclusions from work by Gruenberg (1967), who describes "progressive deterioration" that may emerge over a period of years, and evolve from

mild to more extreme forms in small increments. Connolly describes the consequences of neglect as ranging from "no discernible harm" to "modest discomfort"
to "serious deterioration" to "grave physical or psychological injury" to "death"
(Connolly, 2008, p. S244). One model of ESN, developed by Dyer and colleagues
(Dyer et al., 2007), posits a framework predicated on the notion that medical
comorbidities lead to diminishment of executive function, which in turn can worsen
the ability to perform activities of daily living and instrumental activities of daily
living. Combined with an inadequate support system, and influenced by extrinsic
social issues (e.g., poverty) as well as person-specific characteristics, such as lack
of capacity, the result is self-neglect.

Dong et al. (2009) supported this conclusion with evidence that a decline in physical
performance testing and increased impairment in self-reported physical function was
associated with increased risk of self-neglect. In addition to physical and functional
dependency needs and cognitive impairment, Choi, Kim, and Asseff (2009) showed
that self-neglect is also attributable to older adults' lack of economic resources necessary to provide themselves with basic necessities. Complicating determinations of
causality, important when considering interventions, is the problem of capacity. Naik
and colleagues (Naik, Pickens, Burnett, Lai, & Dyer, 2006) note that vulnerability for
self-neglect has been shown to be associated with declines in decision-making capacity
related to the ability to care for oneself. They describe a three-part standard for the assessment of decision-making capacity: first is the elder's ability to comprehend relevant
information related to the condition of self-neglect; second is the ability to appreciate
the significance of that information and use it to evaluate possible consequences or
outcomes of one's choices; and third is the ability to articulate a single choice. Assessing self-neglect is a complicated and often difficult task because there is no agreement
regarding "evidence-based" risk factors or a psychometrically sound screening tool for
clinicians and APS professionals (Dyer, Goodwin, Pickens-Pace, Burnett, & Kelly, 2007;
Kelly, Dyer, Pavlik, Doody, & Jogerst, 2008). One notable attempt to produce such
a tool was undertaken by the Consortium for Research in Elder Self-Neglect faculty
group at Baylor College of Medicine, which developed the Self-Neglect Severity Scale
(SSS; Kelly et al., 2008). Items in the SSS are organized into three domains: personal
hygiene, impaired function, and environmental status, along with duration of current
condition. The tool uses a severity rating scale of 0 to 4 and was designed to be used in
the home setting (Dyer et al., 2006). During a field test of the tool, 23 older adults were
assessed. Although the results indicated that the SSS distinguished self-neglect cases
from a comparison sample of older adults who did not self-neglect, the sensitivity and
specificity of the SSS for self-neglect did not reach the standard range of acceptability,
and the unidimensionality of the scale was unclear (Kelly et al., 2008).

THE ESN ASSESSMENT INSTRUMENT

Iris et al. (2010) addressed the need for a validated, psychometrically reliable assessment tool that utilized measurement theory not only to substantiate the presence of
self-neglect, but also to assess the degree of severity (see Iris et al., 2010 for a detailed
description of the methods and findings of this study). In phase 1 of the study, they
used concept-mapping methodology (Kane & Trochim, 2007) to establish a set of
ESN indicators, their importance to the concept, and the underlying conceptual
organization of the construct. The product was a 73-item assessment measure. In

phase 2, a field test of the measure to determine its psychometric properties was conducted, using Rasch analysis methods (Conrad & Smith, 2004). The CJE SeniorLife Institutional Review Board approved both phases of the project.

In phase 1, a total of 50 academicians, policy and planning professionals, APS practitioners, and older adults brainstormed lists of ESN indicators that the research team then consolidated into a set of 73 items. Next, a subset of the participants sorted the items into groupings based on the principle of "likeness." Using multidimensional scaling and hierarchical cluster analysis (see Kane & Trochim, 2007), seven conceptual domains emerged from the sorting (see Iris et al., 2010 for details of the concept-mapping exercises). The domains were (1) personal endangerment, (2) physical living conditions, (3) financial issues, (4) mental health, (5) personal living conditions, (6) physical health risk, and (7) social network. Figure 20.1 shows a two-dimensional point map of the conceptual domain, with two broad regions of meaning; physical and psychosocial aspects of ESN and environmental aspects of ESN. Numbers indicate the item number from the list of 73 items (see Iris et al., 2010, for a full list of items).

The final product of this first phase of the research was the 73-item observational measure of ESN, the ESNA (ESNA is described in Iris, Conrad, & Ridings, 2014). The ESNA assesses an older adult's status in each of the seven conceptual areas listed previously, using indicators generated through the concept-mapping exercise. There are five possible responses: Yes (problem exists), No (problem does not exist), Suspected problem (problem believed to exist but no firm evidence based on observation), Don't know (no ability to conduct an observation), and Not applicable (problem does not apply to this individual). The two broad regions of meaning, environmental aspects

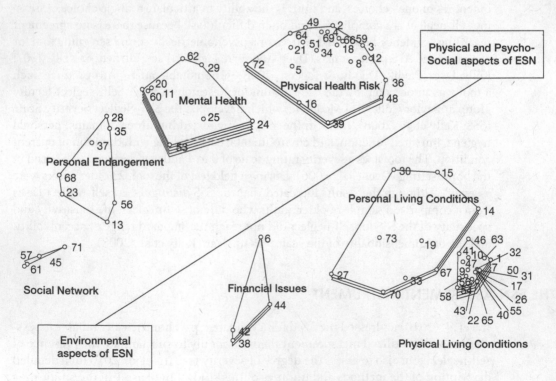

Figure 20.1   Seven-cluster conceptual map of elder self-neglect with items and two regions of meaning.

Source: From Iris, Ridings, and Conrad (2010). Used with permission of Oxford University Press.

TABLE 20.1　Conceptual Model of Elder Self-Neglect

Physical and Psychosocial Region of Meaning	Consequences for the Older Adult	Environmental Region of Meaning
ELDER SELF-NEGLECT		
Mental Health: May abuse substances, experiences cognitive deficits such as Alzheimer's disease *Physical Health Risk*: Ignores signs and symptoms of disease or illness, Does not take medications as instructed, Has no primary care provider	Life-altering or life-threatening conditions, including eviction, relocation, exposure, homelessness, institutionalization, serious illness, death	*Physical Living Conditions*: Appliances not working, utilities turned off, housing code violations
Social Network: Poor social support network, lack of family members and friends, no one to turn to for help	Lack of social support, risk of abuse or exploitation	*Financial Issues*: No money for home improvement or maintenance, unpaid bills
Personal Endangerment: Refuse to accept help, noncompliant with medical directives	Poor health, dangerous and/or substandard living conditions	*Personal Living Conditions*: Hoarding (pets, garbage, papers, etc.), blocked pathways to exits/bathroom/kitchen
NORMAL AGING		

Source: From Iris, Ridings, and Conrad (2010). Used with permission of Oxford University Press.

of ESN and physical, and psychosocial aspects of ESN, guided the development of a conceptual model of ESN, as shown in Table 20.1.

This model incorporates the seven conceptual domains in a hierarchical layout ranging from frequent aspects of normal aging at the low end of severity, and behavioral characteristics and aspects of living conditions specifically associated with ESN at the high end of severity. The model also shows the possible consequences for the older adult that may result from the interaction of specific indicators in each region of meaning. Iris et al. (2010) include a more complete discussion of this conceptual model.

In the next phase of the research, a full-scale field test of the ESNA was conducted. Thirteen agencies responsible for conducting assessments of older adults seeking home- and community-based services participated in the field test along with one municipal department that conducted its own self-neglect screenings, and one social service agency that offered counseling and support services to older adults already identified as experiencing self-neglect. Each organization incorporated the ESNA into its usual assessment procedures for older adults believed to be self-neglecting. We received 215 completed assessments over a period of approximately 10 months.

THE SHORT-FORM ESNA INSTRUMENT

Using the results of our analysis of the ESNA, we found the measure to be unidimensional, confirming that the measure assessed a single construct, with high internal consistency reliability. We then conducted a second round of analyses, in order to develop a shorter version, the SF-ESNA. Using a multistep iterative procedure, we ended up with a set of 25 items that had good person reliability (.83) and a Cronbach's alpha of .87. For detailed descriptions of the methodology used to create the 25-item SF-ESNA and the psychometric properties of the long and short versions, see Iris et al. (2014). The analysis provided good evidence of unidimensionality, although there appeared to be two somewhat distinct aspects, which we have labeled Behavioral Characteristics and Environmental Conditions, corresponding to the two regions of meaning (psychosocial aspects and environmental aspects of ESN) shown in Figure 20.1.

These findings supported the construct validity of the theoretical model presented in Table 20.1. Rasch analysis generates a hierarchy of item severity based on an estimate of item difficulty. In the findings, frequency of occurrence corresponds to the severity of each self-neglect indicator: that is, difficult items, believed to indicate more severe self-neglect, are posited to occur less often than easier items, or those thought to be less severe. Using the importance ratings produced in phase 1, we compared the mean scores for each of the seven conceptual components of ESN: physical living conditions (3.99); mental health (3.92); financial issues (3.76); personal living conditions (3.73); physical health risk (3.66); social network (3.45); and personal endangerment (3.44), as mapped in Figure 20.1. We found the order (in descending importance from high to low) corresponded with the hierarchy of items generated by the Rasch analysis. This concurrence provided further evidence of construct validity and confirmed the findings from our prior work developing the ESNA (Iris et al., 2010).

A formal version of the 25-item SF-ESNA is now available and is included here as Appendix 20.1. In this version, items are marked as denoting either the environmental aspects of ESN (marked with an E for Environmental) or the physical and psychosocial aspects of ESN (marked with a B for Behavioral). The short form has 12 items in the behavioral category and 13 items in the environmental category and includes scoring instructions as follows: "Yes" for any item equals 2 points; "Suspected" equals 1 point; "No" "Don't know " or "Not applicable" equals 0. Thus, for the 12 items in the behavioral category, the highest possible score is 24, whereas for the environmental category the highest possible score is 26, yielding a total possible highest score of 50. We suggest that assessors create subtotals for behavioral and environmental indicators, in order to prioritize interventions according to the most significant type of self-neglect problems found. We propose that a high score in the behavioral category indicates a high risk of ESN. If the score is high in the environmental category, but not in the behavioral category, then intentional self-neglect may be occurring. If scores are high in both categories, then severe, nonintentional self-neglect may exist. In turn, low scores may reflect changes commonly associated with the aging process, but they may also indicate that individuals are at risk for more significant self-neglect in the future.

The SF-ESNA is now being used by several organizations that assess ESN. For example, the City of Chicago Department of Family & Support Services, which includes senior services, sponsors a project called Intensive Case Advocacy and Support (ICAS). The ICAS program contracts with a variety of service providers throughout the city, some specializing in specific populations and interventions, in order to reach as diverse a group of clients as possible. Services offered include home repair, counseling, housing assistance, cleanup services, and so forth (see Chapter 16 for more information). ICAS providers use the SF-ESNA as part of their initial assessment process.

In western Illinois, a multiservice organization, Alternatives for the Older Adult (hereafter Alternatives), adopted the tool in late 2014, following reauthorization of Illinois's elder abuse statute, amended to include self-neglect as a type of elder abuse. Alternatives is headquartered in Moline, Illinois, a city of approximately 43,500, with over 381,000 people living in the greater metro area. According to the 2010 census, over 86% of residents were White, and only 4.6% were African American; just 9.4% of the population identified as Hispanic or Latino. In addition, 12.6% of households included someone at least 65 years of age, although 15.4% of the population as a whole was 65 or older. The median income for all households was $47,970 and approximately 2.1% of the older adult population lived below the federal poverty line.

The Alternatives provided the author with 52 "deidentified" assessments completed between August 2015 and December 2015. These represent 38% of all the self-neglect referrals received by the agency during that time. The sample included five clients younger than 60 years of age, as in 2013 Illinois's elder abuse program became a full APS program, which now included assessment and intervention services for people 18 to 59 years of age if they are believed to have a disability. Those 60 and older automatically qualify by age alone. Illinois uses the following definition for self-neglect:

> "Self-neglect" means a condition that is the result of an eligible adult's inability, due to physical or mental impairments, or both, or a diminished capacity, to perform essential self-care tasks that substantially threaten his or her own health, including: providing essential food, clothing, shelter, and health care; and obtaining goods and services necessary to maintain physical health, mental health, emotional well-being, and general safety. The term includes compulsive hoarding, which is characterized by the acquisition and retention of large quantities of items and materials that produce an extensively cluttered living space, which significantly impairs the performance of essential self-care tasks or otherwise substantially threatens life or safety. (State of Illinois Department on Aging, 2011, p. 38)

In addition to the completed SF-ESNA, information on the client's age, gender, type of residence, race, primary language, cognitive status, and mental health status was provided. Investigators also indicated whether there was any suspicion of elder abuse.

DEMOGRAPHICS FROM THE ALTERNATIVES SAMPLE

Clients assessed by Alternatives were relatively young, with a mean age of just 70.7 years, and a range of 43 to 94 years; only five of the 52 people were younger than 60; just over half the clients (53.9%) were men, and most individuals owned their own homes, where they resided. In addition, the majority was White (84%), in keeping with the overall demographic makeup of the area, and just one person was reported to be of Hispanic origin. Twenty-four of the 52 clients (46.2%) were judged to have some type of cognitive impairment, 14 (26.9%) did not, and another 14 clients (26.9%) could not be assessed. Mental illness was also prevalent: 22 people (42.3%) were thought to have some type of mental illness; 16 (30.8%) did not, and 14 people (26.9%) could not be assessed. Note that the terms *cognitive impairment* and *mental illness* were used without a clinical definition, and presence or absence of either condition was based on the investigator's judgment. Only eight people were thought to be

TABLE 20.2 Demographic and Other Characteristics of the Alternatives Sample

Mean age (n = 51) SD = 10.85	70.69		
Age range	43–94		
Mean age persons 60 and older (n = 44) SD = 9.57	72.61		
Persons younger than 60	5		
Gender	29 (55.76%) male		
	23 (44.20%) female		
Residence	Owns own home: 27 (52.90%)	Rents: 4 (7.80%)	Lives in someone else's home: 4 (7.80%)
Race (n = 49)	White: 42 (84.0%)	African American: 7 (14.0%)	
Hispanic/Latino origin	1 (0.96%)		
Cognitive impairment (n = 36)	Yes = 24 (46.2%)	No = 14 (26.9%)	Don't know/Not able to assess = 14 (26.9%)
Mental illness (n = 34)	Yes = 22 (42.3%)	No = 16 (30.8%)	Don't know/Not able to assess = 14 (26.9%)
Elder abuse suspected	Yes = 8 (15.38%)		

SD, standard deviation.

victims of elder abuse as well as self-neglect. Table 20.2 provides a summary of the sample characteristics. Note that sample sizes vary due to missing data for some items.

Two clients were dropped from further analyses; one client scored 0, as no evidence of self-neglect was found and a second person was unable to be assessed, because he was homeless and could not be found following discharge from the hospital. Across the remaining sample of 50 cases, SF-ESNA total scores ranged from a low of 1 (2.1%) to a high of 38 (75%). The total mean score for all 25 items was 16.75 (33.97%) out of a possible 50. By subtype, mean scores were 10.6 (41.8%) for behavioral aspects and 6.1 (24.8%) for environmental aspects.

Because of the small sample size, we did not attempt to test the results using Rasch methodology. Instead, using frequency of endorsement across the 50 assessments for those individuals suffering from some type of self-neglect, we determined which problems were most common, such as the least severe according to Rasch theory, and those which were least common, that is, more or most severe. Table 20.3 shows the items in hierarchical order, from low to high frequency, that is most severe to less severe.

TABLE 20.3 Hierarchy of Items From Less Frequent to Most Frequent

Item and Subtype	Total # of Endorsements
B22: Majority of OA's medications out of date E24: Toilet not in working order	2
E25: OA has lice or other parasites	5
E21: OA is eating spoiled food	7
E17: Human/animal feces/urine on the floors/ walls in OA's home E19: OA lacks access to needed areas of the home (bathtub, sinks, bed) E20: Sinks in the home are in poor or nonworking condition E23: Temperature in home not appropriate for summer/winter conditions	10
B13: No primary care physician	12
B18: OA shows signs of malnourishment or dehydration	17
E14: Bathing facilities are unsafe, unsanitary, or inoperable E16: Evidence of vermin in home	18
E15: Accumulation of garbage in OA's home	20
B7: Odors in the home raise concerns (urine, feces, garbage)? B12: OA generally uncooperative	22
B6: OA ignores signs and symptoms of disease	25
B8: OA wears dirty clothes B9: OA exhibits poor personal hygiene E11: OA's home at risk for fire hazards	26
E2: Condition of house/apartment or yard appears unsafe or unsanitary	30
B1: OA fails to follow through with preventive or diagnostic testing related to health conditions	35
B3: OA lacks sufficient care to meet his/her needs B10: OA's behaviors likely to cause him/her imminent physical harm	39
B4: OA fails to engage in adequate preventive practices	40
B5: Isolation putting OA at risk	42

OA, older adult.

VALIDATION OF THE THEORETICAL MODEL

The hierarchy of severity based on these frequencies can be compared to the severity hierarchy generated by our original Rasch analysis (Iris et al., 2014) and validates our conclusion that self-neglect falls into two types: behavioral characteristics and environmental conditions. For example, for both the original SF-25 sample and the Alternatives sample, we find almost identical results; the same items appear in the top 10 most severe indicators of self-neglect for both samples. Of these, for the 10 most common or least severe indicators, nine out of 10 items fall into that grouping for both samples.

Looking at the order of indicators on Table 20.2 we find that behavioral indicators occur more frequently than environmental indicators. Among the least severe or most common indicators, eight out of 10 are behavioral characteristics for both the Alternatives and the original SF-ESNA samples. In contrast, for the Alternatives sample among the 10 most severe indicators, seven out of 10 fall into the environmental category, as do eight out of 10 for the original SF-ESNA analysis (see Iris et al., 2014).

To better understand the conditions under which self-neglect may occur, we explored the relationship between the presence or absence of cognitive impairments, mental illness, or both, and SF-25 scores, based on investigators' opinions. First, working with the total sample of 52 clients, we examined the frequencies of cases where both conditions were indicated, where neither was indicated, and where the investigator could not assess for one or both conditions.

As Table 20.4 shows, almost one quarter (12, 23%) of the clients had both cognitive impairment and mental illness. Fourteen (26.9%) clients were determined to have either cognitive impairment or mental illness, but not both. Only four clients (7.7%) were found to have no indication of both conditions. However, the number of clients who could not

TABLE 20.4 Frequency of Identification of Cognitive Impairment and Mental Illness (*n* = 52)

Condition	Number of Times Indicated	Percentage
Cognitive impairment and mental illness indicated	12	23.0
Cognitive impairment, no mental illness indicated	8	15.4
Cognitive impairment, can't assess mental illness	4	7.7
Can't assess cognitive impairment, mental illness indicated	4	7.7
Can't assess cognitive impairment, no mental illness indicated	4	7.7
No cognitive impairment, mental illness indicated	6	11.5
No cognitive impairment, can't assess mental illness	4	7.7
No cognitive impairment and no mental illness indicated	4	7.7
Can't assess either condition	6	11.5
	52	100

be assessed for one or both conditions was high: there were 16 (30.8%) cases in which clients had indications of either cognitive impairment or mental illness but could not be assessed for the other condition, and there were an additional six (11.5%) cases in which the clients could not be assessed for both conditions, for a total of 22 cases (42.5%) where information on a client's cognitive status or mental health could not be ascertained. Most of the time, no reasons were given for inability to assess. It is important to note that only six clients (11.5%) were found to have no indications of either cognitive impairment or mental illness. These numbers indicate that cognitive impairment and mental illness, either alone or in combination, are significant problems for many of the older adults in this sample, but the inability to assess clients is very problematic.

Next, to examine the association among cognitive impairment, mental illness, and self-neglect severity, we selected 50 cases in which at least one indicator of some type of self-neglect was checked, used total self-neglect scores (behavioral and environmental indicators) to split the sample into two groups. Group 1 comprised individuals who had a total self-neglect score of 50% ($n = 12$) or higher and Group 2 contained individuals with self-neglect scores of 49% or lower ($n = 38$). Table 20.5 includes a breakdown of cases for each group in which cognitive impairment and mental illness together were present, neither condition was indicated, cognitive impairment or mental illness alone was indicated, and the older adults could not be assessed for one or both conditions.

For those with total self-neglect scores of 50% or higher ($n = 12$), only three clients had both cognitive impairment and mental illness (25%), whereas seven (58.3%) could not be assessed for one or both conditions. This compares to those with scores of 49% or lower ($n = 38$), of which nine individuals (23.7%) were found to have both cognitive impairment and mental illness. In both groups, much smaller percentages of

TABLE 20.5 Total Scores and Presence or Absence of Cognitive Impairment and Mental Illness ($n = 50$)

Condition	Number of Times Indicated	Percentage
Those with total scores of 50% or higher (n = 12)		
Cognitive impairment and mental illness	3	25.0
Cognitive impairment only	1	8.3
Mental illness only	1	8.3
No cognitive impairment or mental illness	0	0
Unable to assess one or both conditions	7	58.3
Those with total scores of 49% or lower (n = 38)		
Cognitive impairment and mental illness	9	23.7
Cognitive impairment only	5	13.2
Mental illness only	5	13.2
No cognitive impairment or mental illness	4	10.5
Unable to assess one or both conditions	15	39.5

people had only one condition, although a larger percentage of individuals in Group 2 had either cognitive impairment or mental illness alone. All the older adults in Group 1 had at least one condition, as compared to four people in Group 2 (10.5) who were found to not have either problem. However, seven people (58.3%) in Group 1 and 15 (39.5%) older adults in Group 2 could not be assessed for one or both conditions.

In the next analysis, we examined those cases in which at least one behavioral self-neglect indicator was checked. Using the same groupings described previously, Table 20.6 shows the distribution of cases vis-à-vis findings of cognitive impairment, mental illness, or both.

Of the 50 cases in this subsample, 19 had scores of 50% or higher (Group 1) and 31 had scores of 49% or lower (Group 2). In Group 1, seven (36.8%) had cognitive impairment and mental illness, one (5.2%) had cognitive impairment alone, three (15.8%) had mental illness alone, and just one person (5.2%) had neither condition, whereas seven more (36.8%) could not be assessed. In Group 2 ($n = 31$), five people (16.1%) had both cognitive impairment and mental illness, whereas six (19.4%) had cognitive impairment alone, and three (9.6%) had mental illness alone. Only three people (43.8%) were reported to have no cognitive impairment and no mental illness, but almost half of the clients in this category (14, 45.2%) could not be assessed.

Clearly, those in Group 1 were more impaired as compared to those in Group 2, as a larger percentage of those in Group 2 (9.6%) had no cognitive impairment or mental illness, although a larger proportion of people in Group 2 could not be assessed (45.2%).

Table 20.7 displays findings regarding those cases in which environmental indicators of self-neglect were seen. For those with scores above 50% ($n = 10$), two people (20%) had both cognitive impairment and mental illness, one person had cognitive impairment only or mental illness only (10% each), and no one was found not

TABLE 20.6 Behavioral Self-Neglect and Presence or Absence of Cognitive Impairment and or Mental Illness ($n = 50$)

Condition	Number of Times Indicated	Percentage
Those with behavioral self-neglect scores of 50% or higher (n = 19)		
Cognitive impairment and mental illness	7	36.8
Cognitive impairment only	1	5.2
Mental illness only	3	15.8
No cognitive impairment or mental illness	1	5.2
Unable to assess one or both conditions	7	36.8
Those with behavioral self-neglect scores of 49% or less (n = 31)		
Cognitive impairment and mental illness	5	16.1
Cognitive impairment only	6	19.4
Mental illness only	3	9.6
No cognitive impairment or mental illness	3	9.6
Unable to assess one or both conditions	14	45.2

TABLE 20.7 Environmental Self-Neglect and Presence or Absence of Cognitive Impairment or Mental Illness (*n* = 50)

Condition	Number of Times Indicated	Percentage
Those with environmental self-neglect scores of 50% or higher (n = 10)		
Cognitive impairment and mental illness	2	20
Cognitive impairment only	1	10
Mental illness only	1	10
No cognitive impairment or mental illness	0	0
Unable to assess one or both conditions	6	60
Those with environmental self-neglect scores of 49% or less (n = 40)		
Cognitive impairment and mental illness	10	25
Cognitive impairment only	6	15
Mental illness only	5	12.5
No cognitive impairment or mental illness	4	10
Unable to assess one or both conditions	15	37.5

to have either condition. However, six (60%) of the older adults in this group could not be assessed. For those in Group 2 (*n* = 40), 10 people (25%) had both cognitive impairment and mental illness, six (15%) had cognitive impairment alone, five (12.5%) had mental illness alone, and four (10%) had neither condition. However, 15 (37.5%) of this subsample could not be assessed.

The statistics presented in Tables 20.6 and 20.7 do not present a clearly defined picture of the impact of severity on cognitive impairment and/or mental illness for either behavioral or environmental self-neglect, and it is difficult to identify any consistent trend. However, for both types of ESN, the inability to assess for cognitive impairment and mental illness limits the conclusions that can be drawn regarding the influence of these conditions on self-neglect.

The SF-ESN is a "stand-alone" measure, but the findings described previously highlight the need for including a standardized assessment of both cognitive impairment and mental illness when investigating cases. Used together, the information collected should direct attention to the need for specific types of interventions and services. In addition, investigators should also assess functional deficits in both activities of daily living and instrumental activities of daily living, as these are likely to also play a role in increasing the risk of greater severity.

CONSIDERATIONS OF FINANCIAL STATUS WHEN ASSESSING ESN

In our conceptual model (Table 20.1), we show that financial issues may play a role in contributing to self-neglect, in that older adults with limited or no income are likely to be unable to maintain their home environments and pay for the basics of daily life, such as medications, food, laundry, and so on. However, items in the original ESNA that targeted financial issues were not included in the SF-ESNA, as they did not perform well in terms of fit to the Rasch model, and, unfortunately, in our original ESNA sample the information we did have regarding financial status was unreliable or incomplete (Iris et al., 2014). The Alternatives dataset did not include any information on income or assets.

CONCLUSION

It is clear that in practice settings some sort of determination of financial resources is important when planning interventions, identifying eligibility for public benefits, and for securing resources for the older adult. For research purposes, strategies for attaining income information should be devised, and the importance of this information for understanding the underlying causes of ESN should be stressed in the study design and training of data collectors.

The development of the SF-ESNA and its validation provides self-neglect investigators and other practitioners with a brief, standardized assessment tool that applies indicators of self-neglect across a continuum from least to most severe. Using the recommended scoring, it is possible for practitioners to devise tailored care plans that address the range of problems found, and prioritize services and interventions in accordance with the hierarchy of severity described here. Behavioral indicators of ESN may be precursors or risk factors for more severe environmental declines later. Hence, early intervention with older adults exhibiting self-neglect associated with behavioral indicators could forestall later and more severe environmental harm. In addition, identification of cognitive decline or onset of depression in an older adult should serve as a warning sign for possible self-neglect. Addressing the self-care capacity and mental health of such individuals early on may help to prevent or at least lessen the negative impact of ESN.

IMPLICATIONS FOR RESEARCH AND PRACTICE

- The findings described in this chapter provide evidence for thinking about ESN as a continuum of decline, from a position of well-being (good self-care and an adequate home environment) characterized by the notion of "normal aging," to a situation of increasing severity of deficits with respect to self-care practices and environmental conditions.
- At their most extreme, that is, most severe, the practices and conditions captured by the SF-ESNA indicators constitute significant threats to the older adult, and, in the absence of intervention, can result in removal from the home, institutionalization, or death.
- To test this theory a naturalistic, longitudinal design that follows individuals over time, from the early identification of risk of self-neglect (indicated by the endorsement of several of the most common indicators) through individual end points (i.e., placement, hospitalization, death) would be the ideal. However, because such a study would violate ethical and professional standards, an alternative would be to utilize an epidemiologic approach to identify a population-wide sample that would include individuals without self-neglect, those who are self-neglecting but accept interventions and services, and those who are self-neglecting but refuse assistance.

REFERENCES

Choi, N. G., Kim, J., & Asseff, J. (2009). Self-neglect and neglect of vulnerable older adults: Reexamination of etiology. *Journal of Gerontological Social Work, 52*(2), 171–187.

Connolly, M. T. (2008). Elder self-neglect and the justice system: An essay from an interdisciplinary perspective. *Journal of the American Geriatrics Society, 56*, S244–S252.

Conrad, K., & Smith, E. (2004). International conference on objective measurement: Applications of Rasch analysis in health care. *Medical Care, 42*(Suppl. 1), 1–6.

Dong, X. (2014). Elder abuse: Research, practice, and health policy: The 20212 GSA Maxwell Pollack Award Lecture. *The Gerontologist, 54*(2), 153–162.

Dong, X., Simon, M. A., Mendes de Leon, C., Fulmer, T., Becks, T., Herbert, L., . . . Evans, D. (2009). Elder self-neglect and abuse and mortality risk in a community-dwelling population. *Journal of the American Medical Association, 302*(5), 517–526.

Dyer, C., Goodwin, J., Pickens-Pace, S., Burnett, J., & Kelly, P. (2007). Self-neglect among the elderly: A model based on more than 500 patients seen by a geriatric medicine team. *American Journal of Public Health, 97*(9), 1671–1676.

Dyer, C., Kelly, P., Pavlik, V., Lee, J., Doody, R., Regev, T., . . . Smith, S. M. (2006). The making of a self-neglect severity scale. *Journal of Elder Abuse & Neglect, 18*, 13–21.

Gibbons, S., Lauder, W., & Ludwick, R. (2006). Self-neglect: A proposed new NANDA diagnosis. *International Journal of Nursing Terminologies and Classification, 17*(1), 10–18.

Gruenberg, E. M. (1967). The social breakdown syndrome: Some origins. *American Journal of Psychiatry, 123*(12), 1481–1489.

Iris, M., Conrad, K. J., & Ridings, J. (2014). Observational measure of elder self-neglect. *Journal of Elder Abuse & Neglect, 26*(4), 365–397.

Iris, M., Ridings, J., & Conrad, K. J. (2010). The development of a conceptual model for understanding elder self-neglect. *The Gerontologist, 50*(3), 303–315.

Kane, R., & Trochim, W. (2007). *Concept mapping for planning and evaluation.* Thousand Oaks, CA: Sage.

Kelly, P., Dyer, C., Pavlik, V., Doody, R., & Jogerst, G. (2008). Exploring self-neglect in older adults: Preliminary findings of the self-neglect severity scale and next steps. *Journal of the American Geriatrics Society, 56*, S253–S260.

Lauder, W., Anderson, I., & Barclay, A. (2005). Housing and self-neglect: The response of health, social care, and environmental health agencies. *Journal of Interprofessional Care, 19*(4), 317–325.

Naik, A., Pickens, S., Burnett, J., Lai, J., & Dyer, C. (2006). Assessing capacity in the setting of self-neglect: Development of a novel screening tool for decision-making capacity. *Journal of Elder Abuse & Neglect, 18*, 79–91.

Rathbone-McCuan, E., & Fabian, D. (1992). *Self-neglecting elders: A clinical dilemma.* New York, NY: Auburn House.

State of Illinois Department on Aging. (2011). Elder Abuse and Neglect Act and Related Law. Springfield, IL: Author.

APPENDIX 20.1

DIRECTIONS: Please mark all responses with an X or use the space provided to enter a written response where applicable.

ID #:_____ Date of first contact: _____ Date of completion: _____

_____

_____

<table>
<tr><td>Source of Information Used for Evaluation:
□ Investigator
□ Older Adult
□ Third Party (who?)</td></tr>
</table>

Has this client been assessed previously? Yes = 1 No = 2

Assessor's Information

Assessor (Last Name Only):

Title/Department:

Name of agency:

Is agency an elder abuse provider agency? Yes   No

Is agency a case coordination unit? Yes   No

Demographics of Older Adult

Age of the older adult: _____   Gender: □ Female   □ Male   □ Unknown

Address: _____

_____

Does the older adult own or rent his or her home or apartment?

□ Owns   □ Rents   □ Someone else owns/rents

Is the older adult of Hispanic/Latino origin?   □ Yes = 1   □ No = 2

Race or ethnicity? (If biracial, circle all that apply)

□ White = 1

□ Black = 2

□ American Indian/Alaskan Native = 3

□ Asian/Pacific Islander = 4

□ Don't know/Refused = 5

□ Other = 6

Please describe: _____

What language(s) are spoken, if not English?

Is an interpreter needed?   □ Yes   □ No

Risk Assessment

Is elder abuse also suspected?   □ Yes   □ No

Please indicate the overall risk level for this older adult: □ High   □ Moderate   □ Low

Action

☐ Refer to elder abuse   ☐ Refer to case management   ☐ Needs assistance but not case management

Elder Self-Neglect Assessment

Instructions: Please answer each question based upon your professional judgment, reports from the older adult directly, or from a third party. Please complete the assessment as best you can, using currently available information. If you have questions about a specific diagnostic description of a mental illness, please refer to the *Diagnostic and Statistical Manual of Mental Disorders*. There is a comment box at the end of the Elder Self-Neglect Assessment. Please write your comments there, and indicate which questions they relate to.

Note that items are arranged in order of severity, from low to high. Clustering of items at the low, middle, or high end of the assessment should help you determine the overall severity of the self-neglect.

Elder Self-Neglect Rating Scale

Circle the appropriate number for each question. If completing this electronically, insert an X in front of the correct response. Yes = 2, Suspected problem (SusP) = 1, No = 0, Don't know (DK) = 0, Not applicable (N/A) = 0

No.	Elder Self-Neglect Indicator	Yes	SusP	No	DK	N/A
1	Does the older adult fail to follow through with preventive or diagnostic testing related to health conditions? (B)	☐	☐	☐	☐	☐
2	Does the condition of the older adult's house, apartment, or yard appear unsafe or unsanitary? (E)	☐	☐	☐	☐	☐
3	Does the older adult lack sufficient care to meet his or her needs? (B)	☐	☐	☐	☐	☐
4	Does the older adult fail to engage in adequate preventive practices (e.g., diet, exercise, smoking cessation)? (B)	☐	☐	☐	☐	☐
5	Is the older adult's isolation putting him or her at risk? (B)	☐	☐	☐	☐	☐
6	Does the older adult ignore signs and symptoms of disease? (B)	☐	☐	☐	☐	☐
7	Are there odors in the home that raise concerns (urine, feces, garbage)? (E)	☐	☐	☐	☐	☐
8	Does the older adult wear dirty clothes? (B)	☐	☐	☐	☐	☐
9	Does the older adult exhibit poor personal hygiene as evidenced by a noticeable odor, long and dirty fingernails, and so on? (B)	☐	☐	☐	☐	☐
10	Are the older adult's behaviors likely to cause him or her imminent physical harm? (B)	☐	☐	☐	☐	☐
11	Is the older adult's home at risk for fire hazards? (E)	☐	☐	☐	☐	☐
12	Is the older adult generally uncooperative? (B)	☐	☐	☐	☐	☐
13	Does the older adult lack a primary care physician?(B)	☐	☐	☐	☐	☐
14	Are the bathing facilities unsafe, unsanitary, or inoperable? (E)	☐	☐	☐	☐	☐
15	Is there an accumulation of garbage in the older adult's house/apartment? (E)	☐	☐	☐	☐	☐
16	Is there evidence of vermin (e.g., rodents or insects) in the older adult's home? (E)	☐	☐	☐	☐	☐

No.	Elder Self-Neglect Indicator	Yes	SusP	No	DK	N/A
17	Is there human/animal feces/urine on the floors/walls in the older adult's home? (E)	☐	☐	☐	☐	☐
18	Does the older adult show signs of malnourishment or dehydration? (B)	☐	☐	☐	☐	☐
19	Does the older adult lack access to needed areas of the home (bathtub, sinks, bed)? (E)	☐	☐	☐	☐	☐
20	Are the sinks in the older adult's home in poor or nonworking condition? (E)	☐	☐	☐	☐	☐
21	Is there evidence the older adult is eating spoiled food? (E)	☐	☐	☐	☐	☐
22	Are the majority of the older adult's medications out of date? (B)	☐	☐	☐	☐	☐
23	Is the temperature in the older adult's home not appropriate for summer/winter conditions? (If the older adult is not responsible for the temperature of the home, please indicate this in the comment box at the end of the form.) (E)	☐	☐	☐	☐	☐
24	Is the older adult's toilet not in working order? (E)	☐	☐	☐	☐	☐
25	Does the older adult have lice or other parasites? (E)	☐	☐	☐	☐	☐

Scoring Instructions

1. Score each item as follows:

   Yes = 2
   Susp = 1
   No = 0
   DK = 0
   N/A = 0

2. Add up the total to indicate severity of ESN.

   You can create totals for the two subsections: Social–Behavioral Self-Neglect (B) and Environmental Self-Neglect (E) by totaling items with a B or E separately.

Suggested interpretations: If high B, not E, then high risk for ESN.

If high in both, then severe ESN (unintentional).

If high in E, not B, then intentional ESN.

Please enter detailed comments on the next page.

Comments:

_____

_____

_____

_____

_____

_____

_____

_____

_____

_____

_____

_____

_____

_____

_____

_____

_____

_____

_____

_____

_____

_____

_____

_____

_____

_____

_____

_____

_____

CHAPTER 21

MAKING AND EXECUTING DECISIONS FOR SAFE AND INDEPENDENT LIVING (MEDSAIL): A SCREENING TOOL FOR COMMUNITY-DWELLING OLDER ADULTS

Whitney L. Mills and Aanand D. Naik

Older adults prefer to remain independent in the community for as long as possible, often resisting needed additional services and supports. When everyday competence is not in balance with the demands and supports of the environment, an older adult can be at risk for self-neglect and other poor outcomes (e.g., institutionalization, morbidity, health services utilization, and mortality). Everyday competence is an individual's ability to solve the problems encountered in everyday life. Few tools exist for nurses and other health and social service providers to quickly screen older adults for everyday competence. Using widely accepted standards for assessing medical decision making, we developed the Making and Executing Decisions for Safe and Independent Living (MEDSAIL) tool to fill this gap. This chapter briefly highlights the literature around assessment of everyday competence; describes our development, validation, and refinement of MEDSAIL; and provides a case study demonstrating how MEDSAIL can be used in practice.

In this chapter, we discuss the assessment of everyday competence for safe and independent living in the community. Impairments in everyday competence can put people at risk for poor outcomes, including self-neglect. Health and social service providers, especially those working in the community, lack simple and effective tools to quickly identify older adults who are at risk of losing their ability to live safely and independently in the community. To address this gap, we have developed a screening tool of everyday competence. MEDSAIL was initially designed for use among community-based health and social service providers, but it is equally useful for nurses and other health care providers based in clinical settings. We describe our development of the tool and present a case study to illustrate how the tool can be used in practice.

BACKGROUND LITERATURE

Overwhelmingly, older adults prefer to live independently in the community for as long as possible (Naik, Schulman-Green, McCorkle, Bradley, & Bogardus, 2005). Because the familiar surroundings of the home and neighborhood provide feelings of comfort, control, and independence, older adults may not seek additional supports even when the environment no longer meets their needs (Golant, 2008). The model of person–environment fit examines the relationship between an individual's everyday competence and the residential environment, seeking an equilibrium that allows the individual to reside in the least restrictive environment possible (Lawton & Nahemow, 1973). *Everyday competence* has been simply defined as an individual's ability to solve problems associated with everyday life (Schaie, Boron, & Willis, 2005) and the ability to perform "a broad array of activities considered essential for independent living" (Diehl, 2008). For this chapter, we will use the term everyday competence, although this concept has been referred to by a number of terms, such as *everyday problem solving, everyday decision making, functional cognition,* and *capacity for safe and independent living.*

The cumulative burden of functional, psychological, and physical declines can adversely affect an older adult's everyday competence, and thus the ability to live safely and independently in the community. Community-dwelling older adults with low levels of everyday competence and absent supports are at risk for poor outcomes, such as frequent hospitalizations and visits to the emergency department, long-term care placement, morbidity, mortality, and myriad forms of abuse (Fulmer, Paveza, Abraham, & Fairchild, 2000; Lachs, Williams, O'Brien, Pillemer, & Charlson, 1998; Pavlik, Hymen, Festa, & Bitondo-Dyer, 2001; Pavlou & Lachs, 2006; Wolinsky, Callahan, Fitzgerald, & Johnson, 1992). Impairment in everyday competence may begin to appear in the early stages of dementia, but can also be part of the normative changes related to aging (Willis, 1996).

A person may make and execute (what other people might judge to be) risky, odd, or foolish decisions every day, but this alone is not sufficient to determine that the person lacks everyday competence. Living in an environment that is not clean or having poor personal hygiene standards may be signs of self-neglect, but may also be how the person has chosen to live his or her entire life. Disentangling lifelong eccentricities and preferences from impaired everyday competence can be daunting for health and social service providers. To further complicate the issue, many older adults with impaired everyday competence retain appropriate communication and social skills, even making claims about capabilities that do not mirror actual performance.

In the absence of neuropsychological diagnoses, providers in health care settings may initially notice frequent emergency room visits; poor social support; and difficulties with personal care, nutrition, and medication management (Dyer, Pickens, & Burnett, 2007). In the health care setting, a clinician may consult another clinical expert to make a determination about capacity. Outside the clinical environment, it is more challenging to identify older adults who are struggling to maintain independence. The first contact with the health or social service systems may occur at the behest of a concerned family member or acquaintance owing to difficulty managing tasks such as bill paying, home care, or transportation (Naik, Kunik, Cassidy, Nair, & Coverdale, 2010). Even when suspicions of impairment arise, health and social service providers do not have many options for conducting an assessment of an older adult's everyday competence (Law, Barnett, Yau, & Gray, 2012).

Evaluations of older adults have relied too heavily on unverified verbal claims in the absence of valid and reliable assessment instruments (Agich, 1993; Collopy, 1988; Lidz, Fischer, & Arnold, 1992; Stang, Molloy, & Harrison, 1998). Health and human service providers often lack the training to conduct such assessments and do not feel comfortable making a referral for a formal comprehensive capacity evaluation until something egregious occurs. This hesitation can result in an older adult remaining in an environment that does not have the necessary supports in place to maintain safety. Therefore, it is critical that health and social service providers have tools to quickly and reliably screen for everyday competence to determine whether a referral for a formal comprehensive capacity evaluation is warranted (Naik, Teal, Pavlik, Dyer, & McCullough, 2008).

Everyday competence for safe and independent living is multidimensional and requires assessment across the domains of function, cognition, and judgment (Appelbaum & Grisso, 1988; Brandt et al., 2009; Dyer, Goodwin, Pickens-Pace, Burnett, & Kelly, 2007; Lai & Karlawish, 2007; Marsis & Willis, 1995; Mosqueda & Dong, 2011; Willis, 1996). Assessment of everyday competence is invaluable for timely interventions or discharge planning to ensure optimal person–environment fit, which would mean the individual functions at his or her full potential in the least restrictive environment possible. Despite the importance of this type of assessment, there are few options for screening everyday competence (Law et al., 2012). Common assessments focus primarily on the cognitive aspects of everyday competence, including short-term memory, spatial orientation, and attention/concentration without consideration of the other domains. If the individual performs well on cognitive tests, function beyond those abilities is typically not addressed. Understanding an older adult's cognitive function is necessary but not sufficient to assess everyday competence. These types of assessments do not adequately reflect how the individual would perform in a real-life situation because they do not allow for the inclusion of wisdom and experiences gained over the life course (Marsis & Willis, 1995). For example, executive functioning abilities, such as the ability to plan, sequence, initiate, understand abstract concepts, and delay gratification, are critical for problem solving and decision making (Lezak, Howieson, & Loring, 2004). Traditionally, conducting comprehensive evaluations of all these domains requires multidisciplinary teams in a medical setting, which can create barriers in terms of access for patients and time investment for health and social service providers (Mosqueda & Dong, 2011).

THE MEDSAIL SCREENING TOOL

To address these challenges in the literature and in practice, we developed the MEDSAIL screening tool. MEDSAIL evaluates an individual's ability to live safely and independently in a community setting through a brief scenario-based assessment of function, cognition, and judgment. The foundation for MEDSAIL is widely cited standards for assessing medical decision-making capacity (Appelbaum & Grisso, 1988; Dyer et al., 2007; Volicer & Ganzini, 2003) and our team's prior research (Mills et al., 2014; Naik et al., 2010; Naik, Burnett, Pickens-Pace, & Dyer, 2008; Naik, Lai, Kunik, & Dyer, 2008; Naik, Pickens, Burnett, Lai, & Dyer, 2006; Naik, Teal, et al., 2008; Skelton, Kunik, Regev, & Naik, 2010). There are five domains derived from the established theoretical frameworks for evaluating capacity to consent used in medical settings: understanding, appreciation, expressing a choice, reasoning, and generating consequences (American Bar Association/American Psychological Association Assessment of Capacity in Older Adults Project Working Group, 2008; Appelbaum & Grisso, 1988; Lai & Karlawish, 2007; Marson, Ingram, Cody, & Harrell, 1995). Table 21.1 briefly describes each of the domains, including the two types of reasoning: problem solving/consequential and comparative.

In the development of MEDSAIL, we examined the clinical and bioethical literature to identify a comprehensive list of standards used to determine whether

TABLE 21.1 MEDSAIL Domains

Domain	Description
Understanding	Ability to comprehend a situation and explain it in their own words
Appreciation	Ability to recognize the impact of a situation on their own lives
Expressing a choice	Ability to communicate choices and/or plans
Reasoning	
Problem solving/consequential	Ability to perform abstract problem solving in a new hypothetical situation
Comparative	Ability to compare advantages and disadvantages of two options
Generate consequences	Ability to generate ideas about how to prevent a situation from occurring or to prepare in case it does occur

MEDSAIL, Making and Executing Decisions for Safe and Independent Living.

an older adult could make and execute decisions regarding health, safety, and independence (Naik, Teal, et al., 2008). We also conducted a series of five focus groups with community-based health and social service providers to understand how to operationalize these standards for use in the field (Naik et al., 2010). Through an iterative process, the focus group participants helped develop and refine a set of scenarios based on these standards and situations older adults face in the community, which became the basis for MEDSAIL (see Box 21.1). Methods that assess everyday competence in situations similar to those encountered in everyday life are considered to be more ecologically valid and provide sufficient indication of how an older adult would actually perform in the real world (Law et al., 2012).

MEDSAIL differs from traditional cognitive screening tools in key ways. Typically, administrators are expected to follow a given script without deviation, and responses are scored with no additional explanation or probing permitted. For instance, in the St. Louis University Mental State Examination, Question 11 asks: "What work did she do?" If a patient misunderstands this and responds with "she was a housewife" rather

---

BOX 21.1 MEDSAIL SCENARIOS

1. The door to your home is locked and you do not have a key.
2. You run out of a medication that you take regularly.
3. You are at home, and suddenly there is a fire in your kitchen.
4. You notice that the cut on your foot is not healing and has become infected.
5. Someone calls you, saying you've won $100,000 and all they need from you is your Social Security number to verify your identity.
6. You are driving to the grocery store and you get a flat tire.
7. Your heating unit/air conditioner breaks down, and it is very cold/hot outside.

MEDSAIL, Making and Executing Decisions for Safe and Independent Living.

than the expected "stockbroker," the administrator can only repeat the question to attempt to elicit the correct response. With the MEDSAIL tool, however, administrators are able to use probing to encourage respondents to elaborate or clarify their answers. In the scenario presented later, Mr. Smith responds to a question about how he would respond if locked out of his home. His response is to wait for his son to come home. The interviewer knows that this is a superficial response, so she probes deeper ("Does your son live with you full time?") to see whether Mr. Smith can identify a more reasoned solution to this problem (see Table 21.2). This approach is supported by research literature on legal capacity determinations, which suggests that probing within narrow criterion standards is necessary to effectively establish capacity (Appelbaum & Grisso, 1988; Lai & Karlawish, 2007; Marson et al., 1995; Moye, Butz, Marson, Wood, & ABA-APA Capacity Assessment of Older Adults Working Group, 2007).

Validity of MEDSAIL

MEDSAIL has been used in a variety of settings, including a geriatric outpatient clinic (Mills et al., 2014) and by clinical psychologists (Wisniewski et al., 2013). We conducted a validation study of an earlier version of the tool (Mills et al., 2014), but have since added the domain of appreciation to the assessment. Validation testing for the finalized instrument is currently underway. In the initial validation study, MED-SAIL was administered by a social worker to 49 community-dwelling older adults referred to a geriatrics clinic for a comprehensive capacity assessment. The clinic's standardized battery of tests included assessments of cognition (St. Louis University Mental State Examination; Tariq, Tumosa, Chibnall, Perry, & Morley, 2006), depression (Patient Health Questionnaire; Kroenke, Spitzer, & Williams, 2001), functioning and judgment (Independent Living Scales; Loeb, 1996), instrumental activities of daily living (Lawton & Brody, 1969), and activities of daily living (Katz, Downs, Cash, & Grotz, 1970). Medical and neuropsychiatric examinations along with clinical judgment were also used to make final determinations of no, partial, or full capacity. MEDSAIL demonstrated internal consistency (five items; $\alpha = .85$), indicating it was assessing the unitary construct of everyday competence. We also found that MEDSAIL scores correlated with the Independent Living Scales ($r = .573, p \leq .001$) and instrumental activities of daily living ($r = .440, p \leq .01$), demonstrating convergent validity. To test construct validity, a Mann–Whitney U test showed significant differences on MEDSAIL scores between individuals classified by the clinic's comprehensive capacity assessment as having "no capacity" versus those with "partial/full capacity" classifications ($U(48) = 60.5, Z = -0.38, p < .0001$). A receiver operating curve analysis that compared MEDSAIL to the comprehensive assessment demonstrated a high level of performance with an area under the curve of .864 (95% CI = 0.84 to 0.99).

Administering MEDSAIL

The person administering MEDSAIL chooses two or three scenarios most related to the respondent's life or current challenges. If the administrator is uncertain about which scenario would be most appropriate for the respondent, the MEDSAIL training guide (Mills, Regev, Naik, & Kunik, 2012) contains an introductory script and list of questions (e.g., "Do you drive a car?" and "Do you use a key to get into your home?") that may be asked to help with scenario selection. Once the appropriate scenarios have been chosen, the administrator simply presents the scenario and guides the

TABLE 21.2 Mr. Smith's MEDSAIL Responses and Scoring for Scenario 1 ("The door to your home is locked and you do not have a key.")

MEDSAIL Domain and Question/ Prompt/Probe	Mr. Smith's Response	MEDSAIL Score
Understanding		
Please tell me in your own words what I just said.	My door is locked and I don't have the key.	*Proceed*
Appreciation		
Would getting locked out of your home be a problem for you? Why or why not?	Of course. I have to be able to get into my house. All of my important things are in there.	2/2
Expressing a Choice		
What would you do if the door to your home was locked and you did not have a key?	I'd wait for my son. He stays with me and I'd just wait for him to come home.	2/2
Probe: Does your son live with you full time?	Well, no, I guess he doesn't. I could still call him on my cell phone, though. He could bring his key to let me in.	
Problem Solving/Consequential Reasoning		
What would you do if calling your son didn't work?	It would work. He would call me back eventually.	0/2
Probe: What if your cell phone was inside?	I've always got my phone with me. So I'd just keep calling until I got him.	
Comparative Reasoning		
So you told me that you would wait for your son or call your son on your cell phone. Explain what is good and bad about each of these options.	Calling my son would be better than waiting for him.	1/2
Probe: Can you think of one bad outcome for each option to compare?	Oh, I don't know.	
Generate Consequences		
What could you do to prevent yourself from getting locked out of your home?	I still don't think this could happen.	1/2
Probe: Just pretend there is a chance it could happen; what could you do to prevent it?	I will keep my door key with me all the time. That's why I won't have this problem.	
Total MEDSAIL Score		6/10

MEDSAIL, Making and Executing Decisions for Safe and Independent Living.

respondent through a set of questions. These questions are based on the five domains derived from established theoretical frameworks (American Bar Association/American Psychological Association Assessment of Capacity in Older Adults Project Working Group, 2008; Appelbaum & Grisso, 1988; Lai & Karlawish, 2007; Marson et al., 1995) for evaluating capacity to consent used in medical settings: understanding, appreciation, expressing a choice, reasoning, and generating consequences.

Scoring MEDSAIL

To assess the first domain of understanding, the respondent is instructed to repeat the scenario in his or her own words. If the respondent is able to do this, the screening continues. If the respondent cannot successfully demonstrate understanding, the screening does not proceed. For the remaining four domains, items are scored in terms of the logic and completeness of the response on a scale of 0 to 2. A score of 0 indicates that the respondent gave no answer or that the response was incomplete or illogical. Responses that are logical but incomplete receive a score of 1. The highest score of 2 is given to responses that are complete and logical. Each scenario can have a maximum score of 10 points, and the final score is an average of the scores from the two scenarios.

Establishing final cut scores is ongoing, but in our initial validation study (Mills et al., 2014) scores less than 5 were found to be indicative of severe impairment in everyday competence. Scores greater than 6 indicate partial to full everyday competence. The MEDSAIL manual provides examples of responses and corresponding scores to help the administrator calibrate scores. It is important to note that MEDSAIL is not a confirmatory diagnostic tool and scores indicating impairment should not be considered as evidence of significant, irreversible loss of competence. Rather, MEDSAIL is a screening tool that may help health and social service providers take preliminary steps to ensure the individual's safety while making a referral for formal evaluation by a clinician with appropriate training and experience in competence testing (Naik et al., 2006).

APPLICATIONS OF MEDSAIL IN HOSPITAL AND LONG-TERM CARE SETTINGS

MEDSAIL has been implemented and tested in a variety of settings with favorable results (Mills et al., 2014). Although an initial validation study was successful, we are currently conducting further studies with the revised version of the instrument among community-dwelling older adults to establish a finalized set of cut scores. With the pressure to reduce the length of stay and caregiving in the community, we are also testing the use of MEDSAIL during care planning for transitions from residential long-term care settings (e.g., nursing homes) and hospitals. Understanding a person's everyday competence at the time of discharge is crucial for determining whether a return to home is possible or whether the older adult may benefit from more intense residential postacute or nursing home care. If returning to home is the most appropriate option, then everyday competence is useful for ensuring that the necessary services and supports are in place to reduce the risk of readmission, emergency department visits, and permanent institutionalization.

In residential long-term care settings, screening for everyday competence can be useful in deciding who may attempt a transition to the community but may have additional utility to staff for long-stay residents. Nursing home staff rarely have easy

---

CASE STUDY 1: MR. SMITH

Mr. Smith is a 76-year-old Black male who was referred to a geriatrics clinic by a local social services provider because of suspected self-neglect. Adult protective services has also been involved in the case. Once at the geriatric clinic, Mr. Smith was interviewed by members of an interdisciplinary team specializing in the assessment of capacity for safe and independent living.

Social History

Mr. Smith exhibited poor hygiene and personal care, including elongated fingernails and an unkempt appearance. He lives alone in an apartment. Mr. Smith was born in rural Texas and is the only survivor of two children born to his parents. He graduated high school and worked in the construction field his whole life up until 3 years ago. Mr. Smith has been divorced since 1969 and has six children. He was accompanied by his adult son Sam at all of his appointments at the clinic. Sam occasionally stays with his father for a few days at a time to help him with his affairs. Mr. Smith has resisted his son moving in full time, claiming that he is doing fine on his own. Although Mr. Smith claims that he only sips gin each day, he consumes three to four bottles per week, which is consistent with his son's accounting of a long history of alcohol abuse. The team found that Mr. Smith had misplaced his Social Security identification card and did not know whether he qualified for Medicaid, Supplemental Security Income, or any other benefits/entitlements. He was not able to report his annual income, but his son believes he receives approximately $400 per month.

Medical History

Mr. Smith was unable to provide many of the details of his medical history and initially denied having any medical problems. His son was able to provide a more detailed history and stated his father had not received medical care for a number of years. Sam mentioned that he had noticed some problems with his father's thinking and memory. He also stated that his father had previously fallen on several occasions. During a review of symptoms, Mr. Smith indicates that he has numbness and tingling in his right foot and hand. He then acknowledges that he has been diagnosed with hypertension. Mr. Smith is able to perform all of his activities of daily living, although he does not cook. He is dependent on his son for all of his instrumental activities of daily living.

MEDSAIL Evaluation

Mr. Smith completed MEDSAIL scenarios. Because he does not drive or do much cooking, the administrator eliminated scenarios related to those topics. The following two scenarios were chosen: "The door to your home is locked and you do not have a key." and "You run out of a medication that you take regularly." For the purpose of illustration, Mr. Smith's responses to the first scenario are presented in Table 21.2, along with the scoring. In general, he was able to provide cursory responses to the questions, but he struggled to evaluate the consequences of his responses and to create a plan for executing decisions. On the first scenario, Mr. Smith received a score of 6, and on the second scenario he received a score of 7. Averaging these scores yields a total of 6.5 on MEDSAIL, indicating moderate impairment of everyday competence.

Outcomes

After the MEDSAIL finding of moderate impairment, Mr. Smith received a comprehensive workup from the full formal capacity assessment team. Mr. Smith was found to have significant cognitive impairment (Montreal Cognitive Assessment score of 14), no signs of depression, and a need for assistance with bathing and dressing. As a result of these assessments, several interventions were put in place to improve Mr. Smith's person–environment fit. Seeing how his father responded to the MEDSAIL scenarios, Sam realized that his father needed more assistance than he had realized. The team helped Sam talk with his father about why he needs to move in with him full time and take full control over his finances and medical decisions. Because Sam was taking on a significant amount

---

CASE STUDY 1: MR. SMITH (*continued*)

of caregiving, he involved two of his sisters to help provide care for their father and give him respite as needed. His children helped Mr. Smith obtain a new Social Security card, apply for Medicaid benefits, and receive home-delivered meals once per day. They also make sure that he obtains regular checkups and attends all of his medical appointments. Because of these interventions, Mr. Smith has been able to remain in his home as safely and independently as possible.

---

access to a psychologist or psychiatrist who can make determinations about capacity. Nursing home staff are often faced with unexpected situations in which residents make decisions that are in conflict with what the staff think are best. For example, a resident with diabetes decides to forgo the meal offered in the facility dining room and instead eats a box of cookies for dinner. Waiting a week, a month, or longer for a formal capacity assessment may put that resident's life at risk. Thus, one future direction for MEDSAIL is developing scenarios relevant to residential long-term care that may be used by front-line nursing home staff when such situations arise.

CONCLUSION

In the United States, the cultural value of individualism is one that is maintained throughout the life span. Personal and anecdotal stories of older adults in dire situations, struggling to maintain their independence are far too common. Even when it is clear that a residential environment is no longer in balance with older adults' needs and abilities, they frequently do not seek additional supports and may even refuse interventions when offered. Health and social service providers are faced with the challenging task of determining whether a person has made similar types of decisions throughout his or her life or whether impairment in everyday competence is likely. MEDSAIL is an effective tool that health and social service providers can use to quickly screen for everyday competence and then make referrals for comprehensive testing and service planning as needed. By identifying older adults with impaired everyday competence, efforts can be made to rebalance person–environment fit, reducing the risk for poor outcomes, such as self-neglect, and improving the likelihood of safely aging in place.

IMPLICATIONS FOR RESEARCH AND PRACTICE

- Impaired everyday competence for safe and independent living puts older adults at risk for poor outcomes, including self-neglect.
- There are few tools to quickly and effectively screen for everyday competence, thus MEDSAIL was designed to fill this gap.
- MEDSAIL can be used, with minimal training, by a large variety of health and social service providers, such as physicians, social workers, community health workers, and occupational and physical therapists.
- MEDSAIL is not a confirmatory diagnostic tool. Persons with lower MEDSAIL scores should be referred for formal comprehensive capacity testing.
- Additional research is needed to further validate the final version of MEDSAIL in a variety of study populations and settings.

REFERENCES

Agich, G. J. (1993). *Autonomy and long-term care*. New York, NY: Oxford University Press.

American Bar Association/American Psychological Association Assessment of Capacity in Older Adults Project Working Group. (2008). *Assessment of older adults with diminished capacity: A handbook for psychologists*. Washington, DC: Author. Retrieved from http://www.apa.org/pi/aging/capacity_psychologist_handbook.pdf

Appelbaum, P., & Grisso, T. (1988). Assessing patients' capacities to consent to treatment. *New England Journal of Medicine, 319*, 1635–1638.

Brandt, J., Aretouli, E., Neijstrom, E., Samek, J., Manning, K., Albert, M. S., & Bandeen-Roche, K. (2009). Selectivity of executive function deficits in mild cognitive impairment. *Neuropsychology, 23*(5), 607–618.

Collopy, B. J. (1988). Autonomy in long term care: Some crucial distinctions. *Gerontologist, 28*(Suppl. 3), 10–17.

Diehl, M. (2008). Everyday competence in later life: Current status and future directions. *The Gerontologist, 38*, 422–433.

Dyer, C., Goodwin, J. S., Pickens-Pace, S., Burnett, J., & Kelly, P. (2007). Self-neglect among the elderly: A model based on more than 500 patients seen by a geriatric medicine team. *American Journal of Public Health, 97*, 1671–1676.

Dyer, C., Pickens, S., & Burnett, J. (2007). Vulnerable elders: When it is no longer safe to live alone. *Journal of the American Medical Association, 298*, 1448–1450.

Fulmer, T., Paveza, G., Abraham, I., & Fairchild, S. (2000). Elder neglect assessment in the emergency department. *Journal of Emergency Nursing, 26*(5), 436–443.

Golant, S. (2008). Irrational exuberance for the aging in place of vulnerable low-income older homeowners. *Journal of Aging & Social Policy, 20*, 379–397.

Katz, S., Downs, T. D., Cash, H. R., & Grotz, R. C. (1970). Progress in development of the Index of ADL. *The Gerontologist, 10*, 20–30.

Kroenke, K., Spitzer, R. L., & Williams, J. B. (2001). Validity of a brief depression severity measure. *Journal of General Internal Medicine, 16*, 606–613.

Lachs, M. S., Williams, C. S., O'Brien, S., Pillemer, K. A., & Charlson, M. E. (1998). The mortality of elder mistreatment. *Journal of the American Medical Association, 280*(5), 428–432.

Lai, J., & Karlawish, J. (2007). Assessing the capacity to make everyday decisions: A guide for clinicians and an agenda for future research. *American Journal of Geriatric Psychiatry, 15*, 101–111.

Law, L. L., Barnett, F., Yau, M. K., & Gray, M. A. (2012). Measures of everyday competence in older adults with cognitive impairment: A systematic review. *Age and Ageing, 41*(1), 9–16.

Lawton, M. P., & Brody, E. M. (1969). Assessment of older people: Self-maintaining and instrumental activities of daily living. *The Gerontologist, 9*, 179–186.

Lawton, M. P., & Nahemow, L. E. (1973). Ecology and the aging process. In C. Eisdorfer & M. P. Lawton (Eds.), *The psychology of adult development and aging* (pp. 619–674). Washington, DC: American Psychological Association.

Lezak, M. D., Howieson, D. B., & Loring, D. W. (2004). *Neuropsychological assessment* (4th ed.). New York, NY: Oxford University Press.

Lidz, C. W., Fischer, L., & Arnold, R. M. (1992). *The erosion of autonomy in long-term care*. New York, NY: Oxford University Press.

Loeb, P. A. (1996). *Independent Living Scales (ILS) manual*. San Antonio, TX: Psychological Corporation.

Marsis, M., & Willis, S. L. (1995). Dimensionality of everyday problem solving in older adults. *Psychology and Aging, 10*, 269–283.

Marson, D., Ingram, K., Cody, H., & Harrell, L. (1995). Assessing the competency of patients with Alzheimer's disease under different legal standards: A prototype instrument. *Archives of Neurology, 52*, 949–954.

Mills, W. L., Regev, T., Kunik, M., Wilson, N., Moye, J., McCullough, L. B., & Naik, A. N. (2014). Making and Executing Decisions for Safe and Independent Living (MEDSAIL): Development and validation of a brief screening tool. *American Journal of Geriatric Psychiatry, 22*, 285–293.

Mills, W. L., Regev, T., Naik, A. D., & Kunik, M. E. (2012). Comprehensive assessment of capacity to live safely and independently in the community. *MedEdPORTAL, 8*, 9263. doi:10.15766/mep_2374-8265.9263

Mosqueda, L., & Dong, X. (2011). Elder abuse and self-neglect: "I don't care anything about going to the doctor, to be honest..." *Journal of the American Medical Association, 306*, 532–540.

Moye, J., Butz, S., Marson, D., Wood, E., & ABA-APA Capacity Assessment of Older Adults Working Group. (2007). A conceptual model and assessment template for capacity evaluation in adult guardianship. *The Gerontologist, 47*, 591–603.

Naik, A. D., Burnett, J., Pickens-Pace, S., & Dyer, C. (2008). Impairment in instrumental activities of daily living and the geriatric syndrome of self-neglect. *The Gerontologist, 48*, 388–393.

Naik, A. D., Kunik, M., Cassidy, K., Nair, J., & Coverdale, J. (2010). Assessing safe and independent living in vulnerable older adults: Perspective of professionals who conduct home assessments. *Journal of the American Board Family Medicine, 23*, 614–621.

Naik, A. D., Lai, J., Kunik, M., & Dyer, C. (2008). Assessing capacity in suspected cases of self-neglect. *Geriatrics, 63*, 24–31.

Naik, A. D., Pickens, S., Burnett, J., Lai, J., & Dyer, C. (2006). Assessing capacity in the setting of self-neglect: Development of a novel screening tool for decision-making capacity. *Journal of Elder Abuse & Neglect, 18*, 79–91.

Naik, A. D., Schulman-Green, D., McCorkle, R., Bradley, E. H., & Bogardus, S. T. (2005). Will older persons use a shared decision making instrument? *Journal of General Internal Medicine, 20*(7), 640–643.

Naik, A. D., Teal, C., Pavlik, V., Dyer, C. B., & McCullough, L. B. (2008). Conceptual challenges and pratical approaches to screening capacity for self-care and protection in vulnerable older adults. *Journal of the American Geriatrics Society, 56*, S266–S270.

Pavlik, V. N., Hyman, D. J., Festa, N. A., & Bitondo-Dyer, C. (2001). Quantifying the problem of abuse and neglect in adults—Analysis of a statewide database. *Journal of the American Geriatrics Society, 49*(1), 45–48.

Pavlou, M. P., & Lachs, M. S. (2006). Could self-neglect in older adults be a geriatric syndrome? *Journal of the American Geriatrics Society, 54*(5), 831–842.

Schaie, K. W., Boron, J. B., & Willis, S. L. (2005). Intellectual compence. In P. Coleman (Ed.), *Cambridge handbook of adult development and aging*. Cambridge, UK: Cambridge University Press.

Skelton, F., Kunik, M., Regev, T., & Naik, A. (2010). Determining if an older adult can make and execute decisions to live safely at home: A capacity assessment and intervention model. *Archives of Gerontology and Geriatrics, 50*, 300–305.

Stang, D. G., Molloy, D. W., & Harrison, C. (1998). Capacity to choose place of residence: Autonomy vs. beneficence? *Journal of Palliative Care, 14*(1), 25–29.

Tariq, S. H., Tumosa, N., Chibnall, J. T., Perry, M. H., & Morley, J. E. (2006). Comparison of the Saint Louis University mental status examination and the mini-mental state examination for detecting dementia and mild neurocognitive disorder: A pilot study. *American Journal of Geriatric Psychiatry, 14*, 900–910.

Volicer, L., & Ganzini, L. (2003). Health professionals' views on standards for decision-making capacity regarding refusal of medical treatment in mild Alzheimer's disease. *Journal of the American Geriatrics Society, 51*, 1270–1274.

Willis, S. L. (1996). Everyday cognitive competence in elderly persons: Conceptual issues and empirical findings. *The Gerontologist, 36*(5), 595–601.

Wisniewski, K. M., Eichorst, M. K., Allen, R. S., Halli, A., Mills, W. L., & Naik, A. D. (2013). Decision making capacity and social support among community-dwellin golder adults. *The Gerontologist, 53*, 62.

Wolinsky, F. D., Callahan, C. M., Fitzgerald, J. F., & Johnson, R. J. (1992). The risk of nursing home placement and subsequent death among older adults. *Journal of Gerontology, Social Sciences, 47*, S173–S182.

CHAPTER 22

SELF-NEGLECT: DEVELOPMENT AND EVALUATION OF A SELF-NEGLECT (SN-37) MEASUREMENT INSTRUMENT

Mary Rose Day and Geraldine McCarthy[1]

Self-neglect is a global phenomenon, largely hidden, poorly defined, and a serious public health issue. It can be intentional or unintentional and the difference depends on the individual's capacity. Creating a safe living environment for self-neglecting adults can present complex ethical challenges. The purpose of this research was to develop and evaluate the psychometric properties of an instrument to measure professionals' perceptions of self-neglect. A descriptive cross-sectional design was used in this two-stage study. Stage 1 involved the generation of an item pool (90 items), face and content validity; and pilot testing of the instrument. In stage 2, the questionnaire was posted to a national sample of community health and social care professionals (n = 566) across Ireland, with a 60% response (n = 339). Exploratory factor analysis (EFA) was conducted using scale development guidelines to identify scales and subscales of the instrument. Construct validity was established using EFA. The result was a 37-item self-neglect instrument, composed of five factors: environment; social networks; emotional and behavioral liability; health avoidance; and self-determinism, which explained 55.6% of the total variance. Factor loadings were ≥0.40 for all items on each of the five subscales. Cronbach's alpha (α) for four subscales ranged from 0.83 to 0.89 and one subscale was 0.69. The SN-37 can be used not only to measure self-neglect, but also to develop interventions in practice. Further testing of the SN-37 in primary care settings with diverse populations is recommended.

Self-neglect is frequently described as an older person's inability or unwillingness to provide the goods or services required to meet basic needs (Day, 2010). It can be intentional (active neglect) or unintentional (passive neglect; Day, 2010). It encompasses a constellation of behaviors, cumulative self-care deficits (Adams & Johnson, 1998; Braye, Orr, & Preston-Shoot, 2014; Reyes-Ortiz, 2001), and environmental neglect (Iris, Ridings, & Conrad, 2010). The term *domestic squalor* is unique to the Australian context and is applied to households that are extremely cluttered and filthy (Snowdon, Halliday, & Banerjee, 2012). There homes have an accumulation of items, personal objects, waste, excrement, and decomposing food; as a result can the environment jeopardize the health and well-being of the occupant(s)

(Government of South Australia, 2013; Snowdon et al., 2012). Squalor is considered an environmental dimension of self-neglect (Day & McCarthy, 2015). Both domestic squalor and self-neglect are interrelated and conceptualized as the same thing by some researchers (Halliday & Snowdon, 2009; Snowdon et al., 2012). Self-neglect can occur across the life span in both younger and older people. In addition, self-neglect is largely hidden and often co-exists with elder abuse (Bartley, Knight, O'Neill, & O'Brien, 2011; Gunstone, 2003; Health Service Executive, 2013; May-Chahal & Antrobus, 2012).

Definitional issues have created multiple challenges and contributed significantly to a wide disparity in reporting prevalence of self-neglect (Jogerst et al., 2003). Older people's self-care is a multifaceted issue. In the United States, self-neglect is included in the definition of elder abuse in many states (Teaster et al., 2006). However, Australia, England, and Ireland do not include self-neglect as elder abuse (Braye, Orr, & Preston-Shoot, 2013; Department of Health, 2000, 2009; Health Service Executive, 2012; Working Group on Elder Abuse, 2002). The current available data on self-neglect is limited. In the United States it is reported to have a 9% prevalence rate (Dong, Simon, Mosqueda, & Evans, 2012) whereas Korea reported a prevalence of 4.1% (Lee & Kim, 2014). Data from primary care general practitioner caseloads in Scotland suggest that prevalence rates vary from 166 to 211 per 100,000 persons (Lauder & Roxburgh, 2012). This coincides with data from a retrospective review of Community Profile and Health Need Assessments of public health nurses in Ireland, which suggests a prevalence rate for self-neglect of 142 per 100,000 population (Day, Mulcahy, & Leahy-Warren, 2016). Self-neglect cases account for 20% of the referrals received by specialist senior caseworkers who work specifically with elder abuse services (Health Service Executive, 2014).

Available evidence suggests that self-neglect is associated with multiple medical comorbidities: significantly greater mortality (Dong et al., 2009), hospitalization (Dong & Simon, 2015; Dong, Simon, & Evans, 2012a; Dong, Simon, Mosqueda, et al., 2012), hospice use (Dong & Simon, 2013), nursing home placement (Lachs, Williams, O'Brien, & Pillemer, 2002), elder abuse (Dong, Simon, & Evans, 2013), and risk for homelessness (Snowdon, 2011). Self-neglect was associated with reduced physical function, depression, executive dysfunction, and drug and alcohol abuse (Dong, Simon, Fulmer, et al., 2010; Dong, Simon, Beck, & Evans, 2010; Dyer, Pickens, & Burnett, 2007; Gibbons, 2009; Pickens et al., 2013).

Aging populations and medical advances will result in more people living longer in the community with complex comorbidities. Living alone, isolation, poor social networks, helplessness, and economic decline all have the potential to impact on self-care and create vulnerabilities in relation to self-neglect, self-protection, and living independently and safely in the community (Burnett et al., 2006; Lee & Kim, 2014; Spensley, 2008; World Health Organization & National Institute on Aging, 2011). Research suggests a link between social isolation (Spensley, 2008), lack of access to health services (Choi, Kim, & Asseff, 2009), poor coping (Gibbons, 2009), medical neglect (Burnett et al., 2014), noncompliance with medication (Turner, Hochschild, Burnett, Zulfiqar, & Dyer, 2012), risk for harm (Tierney et al., 2004), homelessness (Snowdon, 2011), and self-neglect. Not all self-neglecting adults demonstrate definite risk factors. Cultural issues and a person's life history can influence intention to self-neglect (Band-Winterstein, Doron, & Naim, 2012; Day, Leahy-Warren, & McCarthy, 2013). All of the these present complex triggers and vulnerabilities, which may lead to self-neglect and an array of interrelated social, community, and professional issues. Self-neglect cases can present along a continuum of severity and are enormously complex and ethically challenging.

Based on the literature, it is clear that self-neglect is a complex multidimensional concept that lacks clarity and is conceptualized in many different ways by researchers, professionals, and communities (Bohl, 2010; Day, McCarthy, & Leahy-Warren, 2012; Gunstone, 2003; Lauder, Scott, & Whyte, 2001; May-Chahal & Antrobus, 2012; McDermott, 2010). Mental health and community nurses play a key role in the identification of self-neglecting adults. Safety and support of vulnerable adults at risk for self-neglect can present complex ethical challenges (Day, Leahy-Warren, & McCarthy, 2016). Safeguarding and protective measures, proportionate to assessed risk, must be initiated by professionals. However, there is a dearth of self-neglect instruments, which has led to subjectivity in the measurement of self-neglect (Day et al., 2012; Dyer et al., 2006). Previously, three instruments were used to measure self-neglect: Self-Neglect Severity Scale (SSS; Kelly, Dyer, Pavlik, Doody, & Jogerst, 2008) and two squalor instruments: Living Conditions Rating Scale (LCRS; Samios, 1996) and the Environmental Cleanliness and Clutter Scale (ECCS; Halliday & Snowdon, 2009; Snowdon, Halliday, & Hunt, 2013).

The 28-item SSS was developed by the Consortium for Research in Elder Self Neglect at Baylor College of Medicine (Kelly et al., 2008). The format encompasses pictorial and risk evaluation to assess three domains: hygiene, functioning, and environment (Dyer et al. 2006; Kelly et al., 2008). Field testing of SSS with 23 community-dwelling adults has discriminated between older adults reported as self-neglecting and adults with no history of self-neglect. Statistical evidence has shown that sensitivity and specificity of the SSS were not within the standard range of acceptability and the unidimensionality of the scale was unclear (Kelly et al., 2008). No further research on the use of this scale has been reported.

Two other scales have relevance as they measure environmental dimensions of self-neglect and squalor. The 20-items LCRS was first presented in an unpublished master's thesis (Samios, 1996). Subsequently, the LCRS was used in five studies to measure and assess the home living environments of 83 older adults (Samios, 1996), 87 younger and older adults (Snowdon, 1987), 81 adults living in local authority housing (Halliday & Snowdon, 2009), 173 adults living in squalor (Snowdon & Halliday, 2011), and 108 self-neglecting adults (Leibbrandt, 2007) living in low-income housing. Leibbrandt (2007) reported a Cronbach's α reliability of .89 but few recommendations were made on the utility and reliability of LCRS.

Halliday and Snowdon (2009) developed the 10-item ECCS to measure and observe the severity of domestic squalor and hoarding. Homes ($n = 55$) were rated by specialists ($n = 2$) in geriatric psychiatry using both the ECCS and the LCRS (Samios, 1996). Cronbach's α for LCRS was .89 and Cronbach's α for ECCS was .87. Exploratory factor analysis (EFA) was conducted on ECCS scores collected by the squalor project team on younger and older people ($n = 186$) with the mean age of 61.5 years. EFA of the ECCS reported a two-factor structure (squalor and accumulation of items; Snowdon et al., 2013).

In summary, the SSS, LCRS, and ECCS focus on self-neglect severity, squalor, and hoarding. These tools fail to capture the contextual and complex physical–psychosocial and environmental risk factors that coexist with self-neglecting cases. Community nurses have a critical role in home visiting, early identification, support, and management of adults at risk for self-neglect. One of the primary reasons why self-neglect is underreported is the lack of a comprehensive, psychometrically evaluated instrument that can assist the identification of self-neglect. An objective self-neglect measurement instrument can guide the assessment and interventions in relation to self-neglect (Day, 2014).

The literature synthesis was underpinned by the elder self-neglect (ESN) conceptual framework that includes two key dimensions and seven subcategories: physical/psychosocial (physical health risks, mental health, personal endangerment, and social networks) and environmental (physical living conditions, personal living conditions, and financial issues; Iris et al., 2010). The current study draws on the original work of Iris et al. (2010) in its underpinnings; it also draws on qualitative research (Day et al., 2012, 2013) and an extensive literature review for the development of items. The instrument measure is supported by the ESN conceptual framework that challenges characterization of self-neglect as a medical syndrome (Day, 2014; Iris et al., 2010). The purpose of this research is to develop and evaluate the psychometric properties of an instrument to measure professional perceptions of self-neglect. Ethical approval was obtained from the Clinical Research Ethics Committee of the University Teaching Hospitals.

DESIGN AND METHODS

A quantitative, descriptive cross-sectional design was used in this two-stage study. Stage 1 involved the item generation, face and content validity, and review and field testing of instruments. Stage 2 involved psychometric evaluation of the newly developed instrument. The methods used to validate the self-neglect instrument include content validity and face validity (stage 1), construct validity, exploratory factor analysis (EFA; stage 2), and reliability tests: internal consistency (Cronbach's α; stage 2).

An extensive item pool was generated from three sources: literature review; items from ESN conceptual framework (Iris et al., 2010), previous qualitative research (Day et al., 2012, 2013), and the appraisal of existing instruments (Day, 2014). The 90 items generated were organized under the dimensions and the categories of the ESN conceptual framework (Iris et al., 2010).

In stage 1, content validity was established by a panel of eight purposely selected experts who came from a variety of professional backgrounds: public health nurses (PHNs), social workers (SWs), senior caseworkers (SCWs), safeguarding and protection workers, doctors, gerontologists, and rehabilitation therapists, as well as expertise related to clinical practice, research, leadership and management, academic education, and instrument development. The validity of items was estimated using the Content Validity Index (CVI; Polit & Beck, 2006). Face validity is based on assessment of experts of how clearly items on the scale reflected the concept being measured (Devon et al., 2007; Polit & Beck, 2010).

The decision was made to rule out any items that had not been classified by at least six of the eight experts, I-CVI ≥.75 based on literature from Polit, Beck, and Owen (2007) and Lynn (1986), who identified that a minimum score of .75 for I-CVI is good when there are eight experts.

Corrected CVI for each subscale (S-CVI) ranged from .75 to 1.00 and overall CVI was .875 after removing 28 items. The CVI of the 28 items deleted ranged from .125 to .625; these deleted items were related to six dimensions: physical health risks, mental health, personal endangerment, social networks, personal living conditions, and financial issues. Examples of items deleted included: individual chooses to use acupuncture or exercise rather than see a doctor, individual's income is less than $800, and individual is from a lower social class group. The final revised self-neglect instrument contained 62 items (SN-62) for field testing.

FIELD TESTING

Field testing was conducted with a convenience sample of nine community health and social care professionals (PHNs [$n = 5$], SWs [$n = 3$], community nurses [$n = 1$]) using a postal survey. These individuals who received the survey were identified by the directors and managers of public health nursing and SW services in the Health Service Executive (HSE) South. The questionnaire packet included socio demographic data and a 62-item self-neglect instrument (SN-62). Participants were asked to indicate the relevance of each item to self-neglect. Each of the 62 items was rated on a 5-point Likert scale ranging from 1 (unimportant) to 5 (very important). Subscales showed good Cronbach's α (physical health risks: .88; mental health: .87; personal endangerment: .91; social networks: .95; physical living conditions: .86; personal living conditions: .84, and financial issues: .84) and mean interitem correlations were between .38 and .73. No changes were made as a result.

PARTICIPANTS AND DATA COLLECTION

A letter explaining purpose, risks, and benefits of the study and the voluntary nature of participation was sent via email to directors and managers (PHNs), community registered general nurses (CRGNs), community mental health nurses (CMHNs) SCWs, and SWs identified by the researcher across four HSE regions nationally (HSE South, HSE West, Dublin Mid Leinster, and Dublin North East). This included a request to access the sample and support to facilitate the distribution of a letter of invitation and postal survey to front-line staff. A total of 566 questionnaires were distributed to a convenience sample of health and social care professionals (PHNs [$n = 340$], CRGNs [$n = 78$], CMHNs [$n = 90$], SCWs [$n = 2$]) and SWs [$n = 30$]) a subset of the population of community professionals across four regions. The sample size was larger than the previous studies on the development of self-neglect measurement instruments. Participation was voluntary and confidentiality was maintained by not seeking personal details or names. Returning the questionnaire implied consent.

DATA ANALYSIS

Each questionnaire response was coded and statistical analyses were performed using the Statistical Package for Social Science (SPSS). Descriptive statistics were used to analyze characteristics of the sample and responses to self-neglect (see Table 22.1). A total of 336 (out of a possible 566) participants completed the questionnaire, giving a response rate of 60%. Table 22.1 summarizes the socio-demographic information.

TABLE 22.1 Sample Characteristics

	n (%)
Gender (n = 336)	
Male	25 (7.4)
Female	311 (92.6)
Age group (n = 336)	
25–34 years	44 (13.1)
35–49 years	183 (54.5)
50–64 years	109 (32.4)
Professional group (n = 339)	
Public health nurse	215 (63.4)
Community registered general nurse	46 (13.6)
Senior case worker	18 (5.3)
Social worker	16 (4.7)
Community mental health nurse	44 (13.0)
Highest level of education completed (n = 324)	
Diploma	46 (14.2)
Bachelor Degree	30 (9.3)
Postgraduate Diploma	188 (58.0)
Master's	60 (18.5)
HSE region (n = 340)	
HSE South	168 (49.4)
HSE West	47 (13.8)
HSE Dublin Mid Leinster	86 (25.3)
HSE Dublin North East	39 (11.5)
Years experience in current position/post (n = 334)	
1–5 years	73 (21.9)
5–15 years	209 (62.6)
15+ years	52 (15.6)
Number of self-neglect cases you had contact within last 12 months (n = 331)	
0	38 (11.5)
1–2	104 (31.4)
3–5	112 (33.8)

(continued)

TABLE 22.1 Sample Characteristics (continued)

	n (%)
5–15	60 (18.1)
16–25	7 (2.1)
25+	10 (3.0)

HSE, Health Service Executive.

The decisions in relation to the removal of items(s) were based on the following factors: items with high ceiling–floor effects (i.e., >70%; Polit & Hungler 1999); a large amount of missing responses; interitem correlations >0.7; corrected item-total correction of at least 0.2 (Clarke & Watson 1995), and less than three items loading on a factor and loading >0.3 (Kline, 1994; Polit & Hungler, 1999).

EXPLORATORY FACTOR ANALYSIS

EFA is a statistical method used when there are multiple items to determine construct validity during instrument development. EFA was used to determine the underlying structure and dimensions of self-neglect and sequential steps were guided by Williams, Brown, and Onsman's (2012) five-step-analysis protocol. These included suitability of data for factor analysis, factors to be extracted, criteria to use in factor extraction, selection of rotational method, and interpretation. A total of 339 participants completed the SN-51 measure; 34 participants (10.6%) had missing data so were excluded from data analysis.

Thus, 305 respondents were included in this EFA for the instrument. The Kaiser–Meyer–Olkin (Kaiser, 1974) measure of sampling adequacy was .92, which would be considered good by Field (2005), suggesting that factor analysis will yield distinct and reliable factors. The Bartlett's test of sphericity (1275, degree frequency [Df] 0.001) provided support for the factorability of the correlation matrix.

Multiple heuristics were used to determine factor extraction, including Kaiser's criteria (eigenvalue N 1 rule; Kaiser, 1960), Cattell's Scree Test (Cattell, 1966), parallel analysis (PA), and cumulative percentage of variance extracted (Horn, 1965). In this study, the elbow of the scree plot (Figure 22.1) indicated that one to five factors would be extracted.

When Kaiser's criterion (eigenvalue >1) was applied to the draft SN-51, 11 factors had eigenvalues ≥1.00 in the first run of the principal component analysis (PCA), accounting for 65% of the variance (see Table 22.2). Eigenvalues are considered to be one of the most unreliable sources in determining factors. PA is often recommended as the method to assess the true number of factors. Based on PA, five factors were extracted (Table 22.3). Oblique (promax) rotation was undertaken as it was determined to be the best solution because all correlations between the factors were >.15 (Table 22.4). The result was a 37-item self-neglect instrument, composed of five factors labeled by experts as *environment, social networks, emotional and behavioral liability, health avoidance,* and *self-determinism* (Table 22.5; Figure 22.2), which explained 55.6% of the total variance. The five-factor solution with accompanying items is presented in Table 22.5.

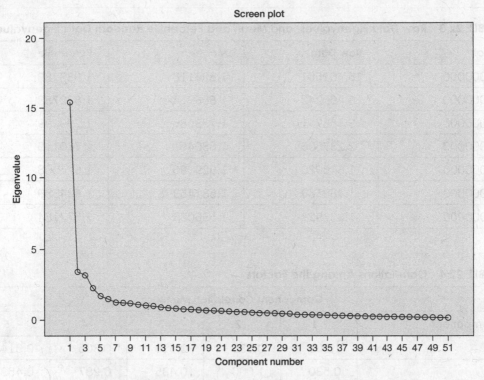

Figure 22.1 Scree plot of 51-item exploratory factor analysis.

TABLE 22.2	Total Variance Explained					
Component	Initial Eigenvalues			Extraction Sums of Squared Loadings		
	Total	Percentage of Variance	Cumulative Percentage	Total	Percentage of Variance	Cumulative Percentage
1	15.408	30.211	30.211	15.408	30.211	30.211
2	3.409	6.685	36.896	3.409	6.685	36.896
3	3.157	6.190	43.085	3.157	6.190	43.085
4	2.238	4.387	47.473	2.238	4.387	47.473
5	1.677	3.288	50.761	1.677	3.288	50.761
6	1.489	2.920	53.681	1.489	2.920	53.681
7	1.238	2.427	56.108	1.238	2.427	56.108
8	1.203	2.358	58.466	1.203	2.358	58.466
9	1.185	2.323	60.790	1.185	2.323	60.790
10	1.081	2.120	62.910	1.081	2.120	62.910
11	1.018	1.996	64.907	1.018	1.996	64.907
12	0.966	1.894	66.800			
51	0.141	0.277	100.000			

Note: Extraction method: Principal component analysis.

TABLE 22.3 Raw Data Eigenvalues, and Mean and Percentile Random Data Eigenvalues

Root	Raw Data	Means	Percentile
1.000000	15.407501	1.896118	1.983789
2.000000	3.409242	1.806964	1.872783
3.000000	3.156741	1.738586	1.799299
4.000000	2.237506	1.680451	1.730119
5.000000	1.676920	1.629396	1.676908
6.000000	1.489160	1.581459	1.624389
7.000000	1.237927	1.536088	1.577184

TABLE 22.4 Correlations Among the Factors

Component Correlation Matrix					
Component	1	2	3	4	5
1	1.000	0.530	0.516	0.305	0.314
2	0.530	1.000	0.435	0.287	0.452
3	0.516	0.435	1.000	0.318	0.206
4	0.305	0.287	0.318	1.000	0.265
5	0.314	0.452	0.206	0.265	1.000

Note: Extraction method: Principal-component analysis; Rotation method: Promax with Kaiser normalization.

TABLE 22.5 Results of the Final Five-Factor Solution of the SN-37 According to the Principal Component Analysis With Promax Rotation

Factors 1: Environment (12 items)

Individual has no way to obtain and/or prepare meals.	0.771
Individual lives in a house/apartment that does not have all the equipment/facilities to fit the individual's physical needs (i.e., wheelchair, bars in the bathroom or hallway or ramps, poor lighting, fuel poverty).	0.705
Individual has an accumulation of items that presents a safety hazard.	0.696
Individual lives in a house/apartment that is very cold.	0.695
Individual lives in a house/apartment that is unsafe (i.e., fire hazards, reduced)	0.694
Individual is hoarding animals.	0.693
Individual is eating spoiled food.	0.682
Individual has no access to bathing facilities.	0.635
Individual lacks funds/money to pay bills (i.e., utilities, structural, household repairs etc.).	0.629
Individual lives in a house/apartment where there is evidence of vermin.	0.615
Individual does not pay household bills despite having adequate income to pay them.	0.489
Individual lives in a house/apartment where appliances are not working (sinks, refrigerator, lighting, phone etc.).	0.436

(continued)

TABLE 22.5   Results of the Final Five-Factor Solution of the SN-37 According to the Principal Component Analysis With Promax Rotation (*continued*)

Factor 2: Social networks (7 items)

Individual is socially disconnected/or has limited social relations with neighbors.	0.867
Individual has not talked to someone in the past week.	0.838
Individual is living alone.	0.784
Individual lacks social contact (family, friends, neighbours) to turn to in an emergency.	0.777
Individual avoids friends, family, religious or social events.	0.718
Individual's contact with family members, friends, and neighbors is less frequent than necessary to attend to his or her needs.	0.672
Individual does not have anyone to provide him/her with the assistance he or she needs.	0.603

Factor 3: Emotional and behavioral liability (8 items)

Individual displays fear in daily situations.	0.785
Individual expresses fear of certain people who are close to him or her.	0.764
Individual demonstrates aggressive, hostile behavior.	0.717
Individual is placing trust in people who have proven not to be trustworthy.	0.717
Individual's behaviors are likely to cause physical harm to others.	0.659
Individual has not left his or her house/apartment for more than 1 month.	0.496
Individual appears sad (i.e., unhappy, gloomy, mournful).	0.468
Individual is overusing drugs/alcohol.	0.443

Factor 4: Health avoidance (6 items)

Individual has unattended foot problems.	0.786
Individual ignores signs and symptoms of disease.	0.757
Individual lacks follow-through with preventive or diagnostic testing related to health conditions.	0.724
Individual does not comply with the prescribed medical treatment (under/over medication, or the consumption of medication that was not prescribed) despite a clear understanding of the rationale for regiment recommendations).	0.722
Individual hoards medication.	0.672
Individual presents with recent unplanned weight loss.	0.482

Factor 5: Self-determinism (4 items)

Individual is not cooperative or willing to accept assistance.	0.706
Individual has displayed self-neglectful behavior at other times in his or her life.	0.667
Individual is reluctant to receive help for daily care.	0.625
Individual neglects personal hygiene (dirty clothing, bad odour, disheveled appearance).	0.606

DISCUSSION

Self-neglect is a complex multifaceted issue that is defined in many different ways and perceptions of self-neglect are often subjective. The purpose of this chapter is to describe the two-stage processes used in developing the self-neglect instrument SN-37 and to report on psychometric testing.

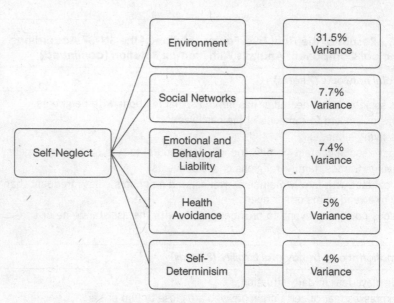

Figure 22.2 Self-neglect factors: contribution to total variance.

The findings affirm that the items reflect the important risks and vulnerabilities factors involved in self-neglect. EFA revealed a five-factor, 37-item instrument, which accounted for 56.5% of total explained variance. Validity and reliability of the study were ensured by EFA. Cronbach's α for four subscales ranged from .83 to .89 and subscale 5 was .69.

As presented in Table 22.5, the 12 items loading on Factor 1: Environment are related to deficiencies, hazards, and neglect within home accommodation that can lead to health and safety concerns, lack of funds and behaviors of person such as hoarding, eating spoiled food, and failure to pay bills. The items demonstrated the importance of assessment of the home environment. High prevalence of unsanitary home conditions, inadequate utilities, and house needing repair were associated with self-neglect (Dong, Simon, & Evans, 2012b); and risk for harm has been attributed to nutritional status and not eating or drinking (McDermott, 2010; Tierney, Snow, Charles, Moineddin, & Kiss, 2007).

Factor 2: Living alone, existence of social networks/level of social contacts to provide and meet changing needs. Social networks items ($n = 7$) demonstrated the importance of social networks and ties and social support as self-care needs change. Lower levels of social engagement and support are associated with significantly greater self-neglect (Dong, Simon, Fulmer, et al., 2010).

Factor 3: Mental health and well-being, risky hostile behaviors, abusing alcohol/drugs, and behaviors that put personal safety of self and others at risk. Mental and behavioral liability items ($n = 8$; Table 22.5) demonstrate that mental health issues, depression, alcohol and drug abuse, and hostility and fear can push misguided trust and dangerous safety concerns for self and others. Greater risk for reporting of self-neglect is associated with impaired decision making (Naik, Pickens, Burnett, Lai, & Dyer, 2006), frontal lobe dysfunction, and Alzheimer's disease (Dong, Simon, Beck, et al., 2010; Gregory, Halliday, Hodges, & Snowdon, 2011).

Factor 4: Avoidance of health care needs. Health avoidance items ($n = 6$; Table 22.5) demonstrate cumulative behavioral characteristics that can potentially increase risk for self-neglect.

Factor 5: Refusal/reluctance to accept assistance, history of self-neglecting behaviors, and personal neglect. Self-determinism items ($n = 4$) demonstrate choice factors and past self-care behaviors. The marginally low α value for factor 5 (0.69) could be due to fewer items ($n = 4$) on this subscale.

Clinical decisions and judgment of risk on safeguarding and protection of self-neglecting older adults are subjective and influenced by culture, beliefs, knowledge, experience, education, and organization (Day et al., 2013). The SN-37 measure offers an objective systematic approach to measuring self-neglect. The application of a scoring scale (yes = 1; no = 0) to the SN-37 for use in practice would provide an objective self-neglect assessment instrument. The SN-37 has the potential to address preventive measures and interventions within primary care and can be used to make appropriate service referrals to community nursing services, adult protective services (APS), SWs, or community organizations (Day, 2014). This information provides researchers with a new self-neglect measurement instrument. Higher level statistical analysis, including confirmatory factor analyses, would contribute to further theory development.

Strengths, Limitations, and Recommendations

This study used a detailed two-stage process that was rigorous to develop the SN-37. The item pool was constructed in a thorough manner. A major strength of the SN-37 instrument is that it is the first study to involve 305 front-line community professionals in the development of a self-neglect instrument. In addition, 57% of the participants had contact with three to 25+ cases in the previous 12 months. The limitations included convenience sampling and descriptive cross-sectional design. Validity and reliability of the study were ensured by exploratory factor analyses and Cronbach's α values.

The key strengths of the SN-37 instrument are comprehensiveness of items, underpinned by the ESN conceptual framework, and construct validity was established using EFA. In addition participants were drawn from a national sample and were experts who worked with self-neglecting individuals.

CONCLUSION

In conclusion, this research addresses a gap in the literature by developing a self-neglect measurement for use by community nurses, health and social care professionals, clinicians, and researchers. A systematic approach was used to develop SN-37, which contained five subscales: environment, social networks, emotional and behavioral liability, health avoidance, and self-determinism. The key strengths of the SN-37 instrument are comprehensiveness of items, underpinned by the ESN conceptual framework, and construct validity was established using EFA. In addition participants were drawn from a national sample and were experts who worked with self-neglecting individuals.

IMPLICATIONS FOR RESEARCH AND PRACTICE
• Confirmatory factor analysis could be used to further test the five-factor structure established in this study.
• The 37-item self-neglect instrument (SN-37) has several potential applications involving research on self-neglect.
• The 37-item self-neglect instrument (SN-37) can be used in the practice field for the identification of self-neglect in various environments as well as in different countries.
• The 37-item self-neglect instrument (SN-37) offers opportunities to measure the self-neglect trajectory pre- and postintervention of APS and safeguarding teams.

REFERENCES

Adams, J., & Johnson, J. (1998). Nurses' perceptions of gross self-neglect amongst older people living in the community. *Journal of Clinical Nursing, 7*(6), 547–552.

Band-Winterstein, T., Doron, I., & Naim, S. (2012). Elder self-neglect: A geriatric syndrome or a life course story? *Journal of Aging Studies, 26*(2), 109–118.

Bartley, M., Knight, P. V., O'Neill, D., & O'Brien, J. G. (2011). Self-neglect and elder abuse: Related phenomena? *Journal of the American Geriatrics Society, 59*(11), 2163–2168.

Bohl, B. (2010). *Investigating elder self-neglect: Interviews with adult protective service workers* (Unpublished doctoral thesis). Ohio State University, Columbus, OH. Retrieved from http://rave.ohiolink.edu/etdc/view?acc_num = osu1281633493

Braye, S., Orr, D., & Preston-Shoot, M. (2013). *A scoping study of workforce development for self-neglect work.* University of Sussex and the University of Bedfordshire. Leeds, UK: Skills for Care.

Braye, S., Orr, D., & Preston-Shoot, M. (2014). *Self-neglect policy and practice: Building an evidence base for social care* (Vol. 17). London, UK: Social Care Institute for Excellence.

Burnett, J., Dyer, C. B., Halphen, J. M., Achenbaum, W. A., Green, C. E., Booker, J. G., & Diamond, P. M. (2014). Four subtypes of self-neglect in older adults: Results of a latent class analysis. *Journal of the American Geriatrics Society, 62*(6), 1127–1132.

Burnett, J., Regev, T., Pickens, S., Prati, L. L., Aung, K., Moore, J., & Dyer, C. B. (2006). Social networks: A profile of the elderly who self-neglect. *Journal of Elder Abuse & Neglect, 18*(4), 35–49.

Cattell, R. B. (1966). The scree test for the number of factors. *Multivariate Behavioral Research, 1,* 245–276.

Choi, N. G., Kim, J., & Asseff, J. (2009). Self-neglect and neglect of vulnerable older adults: Reexamination of etiology. *Journal of Gerontological Social Work, 52*(2), 171–187.

Clarke, L. A., & Watson, D. (1995). Constructing validity: Basic issues in objective scale development. *Psychological Assessment, 7*(3), 309–319.

Day, M. R. (2010). Self-neglect: A challenge and a dilemma. *Archives of Psychiatric Nursing, 24*(2), 73–75.

Day, M. R. (2014). *Self-neglect: Development and evaluation of a self-neglect (SN-37) measurement instrument* (Unpublished doctoral dissertation). University College Cork, Ireland.

Day, M. R., Leahy-Warren, P., & McCarthy, G. (2013). Perceptions and views of self-neglect: A client centered perspective. *Journal of Elder Abuse & Neglect, 25*(1), 76–94.

Day, M. R., Leahy-Warren, P., & McCarthy, G. (2016). Self-neglect: Ethical considerations. *Annual Review of Nursing Research, 34*(1), 89–107.

Day, M. R., & McCarthy, G. (2015). A national cross-sectional study of community nurses and social workers knowledge of self-neglect. *Age and Ageing, 44*(4), 717–720.

Day, M. R., McCarthy, G., & Leahy-Warren, P. (2012). Professional social workers' views on self-neglect: An exploratory study. *British Journal of Social Work, 42*(4), 725–743.

Day, M. R., Mulcahy, H., & Leahy-Warren, P. (2016). Prevalence of self-neglect on public health nurses caseloads. *British Journal of Community Nursing, 21*(1), 31–35.

Department of Health. (2000). *No secrets.* London, UK: Author.

Department of Health. (2009). *With respect to age—2009: Victorian government practice guidelines for health services and community agencies for the prevention of elder abuse.* Melbourne, Australia: State Government of Victoria.

Devon, H. A., Block, M. E., Moyle-Wright, P., Ernst, D. M., Hayden, S. J., Lazaro, D. J., . . . Kostas-Polson, E. (2007). A psychometric toolbox for testing validity and reliability. *Journal of Nursing Scholarship, 39*(2), 155–164.

Dong, X., & Simon, M. A. (2013). Association between elder self-neglect and hospice utilization in a community population. *Archives of Gerontology and Geriatrics, 56*(1), 192–198.

Dong, X., & Simon, M. A. (2015). Elder self-neglect is associated with an increased rate of 30-day hospital readmission: Findings from the Chicago Health and Aging Project. *Gerontology, 61*(1), 41–50.

Dong, X., Simon, M., Beck, T., & Evans, D. (2010). A cross-sectional population-based study of elder self-neglect and psychological, health, and social factors in a biracial community. *Aging & Mental Health, 14*(1), 74–84.

Dong, X., Simon, M. A., & Evans, D. (2012a). Elder self-neglect and hospitalization: Findings from the Chicago Health and Aging Project. *Journal of the American Geriatrics Society, 60*(2), 202–209.

Dong, X., Simon, M. A., & Evans, D. (2012b). Prospective study of the elder self-neglect and ED use in a community population. *American Journal of Emergency Medicine, 30*(4), 553–561.

Dong, X., Simon, M., & Evans, D. (2013). Elder self-neglect is associated with increased risk for elder abuse in a community-dwelling population: Findings from the Chicago Health and Aging Project. *Journal of Aging and Health, 25*(1), 80–96.

Dong, X., Simon, M., Fulmer, T., Mendes de Leon, C. F., Rajan, B., & Evans, D. A. (2010). Physical function decline and the risk of elder self-neglect in a community-dwelling population. *The Gerontologist, 50*(3), 316–326.

Dong, X., Simon, M., Mendes de Leon, C., Fulmer, T., Beck, T., Hebert, L., . . . Evans, D. A. (2009). Elder self-neglect and abuse and mortality risk in a community-dwelling population. *Journal of the American Medical Association, 302*(5), 517–526.

Dong, X., Simon, M. A., Mosqueda, L., & Evans, D. A. (2012). The prevalence of elder self-neglect in a community-dwelling population: Hoarding, hygiene and environmental hazards. *Journal of Aging and Health, 24*(3), 507–524.

Dyer, C. B., Kelly, P. A., Pavlik, V. N., Lee, J., Doody, R. S., Regev, T., . . . Smith, S. M. (2006). The making of a Self-Neglect Severity Scale. *Journal of Elder Abuse & Neglect, 18*(4), 13–23.

Dyer, C., Pickens, S., & Burnett, J. (2007). Vulnerable elders: When it is no longer safe to live alone. *Journal of the American Medical Association, 298*(12), 1448–1450.

Field, A. (2005). *Discovering statistics using SPSS* (2nd ed.). London, UK: Sage.

Gibbons, S. W. (2009). Theory synthesis for self-neglect: A health and social phenomenon. *Nursing Research, 58*(3), 194–200.

Government of South Australia. (2013). *A foot in the door.* Canberra, Australia: Department of Health and Ageing and National Library of Australia.

Gregory, C., Halliday, G., Hodges, J., & Snowdon, J. (2011). Living in squalor: Neuropsychological function, emotional processing and squalor perception in patients found living in squalor. *International Psychogeriatric, 23*(5), 724–731.

Gunstone, S. (2003). Risk assessment and management of patients whom self-neglect: A 'grey area' for mental health workers. *Journal of Psychiatric & Mental Health Nursing, 10*(3), 287–296.

Halliday, G., & Snowdon, J. (2009). The Environmental Cleanliness and Clutter Scale (ECCS). *International Psychogeriatrics, 21*(6), 1041–1050.

Health Service Executive. (2012). *Policy and procedures for responding to allegations of extreme self-neglect.* Kildare, Ireland: Author.

Health Service Executive. (2013). *Open your eyes: There is no excuse for elder abuse.* Kildare, Ireland: Author.

Health Service Executive. (2014). *Safeguarding vulnerable persons at risk of abuse: National Policy and Procedures.* Dublin, Ireland: HSE, Social Care Division.

Horn, J. L. (1965). A rationale and test for the number of factors in factor analysis. *Psychometrika, 30*(2), 179–185.

Iris, M., Ridings, J. W., & Conrad, K. J. (2010). The development of a conceptual model for understanding elder self-neglect. *The Gerontologist, 50*(3), 303–315.

Jogerst, G. J., Daly, J. M., Brinig, M. F., Dawson, J. D., Schmuch, G. A., & Ingram, J. G. (2003). Domestic elder abuse and the law. *American Journal Public Health, 93*(12), 2131–2136.

Kaiser, H. F. (1960). The application of electronic computers to factor analysis. *Educational and Psychological Measurement, 20*, 141–151.

Kaiser, H. F. (1974). An index of factorial simplicity. *Psychometrika, 39*, 31–36.

Kelly, P. A., Dyer, C. B., Pavlik, V., Doody, R., & Jogerst, G. (2008). Exploring self-neglect in older adults: Preliminary findings of the Self-Neglect Severity Scale and next steps. *Journal of the American Geriatrics Society, 56*, S253–S260.

Kline, P. (1994). *An easy guide to factor analysis.* London, UK: Routledge.

Lachs, M. S., Williams, C. S., O'Brien, S., & Pillemer, K. A. (2002). Adult protective service use and nursing home placement. *The Gerontologist, 42*(6), 734–739.

Lauder, W., & Roxburgh, M. (2012). Self-neglect consultation rates and comorbidities in primary care. *International Journal of Nursing Practice, 18*(5), 454–461.

Lauder, W., Scott, P. A., & Whyte, A. (2001). Nurses' judgements of self-neglect: A factorial survey. *International Journal of Nursing Studies, 38*(5), 601–608.

Lee, M., & Kim, K. (2014). Prevalence and risk factors for self-neglect among older adults living alone in South Korea. *International Journal of Ageing and Human Development, 78*(2), 115–131.

Leibbrandt, S. M. V. (2007). *Factors associated with self-neglect in community-dwelling older adults.* Cleveland, OH: Case Western Reserve University.

Lynn, M. (1986). Determination and quantification of content validity. *Nursing Research, 35*(6), 382–385.

May-Chahal, C., & Antrobus, R. (2012). Engaging community support in safeguarding adults from self-neglect. *British Journal of Social Work, 42*(8), 1478–1494.

McDermott, S. (2010). Professional judgements of risk and capacity in situations of self-neglect among older people. *Ageing & Society, 30*(6), 1055–1072.

Naik, A. D., Pickens, S., Burnett, J., Lai, J. M., & Dyer, C. B. (2006). Assessing capacity in the setting of self-neglect: Development of a novel screening tool for decision-making capacity. *Journal of Elder Abuse & Neglect, 18*(4), 79–91.

Pickens, S., Ostwald, S. K., Pace, K. M., Diamond, P., Burnett, J., & Dyer, C. B. (2013). Assessing dimensions of executive function in community-dwelling older adults with self-neglect. *Clinical Nursing Studies, 2*(1), 17–29.

Polit, D. F., & Beck, C. T. (2006). The content validity index: Are you sure you know what's being reported? Critique and recommendations. *Research in Nursing & Health, 29*(5), 489–497.

Polit, D. F., & Beck, C. T. (2010). *Essentials of nursing research: Appraising evidence for nursing practice* (7th ed.). Philadelphia, PA: Lippincott Williams & Wilkins.

Polit, D. F., Beck, C. T., & Owen, S. V. (2007). Is the CVI an acceptable indicator of content validity? Appraisal and recommendations. *Research in Nursing & Health, 30*(4), 459–467.

Polit, D. F., & Hungler, B. P. (1999). *Nursing research: Principles and methods.* Philadelphia, PA: Lippincott Williams & Wilkins.

Reyes-Ortiz, C. A. (2001). Diogenes syndrome: The self-neglect elderly. *Comprehensive Therapy, 27*(2), 117–121.

Samios, K. (1996). *In to the loathsome den: The characteristics of persons living in squalor* (Unpublished PhD thesis). Royal Australian and New Zealand College of Psychiatrists, Sydney.

Snowdon, J. (1987). Uncleanliness among persons seen by community health workers. *Hospital Community Psychiatry, 38,* 491–494.

Snowdon, J. (2011). Preventing progression from squalor to homelessness. *Parity, 24*(5), 41–42.

Snowdon, J., & Halliday, G. (2011). A study of severe domestic squalor: 173 cases referred to an old age psychiatry service. *International Psychogeriatrics, 23*(2), 308–314.

Snowdon, J., Halliday, G., & Banerjee, S. (2012). *Severe domestic squalor.* Edinburg, UK: Cambridge University Press.

Snowdon, J., Halliday, G., & Hunt, G. E. (2013). Two types of squalor: Findings from a factor analysis of the Environmental Cleanliness and Clutter Scale (ECCS). *International Psychogeriatrics, 25*(7), 1191–1198.

Spensley, C. (2008). The role of social isolation of elders in recidivism of self-neglect cases at San Francisco adult protective services. *Journal of Elder Abuse & Neglect, 20*(1), 43–61.

Teaster, P. B., Dugar, T., Mendiondo, M., Abner, E. L., Cecil, K. A., & Otto, J. M. (2006). *The 2004 survey of adult protective services: Abuse of adults 60 years of age and older.* Washington, DC: National Center on Elder Abuse, Administration on Aging. Retrieved from http://www.napsa-now.org/wp-content/uploads/2012/09/2-14-06-FINAL-60+REPORT.pdf

Tierney, M. C., Charles, J., Naglie, G., Jaglal, S., Kiss, A., & Fisher, R. H. (2004). Risk factors for harm in cognitively impaired seniors who live alone: A prospective study. *Journal of the American Geriatrics Society, 52*(9), 1435–1441.

Tierney, M. C., Snow, W. G., Charles, J., Moineddin, R., & Kiss, A. (2007). Neuropsychological predictors of self-neglect in cognitively impaired older people who live alone. *American Journal of Geriatric Psychiatry, 15*(2), 140–148.

Turner, A., Hochschild, A., Burnett, J., Zulfiqar, A., & Dyer, C. B. (2012). High prevalence of medication non-adherence in a sample of community-dwelling older adults with adult protective services-validated self-neglect. *Drugs & Aging, 29*(9), 741–749.

Williams, B., Brown, T., & Onsman, A. (2012). Exploratory factor analysis: A five-step guide for novices. *Journal of Emergency Primary Health Care, 8*(3), 1.

Working Group on Elder Abuse. (2002). *Protecting our future.* Dublin, Ireland: Stationery Office.

World Health Organization & National Institute on Aging. (2011). *Global health and aging.* Geneva, Switzerland: Author.

ETHICAL AND EDUCATIONAL ISSUES

CHAPTER 23

SELF-NEGLECT AMONG OLDER ADULTS: PROFESSIONAL EDUCATION AND PREPARATION FOR PRACTICE

Eleanor Bantry White and Julie Bach

Self-neglect is a complex issue that challenges health and social care professionals. Professional education needs to support students to develop a broad range of knowledge and skills, in addition to discipline-specific knowledge, to ensure professional responses to older adults experiencing self-neglect are ethical and effective. This chapter outlines the pedagogical demands placed on professional educators by the complex nature of self-neglect. Attention is paid to the knowledge of self-neglect and the capacity to navigate frameworks, to undertake assessment and plan interventions, to build relationships with older adults and with interdisciplinary teams, and to negotiate the ethical issues that present in this work. Specific attention is paid to reflective models of teaching and learning that center on active, experiential approaches such as team-based learning, role plays, use of case studies, service user engagement, and field-based learning. The chapter ends with the consideration of future areas of research and development in pedagogical approaches to professional education on self-neglect.

The work of health and social care professionals charged with assessing and responding to the needs of older adults who self-neglect is complex. Professionals must navigate the uncertain terrain of self-neglect, a multifaceted and often contested problem, as it relates to a person's unique presentation and circumstances. This chapter examines the role of professional education in supporting practitioners embarking on their professional careers to respond effectively and ethically to the needs of older adults at risk from self-neglect. Although acknowledging the need for discipline-specific knowledge, the chapter is transdisciplinary in focus, examining the practice demands and pedagogical goals and tasks across qualifying professional programs. It begins with an examination of what is demanded of health and social care practitioners and how educators need to prepare students. It then identifies the knowledge, values, and skills that educators must seek to develop so that students can respond to these demands. The pedagogical process and tools that support such development are explored with a particular emphasis on reflective practice. Two case studies are presented to illustrate the case study method used to elicit critical reflection (see Case Studies 1 and 2). The chapter concludes with a discussion of developmental priorities in the field of professional education.

CASE STUDY 1: MR. D

Mr. D, a 76-year-old Italian man, was admitted to a rehabilitation facility after a fall in which he fractured his right hip. He has a long history of asthma, hypertension, and arthritis. He is participating in occupational and physical therapy with the goal of rebuilding his strength and avoiding future falls. Mr. D is a widower of 7 years. He currently lives alone in a large home, which he has owned for 45 years. He had a small antique shop, and he enjoyed chatting with staff members about vintage furniture and jewelry. His shop closed 9 years ago when his wife's illness demanded more of his time.

His only son has a substance abuse problem, and Mr. D has asked him not to visit as he has taken many items from Mr. D's house to sell for drugs. However, neighbors report that his son appears every few months and that Mr. D gives him money. When asked about this, Mr. D closes his eyes and with a pained expression states, "It is hard to deny your only child."

After 2 weeks of therapy, Mr. D's physical therapist, Trish, came to the rehabilitation facility's interdisciplinary team meeting with concerns about his living environment. Trish reports that she suggested Mr. D might use a four-wheel walker in the future to avoid falls. Mr. D protested, saying that he would then not be able to ambulate through his home as the walker would not fit through the narrow space. He describes his home as cluttered and disorganized and says he has several television sets in his entryway as well as furniture in the hallway. He explained that he has difficulty removing items as they remind him of his wife and he also is unsure of the value of many of the items.

Trish also reports that Mr. D often becomes breathless during his exercises and requires the use of oxygen. Mr. D said that his wife had always kept up the home but that he was not a very good housekeeper and rarely uses the third floor. Since her death, he now primarily stays in a bedroom on the main floor. Mr. D also reports he has not organized his paperwork since closing the antique business and thinks he may owe some money to the owner of the building where he ran his shop. Trish is concerned that Mr. D may be living in an unsafe and overcrowded environment, which is particularly worrying due to his severe breathing symptoms.

As Mr. D's social worker, you are responsible for his safe discharge home. Mr. D plans to return home after his rehabilitation stay and has expressed some homesickness and anxiety about not being able to watch over his things. He has also been visited by neighbors who have taken items from his home at his request. His room at the facility is becoming somewhat cluttered and his roommate has complained to staff that Mr. D will sometimes store food in his bedside table and allow it to rot, creating an odor in the room. Trish attempted to approach Mr. D about his living environment but states that he becomes defensive and claims that he plans to sell many of his collected items as soon as he returns home. She and his occupational therapist expect that Mr. D will physically be ready for discharge in approximately 6 weeks.

In an education session questions/reflective prompts can be tailored to the professional disciplinary role specific of the student group.

Sample Questions:
- How would you approach Mr. D's situation?
- How might you consider his wishes while also ensuring his safety?
- What issues might you encounter and how would you address them?

(Sourced and Adapted from the Council on Social Work Education, Gero-Ed Center. *Teaching module*. Retrieved from http://www.cswe.org)

CASE STUDY 2: MS. A

Ms. A is an 83-year-old single woman who has never been married. She lives in the two-story family home where she has lived all her life. She had two siblings who are both deceased. She has several nieces and nephews with whom she has occasional contact. Ms. A was active in her local church until a year ago when she fell and broke her leg. Although she recovered significant mobility after rehabilitation, she is now using a three-prong cane. She is frightened to leave her home due to concerns of falling again. She fell when she was attempting to enter the car of one of her friends on her way to the church.

Her home requires extensive repairs. Her front porch and wooden stairs are rotten and cannot be used for entry. She must enter through the back door. Despite efforts to fix the roof it is still damaged and water enters the upstairs rooms when severe rainfall occurs. She does not use the second floor due to water damage and the 12-step staircase involved. There is no bedroom on the first floor so, since her return from rehabilitation, she has slept on the couch and has moved some of her clothing to the dining room.

Ms. A eats meals she prepares in the microwave or finger foods (such as sandwiches). She has not cleaned her home for several months. She states she must add water to the toilet to get it to flush well and she has asked her nephew whether he can locate a plumber who wouldn't charge much to fix the problem. She adds that her nephew just keeps telling her to move.

Ms. A has had several notices from the local government about her front entry and has been informed her home may be condemned if she does not repair the house. When the inspector came to the home, it was noted the home has a strong odor due to plumbing problems in the bathroom.

Ms. A has informed the authorities she does not plan to move from her family home. It is the only residence she has resided in her whole life. There is no mortgage on the home and taxes are low. She receives Social Security and feels she can afford to live in the home if it weren't for the home repair costs. She also mentioned she owes $3,000 to the gas company for home heating costs. Ms. A explained she wears a coat while indoors during the winter and gloves if it gets so cold that she needs them. She states her heating bill is so high that she tries to heat only a few of the rooms. She explained she pays the gas company $50 a month, so they should leave her alone.

Ms. A presents wearing clothes that appear worn but clean; she has a rash on her arms and face. In the past she used a cream to help with the rash but she can no longer afford to purchase it. She has a history of breast cancer (10 years ago) for which she had a mastectomy and chemotherapy. The holes in her shoes are taped over. Ms. A states, "I lived during World War II and I don't need new shoes or clothes. We had rationing then."

Ms. A has some church members who call her on the telephone and will drop off groceries for her every month. Ms. A is oriented to time, place, and person. She is aware her home has significant problems but states she will not move from it nor can she afford to make improvements.

In an education session questions/reflective prompts can be tailored to the professional disciplinary role specific of the student group.

Sample Questions:
- How would you approach Ms. A's situation?
- How might you consider her wishes while also ensuring his safety?
- What issues might you encounter and how would you address them?

BACKGROUND LITERATURE: EDUCATING FOR THE PROFESSIONAL TERRAIN

Professional education that prepares practitioners to support older adults experiencing self-neglect is an underdeveloped area. A European report by the World Health Organization (2011) identified a dearth of high-quality studies that have described and evaluated educational programs resulting in a limited understanding of the components of effective educational programs. From the available research, education and training with mentored practice experience appears to support professional skills development and the capacity to work with older adults at risk from self-neglect (Braye, Orr, & Preston-Shoot, 2011a, 2011b). Research on professional knowledge in this sphere indicates the need to develop self-neglect as a focus of learning on qualifying-level educational programs to ensure practitioners have baseline competencies to commence practice in their professional field. Day and McCarthy (2015) identified significant gaps in the professional knowledge in a survey of nurses and social workers in Ireland. Their study identified differences by professional background in terms of reliance on formal knowledge and experience. In particular, the study noted a lack of clarity among practitioners as to their professional roles and responsibilities. Their study supports the need for baseline knowledge and skills teaching on qualifying professional programs across the various health and social care professions that encounter the issue of self-neglect.

KNOWLEDGE, VALUES, AND SKILLS

The task of the professional educator is a challenging one: It is not only to teach for understanding but also to teach for application as knowledge is a key resource for practitioners who need to navigate an uncertain terrain. Students must be supported to engage with the complexities of self-neglect. In addition, the professional educator needs to assist and guide the student in understanding his or her own personal reactions to often challenging and complex living situations.

The behaviors and circumstances associated with self-neglect have multifaceted etiologies and presentations. Students must grapple with the various definitions of self-neglect, its conceptual development and the absence of consensus on a standardized definition (Day, Bantry-White, & Glavin, 2010). Conceptual models illustrate the wide range of physical, psychosocial, and environmental factors associated with self-neglect (Iris, Ridings, & Conrad, 2010) and students need to become familiar with a range of risk factors and comorbidities. The case studies presented in this chapter illustrate the issues that do occur.

Indecisiveness is a prominent feature of individuals at risk of self-neglect and many individuals report stressful or traumatic life events preceding their self-neglect (American Psychiatric Association [APA], 2013). For example, in the first case study, Mr. D, an older adult, is widowed and displays difficulty removing items from his home since his wife died. A comorbid condition, such as major acute illness, depressive disorder, social or generalized anxiety, may also be present (APA, 2013). Biography is also significant and the reaction to stress and ability to cope may be related to the type of attachment formed early in life. Mr. D has an acute illness and is attached to many personal effects and artifacts. Attachment theory can be applied to how the older adult reacts to the changes and stress in the environment. If an older adult has an avoidant personality she or he may be wary and distrustful of assistance from others (Council on Social Work Education/Gero-Ed Center, n.d.).

This may impact the ability for health and social care workers to establish a helping relationship. The educator must therefore develop knowledge and skills in the student to ensure the student has the capacity to identify and respond to the wide range of factors that underlie self-neglect, without imposing personal values on the situation.

Central to how self-neglect is conceptualized and responded to is the issue of cognitive ability and inability, which may arise from neurological illness such as Alzheimer's disease and mental health disorders such as obsessive-compulsive disorder and severe depression (Pavlou & Lachs, 2006). Furthermore, executive dysfunction is more common in adults who self-neglect than the general population (Dong et al., 2010) and similar problems with executive function have been found in older adults with hoarding behavior (Ayers et al., 2013). These issues impact on the older adult's activities of daily living (ADL) and safety. In accounting for such skills of daily living, a distinction has been made in the literature between intentional and unintentional self-neglect (Gibbons, 2009). Such a distinction may potentially be useful for students in making sense of and planning a response to the presenting issues.

Although knowledge of the etiology of behaviors associated with self-neglect is essential to its identification, professional education should not adopt a "checklist" approach, which reduces complex human life to a list of observable behaviors. Professional education needs to support students to recognize that all behaviors, housing, objects, relationships, and living circumstances are imbued with meaning that is significant to the older adult (Andersen, Raffin-Bouchal, & Marcy-Edwards, 2008). By recognizing this, practitioners can then develop the skills to elicit deeper phenomenological insights into how the older person experiences his or her circumstances. Professional education needs, therefore, to facilitate students to move beyond the sole focus on identifying behaviors and circumstances to one that elicits understanding of the symbolic representation of these behaviors and circumstances.

Similar to debates about elder abuse and neglect (Eisikovits, Koren, & Band-Winterstein, 2013), self-neglect is arguably a social construct that at some level requires students to deconstruct categories. Self-neglect as a construct has evolved over time and varies across place (Day, Leahy-Warren, & McCarthy, 2016). The practitioner must ask who defines the behaviors as self-neglect and who defines it and experiences it as a problem. This may help practitioners to gain insight into the older adult's perspective on and insight into the issue. For example, historical events such as World War II and experience with rationing impacts how an older adult may respond to limited resources. Case Study 2 of Ms. A illustrates this possible impact. These shared beliefs and experiences, or cohort elements, may be unfamiliar to a younger student.

Supporting students to recognize the tacit assumptions about self-neglect made by professional groups, families, and older adults can enhance their understanding and response to contestation among the key actors about the nature of the problem. Lack of consensus about what constitutes a problem in terms of the older adult's welfare can lead to conflict among professionals, the older person, and the family (Phillips, Ray, & Marshall, 2006). Recognition of conflict and difference of perspectives requires the professional educator to include the skills of negotiation and partnership in curriculum learning outcomes (Day et al., 2010).

All practitioners work within legislative and policy frameworks and students must have the knowledge of these in order to direct their decision making. The key issues students need to develop awareness of are the parameters of their role, including their obligations under the law and their responsibilities set out in the national and local procedural guidelines and policy such as Safeguarding Vulnerable Persons at Risk of Abuse (HSE, 2014) or the Care Act (2014). Therefore, professional educators need to teach for application rather than relay a descriptive knowledge of legislation and policy. Understanding of legislation and policy guides the practitioner in terms of the interventions warranted following identification of particular behaviors, etiological factors, and living circumstances. In the first case study, Mr. D may be experiencing financial abuse from a son. In the second case study, the housing codes may impact Ms. A's choice to remain in her own home. Understanding the legal issues associated with the previous case scenarios is necessary to ensure student practitioners meet their legal and policy obligations and adhere to their professional codes of ethical conduct.

Findings from serious case reviews have repeatedly drawn attention to deficiencies in capacity assessments made by professionals working with older adults who self-neglect (Braye, Orr, & Preston-Shoot, 2015a, 2015b). Across Western legal systems, the right of the competent person to make decisions has been afforded protection. In jurisdictions where functional definitions of capacity exist, capacity is decision specific and incapacity to make a specific decision is only declared if the person is unable to understand the information given, retain it, weigh it, and communicate the decision (Day et al., 2016; Hughes & Baldwin, 2006). Students are likely to need to develop a working knowledge of the decision-making capacity as well as their wider legal obligations. These act as a compass to help students navigate the complex terrain of self-neglect. Awareness of policies also helps students to determine their roles and responsibilities relative to other professional disciplines and is the first step in developing the skills required for interdisciplinary and interagency work.

Assessment and Intervention Skills

Assessment may involve the identification and measurement of quantifiable features (for example, comorbid illness, physical and psychological functions, and environmental issues), specific objective measures of self-neglect (for example, Day & McCarthy, 2016), or qualitative assessment based on understanding of causative themes and ethical principles (Braye et al., 2011a). Students need to be introduced to the signature approach to assessment within their discipline. An awareness of all other aspects of assessment will help students to value interdisciplinary work. Assessment involves qualitative judgments about the significance of identified issues for the older person and the weighting that should be accorded to the various issues in professional decision making. Through reflective inquiry, students must be supported to integrate knowledge. The work requires the practitioner to look inward (for example, health conditions, mental health, etc.), to look outward to the environment and the systems in which the older adult inhabits, backward to the biographical features relevant to present-day behaviors and circumstances, and to look forward to anticipate the range of possible outcomes arising from the behavior and circumstances. This approach to assessment is enriched by reflective practice. It mirrors an approach first developed by Dempsey, Halton, and Murphy (2001) that supports the student to look backward, look inward, look outward, and look forward. Reflective practices can help students to broaden their assessment beyond presenting behaviors and living circumstances.

Older adults considered to be self-neglecting can experience contact with professionals as disempowering (Day, Leahy-Warren, & McCarthy, 2013; Knight, 1986). To support the anti-oppressive practice, it is valuable to introduce students to the conceptual underpinnings of assessment, particularly the conceptual differences between an assessment of need and an assessment of risk. A focus on risk as opposed to need is likely to have different implications for the outcome of assessment and, potentially, the form of intervention applied. Deconstructing risk and how social processes, including ageism, attribute risk and vulnerability to particular groups is important (Sheldon & MacDonald, 2009). It may help to facilitate students to incorporate the positive aspects of risk taking, including enhanced quality of life brought about by exercising autonomy. A helpful framework for students is provided by Culo (2011), who discusses tolerable and intolerable risks. Intolerable risk is described as "dangerous behaviors or circumstances that can cause serious and imminent harm" (Culo, 2011, p. 423). If self-neglect is viewed on a continuum, students need to develop the assessment skills to differentiate between problems that pose a threat and those that are lifestyle decisions. Therefore, wider knowledge of the health and social issues relevant to assessment is required to support student practitioners to balance the older adult's right to self-determination with the professional commitment to reduce the risk of harm.

Older adults assessed as demonstrating self-neglect may be experiencing clinically depressive symptoms (Abrams, Lachs, McAvay, Keohane, & Bruce, 2002; Burnett, Coverdale, Pickens, & Dyer, 2006), a mental health disorder, or a hoarding disorder recently included in the fifth edition of the *Diagnostic and Statistical Manual of Mental Disorders* (*DSM-5*; APA, 2013). If during assessment there are reasons to believe the person has mental health issues, then the practitioner conducting the assessment needs to conduct a relevant assessment (based on his or her professional skills and competence) or refer to another professional.

Awareness of environmental factors as exemplified in Case Studies 1 and 2 is also important to professional competency development. The environment around the older adult may have changed, creating an *environmental press*. This refers to an environmental feature that influences the behavior of the older adult (Hooyman & Asuman Kiyak, 2011). An example may be an older adult who can no longer access the laundry room and is now attempting to wash clothes in a bathtub. This may result in presenting with dirty clothes and lack of cleanliness. Older adults have often lived in their homes for at least 30 years (Hooyman & Asuman Kiyak, 2011). This can create an accumulation of possessions and also a home with deteriorating structures, such as issues with stairs or roofs as seen in Case Study 2. Local resources to assist with repairs may be limited or too costly to the older adult. Student practitioners need the skills to develop creative approaches and collaborative working relationships with, for example, housing agencies, to assist the older adult in securing resources. This would give the older adult the option to remain in the current environment.

The assessment of self-neglect requires decisional capacity. Complicating this assessment, cognitive tests do not measure competency and individuals with cognitive impairment may still be competent (Culo, 2011). Judgment is often impacted by diseases such as Alzheimer's disease. Assessment of executive function is a better predictor of decision-making capacity than global cognitive ability. Abrams and colleagues (2002) found that cognitive impairment predicted self-neglect in community-dwelling older adults. If dementia or severe mental illness is not present, the outcome of assessment is considered a social rather than a medical problem (Culo, 2011). Awareness of cognitive abilities and inabilities is an important learning outcome across professional programs even for professions for whom the skills to conduct a decisional assessment are not required. Decision-making capacity requires an individual to have an understanding of a situation and its consequences. For example, in both case studies presented here there are a number of factors that require a deep understanding of decisions made by Mr. D and Ms. A and the resulting consequences.

Several theories of help-seeking behavior explain an older adult's refusal for assistance. For example, if the older adult perceives the help as increasing dependency or self-threatening, she or he may react defensively. However, if the assistance is perceived as self-supporting, there is a higher agreement to assistance (Wacker & Roberto, 2014). In Case Studies 1 and 2, the factors influencing both Mr. D and Ms. A in their refusal to change their situations could be explored. For example, Mr. D refused the walker and Ms. A refuses to move from her family home. Through reflective discussions, students can consider how the two older adults might perceive the offer of change.

Assessment of the potential underlying causes of self-neglect is a prerequisite step to introducing students to appropriate interventions and approaches. Evidence-based research suggests older adults with self-neglecting behaviors benefit from therapeutic treatments, such as cognitive behavioral therapy, as well as community-based/case management interventions (Bratiotis, Ayers, & Steketee, 2016). Depending on the professional discipline, students can be supported to integrate these models into their work with older adults. Through role play, educators can review and reinforce the techniques and skills connected to these models. Integrating case studies in both the assessment and intervention allows the student to consider how she or he moves forward in his or her relationship with the older adult. In Case Study 1, students could identify specific steps that might help Mr. D to remove some of the cluttered items before he returns home. Students can complete a role play with peers in which the student who is presenting as the practitioner teaches the older adult to evaluate his or her thoughts. In Case Study 2, students might respond to Ms. A's statements about her fear of leaving her home. Also, students can lead relaxation exercises to assist the older adult in remaining calm when discussions turn to areas such as removing objects from the home.

Values

For the professions, education should not be reduced to only developing instrumental knowledge and skills. In addition to research, theory, policy, and legislative frameworks, the professional educator must also attend to the axiological and ethical dimensions of practice. Through reflection, students become aware of their own personal values and can begin to integrate the values of their profession into their emerging professional identity (Lyons, 2010). Values, mediated through sociocultural processes, such as ageism, influence how practitioners construct problems and how these problems become attributed to people and social groups. The interrogation of personal values embedded in personal biography and life experience and their potential impact on the professional role is a key pedagogical goal if professional educators are to support anti-oppressive practice (Thompson, 2006).

It is important that students explore their own beliefs. Sometimes, because older adults are at the end of their lives, the ratio to benefit of providing services is perceived as low (Laidlaw, Thompson, Dick-Siskin, & Gallagher-Thompson, 2003). Life transitions of retirement; the death of a partner; increased chronic illnesses, including Alzheimer's disease, represent unfamiliar areas to younger health and social care students. Ageism is strong internationally and many health and social care professionals do not explore the negative views they have of their own aging and the aging of older adults (Thompson, 2006). The term *professional ageism* coined by Butler and Lewis (1982), continues to impact the desire and expertise of health and social care professionals working with older adults. Attitudes toward older adults and the aging process impact how health professionals interact with this population. Older adults report being treated as children when the mental health professional responds in a paternalistic role or as a powerful authority figure (Knight, 1986; Sheldon & MacDonald, 2009).

There are several factors that impact the resistance to working with older adults. Many younger students have limited exposure with older adults, and there may be negative stereotypes about older adults as sick, unable to change, or dying (Hooyman & St. Peter, 2007). Health and social care professionals may feel that the problems presented by the older adult are neither preventable nor treatable. Older adults may be seen as rigid and unable to change. Health care professionals have been found to assess older adults as less capable or less healthy with a focus on the failure model (Kalish, 1979). The ability of students to assess areas, such as the typical changes associated with aging, environmental press, and sociocultural values, is overwhelming due to the lack of adequate training in working with older adults. Educators need to take heed of ageism to ensure it does not pose a barrier to student learning.

Self-knowledge is therefore an important component of the development of the professional self and the professional educator's task is to enhance self-awareness in students (Dempsey et al., 2001). Of relevance to work in this field, the assessment of risk is central to intervening where there is self-neglect. In decisions and actions in their personal lives, students are likely to range from risk tolerant to the risk averse. Without such awareness of self and one's attitudes toward risk taking, a practitioner's personal values about risk taking may influence his or her assessment of the older adult and construction of his or her risk-taking behaviors.

Interrogation of personal values and support to incorporate professional values into the professional self are the foundations of ethical practice. The professional educator needs to scaffold ethicality by introducing students to ethical principles and associated frameworks used to support ethical practice in decision making and intervention (Hope, Savulescu, & Hendrick, 2008). Ethicality is a central concern within self-neglect work, which often hinges on a resolution of tensions between the imperative to respect autonomy under human rights law while attending to welfare concerns that could result in the older adults sustaining serious harm. The value of an older adult's autonomy is demonstrated through the client's right to self-determination, use of the least restrictive alternative, and avoidance of ascribing blame (Hooyman & Asuman Kiyak, 2011)

Health and social care professionals and older adults may be faced with two undesirable choices: over-care and under-care. Under-care is the need for an older adult to remain in the home and pay for groceries rather than medication due to limited finances. Over-care is the transition from a home in the community to skilled nursing care when moderate home repairs would have allowed the older adult to remain in their own home. The social service gaps result in choices that are not in the best interest of the older adult. Incorporating social justice as an ethical principle, for example, through the widely applied model of Beauchamp and Childress (2001), enables students to consider their professional role in advocating for older adults through wider health and social policy change.

Relationships

Professional practice is relational: It requires the professional to build relationships and partnerships with clients, and where relevant, a support system with other professionals and agencies. Assessment and intervention are predicated on building a relationship in which the older adult sufficiently trusts the professional to enable the professional to take an emic perspective to "see into" his or her world and the meaning that the older adult makes of his or her circumstances. Professional education needs to incorporate an understanding of and the skills to engage with "hard-to-reach" older adults. This may support students to respond to the problem of service refusal, a factor that has been included in a recent measure of self-neglect (Day & McCarthy, 2016). Specifically, to remain in one's own home represents empowerment and allowing outside service providers in may result in a slow loss of power. Empowering older adults requires the professional and the older adult to have a relationship of collaboration based on a balanced and egalitarian partnership (Mahoney, McGaffigan, Sciegaj, Zgoda, & Mahoney, 2017).

Such skills must be founded on a value-system based on respect. Respect necessitates "being present" to, in this instance, what the older adult is seeing and experiencing (Lyons, 2010). Students can be introduced to practical ways in which they can demonstrate respect. Respect for the older adult can be demonstrated through linguistic respect (how the older adult is addressed, and specific words depending on the cultural background), care respect (providing care for the older adult), acquiescence respect (listening to the older adult), and presentational respect (proper manners and professional dress; Sung & Dunkle, 2009).

Relationships and partnerships are also at the core of interdisciplinary and interagency work. A repeated finding of safeguarding inquiries when a death has occurred is inadequate team functioning, including poor communication, a lack of clarity of roles, and leadership that impedes effective case planning, and coordination (Braye et al., 2015a, 2015b). Health and social care students need to be afforded the opportunity to consider how they work in teams, the roles selected by them or prescribed by others, and how they understand the roles and responsibilities of other team members. One component is developing students' understanding of how the self operates within groups to identify learning goals that would make a students' participation in teamwork more effective (Doel, 2006). Opportunities to work with other professional disciplines provides more experiential learning (Day et al., 2010).

PEDAGOGY BASED ON REFLECTION

Reflective thinking requires a person to understand that knowledge is no longer a given, that: "Knowledge must be understood in context within the construct with which it was generated" (Merriam & Caffarella, 1999, p. 145). Reflection allows a person to accept alternative truths or ways of thinking, known as *dialectic thinking*. Utilizing reflection as a teaching tool, educators help build a critically reflective lens for professional practice. "Mature dialectic thought is characterized by an awareness that all thought processes are culturally and historically bound and therefore dynamic and constantly evolving" (p. 153).

Reflective practice includes problem finding and problem solving as part of the process. It means making judgments about what actions will be taken and results in some form of action (Merriam & Caffarella, 1999). In a reflection, the student practitioner will present what steps might be taken in the future for a case scenario or after an experience in an internship. This includes being aware and paying attention to what happened, attending to feelings and evaluating the experience. Reflective practice may help student practitioners to avoid developing a practice based on the habitual, described by Sheldon and MacDonald (2009) as Pavlovian responses in which practitioners intervene in an automatic way without due consideration of the unique needs, circumstances, and wishes of the older adult.

Educating health and social care students has moved from didactic lecture courses to active learning, also described as problem-based or problem-solving methods of learning. Active learning includes information and ideas: reflecting, doing, and observing (Fink, 2003). Much of active learning occurs with others, not individually. In a specific model, such as team-based learning, the students are placed in teams comprising five to seven students, which remain intact for the full class semester. Throughout the course, the teams complete activities first within their own team and then intrateam discussion occurs. This challenges the team to explain its results and allows all students to see the contrast and similarities in the final team results of the activity (Sibley & Ostafichuk, 2014). Students have reported that a team-based learning model allows them to interact with others who held different views and experiences and to learn to communicate their ideas to others (Taylor & Mclendon, 2013). Team-based learning can also be a useful medium for students to gain experience of interdisciplinary teamwork by bringing together students from different professional disciplines to work collaboratively on cases. In Day et al.'s (2010) article, nursing and social work students reported having a greater sense of their own professional role and ethos than those of students from the other discipline. These skills can then transfer to future team experiences such as interdisciplinary meetings.

As stated previously, reflection is the second major component of active learning. Fink (2003) describes how humans make meaning of new experiences or when encountering a new idea. He adds: "The initial meaning may remain buried at the unconscious or subconscious level" (p. 106). There is a need to pull the original meaning to the conscious level or the meaning may be limited or distorted. When students experience self-neglect, there is a need to spend time reflecting on the experience. The student can write a reflection about an experience or may share ideas with others. Fink (2003) adds that when reflecting with others, new and richer meanings may arise. Discussing with others the initial reaction to the environment or appearance of an older adult who hoards or demonstrates self-neglect behaviors can assist the student in processing his or her thoughts and feelings.

Active learning includes applying or integrating the concepts (information and ideas). Application learning engages in one or more kinds of thinking (creative, critical, and practical), developing an important skill or managing a complex project (Fink, 2003). Application involves doing, and, in professional education, this is often accomplished through case studies, as described earlier. This learning allows students to integrate the concepts learned in the course with real-life situations (Owens, Padula, & Hume, 2002). The use of a clinical case (case vignette/case study) leads to an adaptation of common features of problem-based learning. Self-neglect often involves interdisciplinary teams and interdisciplinary case studies bringing together the different values and perspectives of the various health and social care professions (for example, nurse, physician, social worker, pharmacist, dietician; Owens et al., 2002). Case studies can present older adults in settings that reflect self-neglect behaviors, allowing the students to assess and create potential options for the team. Case studies can also allow students to understand how the different disciplines may identify the case and conceptualize the issues.

Role-playing allows health and social care professionals to practice the skills and techniques learned about self-neglect. One student is the health or social care professional, another is the older adult, or in an interdisciplinary meeting, the other professionals. It is important to prepare for the role play by offering instructions, determining the time limit, and monitoring and debriefing after the activity (Friedman, 2008).

Another form of learning brings current professionals and individuals who have experienced self-neglect into the classroom to share their own stories. Benbow, Taylor, Mustafa, and Morgan (2011) describe the process of integrating health and social care professionals and service users into a class. Students reported how hearing the service user's story changed their attitudes and allowed them to work with people more broadly. In the area of self-neglect, the inclusion of individuals who have been "labeled" self-neglecters offers students a clearer understanding of the experience as it is felt and perceived by the older adult and his or her family. It also elicits understanding of the service user's experience of his or her relationships with professionals. Doel and Best (2008) highlight how service user's stories help students to identify the characteristics of professionals that are valued by service users such as trustworthiness and respect.

A final form of learning is the field experience or internship, known in social work as the *signature pedagogy*. In the internship, practitioners in training integrate the theoretical knowledge and skills in a mentored practice setting (Council on Social Work Education, 2015). In the field internships, self-neglect is found in the actual home visits and also experienced in interdisciplinary team discussions of clients.

CONCLUSION

Self-neglect among older adults presents a complex set of issues that often challenge health and social care professionals charged with responding ethically and effectively to the issues. Reflecting a complex etiology, self-neglect does not present uniformly across older adults and therefore teaching to checklists of problem and solutions does not serve students or older adults well. Didactic methods of teaching do not satisfactorily equip students with the necessary skills of sound judgment, ethicality, and creativity in relationship building, assessment, and the identification of intervention responses. Rather, students need to be supported to interpret behaviors and living circumstances by applying and testing out the wide range of available theoretical explanations and empirical knowledge. Students need to develop the skills of relationship building to elicit emic understanding of the issues as a necessary starting point to affecting positive changes. As a multidimensional problem, students should be supported to develop a commitment to and skills for teamwork and interdisciplinary collaboration.

The chapter has sought to contribute to these demands through a discussion of a transdisciplinary knowledge and skills that support professional development. Although there is a need to supplement this with discipline-specific knowledge and understanding of roles, a transdisciplinary focus is timely in view of the ever-more porous professional boundaries and transdisciplinary roles evident in, for example, models of single assessment. Students can consider where their profession is situated in terms of the emphasis placed by the discipline on the wide range of knowledge and skill requirements presented in this chapter, in tandem with developing a respect for the contribution of other disciplines.

Reflective models of teaching and learning can support students in the process of engaging with a complex set of issues, an often "hard-to-reach" client group, the many ethical dilemmas, and in navigating a sense of professional role identity necessary for effective team collaboration. Experiential and active models of learning have been outlined as a means of making the process of learning explicit. These include team-based learning, the case study method, role plays, service user perspectives and field-based learning. In each method, the process of reflective learning requires careful scaffolding by the professional educator. Case studies for use in the classroom have been included to illustrate the reflective discussion that can ensue from these activities. To ensure these teaching methods, which are well established in professional education, are "fit for purpose," research is necessary to examine how these translate into professional knowledge and skills on qualification in terms of quality, sensitivity, and ethicality of supports provided by health and social care professionals to older adults at risk from self-neglect.

IMPLICATIONS FOR RESEARCH AND PRACTICE

- Although there is a need for discipline-specific knowledge and skills in professional education, students benefit from an introduction to a wide set of approaches available for working collaboratively with older adults at risk from self-neglect and with wider interdisciplinary teams.
- Reflective models of teaching and learning can support students to apply knowledge, skills, and values in ways that recognize the unique circumstances, wishes, biography, and issues experienced by older adults.
- As research on self-neglect evolves, so too must research on effective teaching approaches and methods to ensure research evidence is put to good use.
- Further research is needed on the translation of classroom and field-based learning on qualifying programs to professional knowledge, values, and skills postqualification.

REFERENCES

Abrams, R., Lachs, M., McAvay, G., Keohane, D., & Bruce, M. (2002). Predictors of self-neglect in community-dwelling elders. *American Journal of Psychiatry, 159*(10), 1724–1730.

American Psychiatric Association. (2013). *Diagnostic and statistical manual of mental disorders* (5th ed.). Arlington, VA: American Psychiatric Publishing.

Andersen, E., Raffin-Bouchal, S., & Marcy-Edwards, D. (2008). Reasons to accumulate excess: Older adults who hoard possessions. *Home Health Care Services Quarterly, 27*(3), 187–216. doi:10.1080/01621420802319993

Ayers, C. R., Wetherell, J. L., Schiehser, D., Almklov, E., Golshan, S., & Saxena, S. (2013). Executive functioning in older adults with hoarding disorder. *International Journal of Geriatric Psychiatry, 28*(11), 1175–1181. doi:10.1002/gps.3940

Beauchamp, T., & Childress, J. (2001). *Principles of bioethics.* New York, NY: Oxford University Press.

Benbow, S. M., Taylor, L., Mustafa, N., & Morgan, K. (2011). Design, delivery and evaluation of teaching by service users and carers. *Educational Gerontology, 37*, 621–633. doi:10.1080/03601277.2011.559849

Bratiotis, C., Ayers, C., & Steketee, G. (2016). Older adults who hoard. In D. Kaplan & B. Berkman (Eds.), *The Oxford handbook of social work in health and aging* (2nd ed., pp. 407–416). New York, NY: Oxford University Press.

Braye, S., Orr, D., & Preston-Shoot, M. (2011a). Conceptualizing and responding to self-neglect: The challenges for adult safeguarding. *Journal of Adult Protection, 13*(4), 182–193.

Braye, S., Orr, D., & Preston-Shoot, M. (2011b). *Self-neglect and adult safeguarding: Findings from research* (Report No. 46). London, UK: Social Care Institute for Excellence.

Braye, S., Orr, D., & Preston-Shoot, M. (2015a). Learning lessons about self-neglect? An analysis of serious case reviews. *Journal of Adult Protection, 17*(1), 3–18.

Braye, S., Orr, D., & Preston-Shoot, M. (2015b). Serious case review findings on the challenges of self-neglect: Indicators for good practice. *Journal of Adult Protection, 17*(2), 75–87.

Burnett, J., Coverdale, J., Pickens, S., & Dyer, C. B. (2006). Self-neglect associated with depressive symptoms and untreated medical disease. *Journal of the American Geriatrics Society, 54*(Suppl. 4), S101.

Butler, R. N., & Lewis, M. L. (1982). *Aging and mental health*. St. Louis, MO: Mosby.

Council on Social Work Education, Gero-Ed Center. (n.d.). Teaching module. Retrieved from http://www.cswe.org

Culo, S. (2011). Risk assessment and intervention for vulnerable older adults. *BC Medical Journal, 53*(8), 421–425.

Day, M. R., Bantry-White, E., & Glavin, P. (2010). Protection of vulnerable adults: An interdisciplinary workshop. *Community Practitioner, 83*(9), 29–32.

Day, M. R., Leahy-Warren, P., & McCarthy, G. (2013). Perceptions and views of self-neglect: A client-centered perspective. *Journal of Elder Abuse & Neglect, 33*(2), 145–156.

Day, M. R., Leahy-Warren, P., & McCarthy, G. (2016). Self-neglect ethical considerations. *Annual Review of Nursing Research, 34*, 89–107. doi:10.1891/0739-6686.34.89

Day, M. R., & McCarthy, G. (2015). A national cross-sectional study of community nurses and social workers knowledge of self-neglect. *Age and Ageing, 44*(4), 717–720. doi:10.1093/ageing/afv025

Day, M. R., & McCarthy, G. (2016). Self-neglect: Development and evaluation of a self-neglect (SN-37) measurement instrument. *Archives of Psychiatric Nursing, 30*(4), 480–485. doi:10.1016/j.apnu.2016.02.004

Dempsey, M., Halton, C., & Murphy, M. (2001). Reflective learning in social work education: Scaffolding the process. *Social Work Education, 20*(6), 631–641. doi:10.1080/02615470120089825

Department of Health. (2014). Care and support statutory guidance: Issued under the Care Act 2014. London, UK: The Stationery Office.

Doel, M. (2006). *Using group work*. London, UK: Routledge.

Doel, M., & Best, L. (2008). *Experiencing social work learning from service users*. London, UK: Sage.

Dong, X., Simon, M. A., Wilson, R. S., Mendes de Leon, C. F., Rajan, K. B., & Evans, D. A. (2010). Decline in cognitive function and risk of elder self-neglect: Finding from the Chicago Health Aging Project. *Journal of the American Geriatrics Society, 58*(12), 2292–2299.

Eisikovits, Z., Koren, C., & Band-Winterstein, T. (2013). The social construction of social problems: The case of elder abuse and neglect. *International Psychogeriatrics, 25*(8), 1291–1298. doi:10.1017/S1041610213000495

Fink, L. D. (2003). *Creating significant learning experiences: An integrated approach to designing college courses*. San Francisco, CA: Jossey-Bass.

Friedman, B. (2008). *How to teach effectively: A brief guide*. Chicago, IL: Lyceum Books.

Gibbons, S. W. (2009). Theory synthesis for self-neglect: A health and social phenomenon. *Nursing Research, 58*(3), 194–200.

Health Service Executive. (2014). Safeguarding vulnerable persons at risk of abuse: National policy and procedures. Dublin, Ireland: HSE, Social Care Division.

Hooyman, N., & Asuman Kiyak, H. (2011). *Social gerontology: A multidisciplinary perspective* (9th ed.). Boston, MA: Allyn & Bacon.

Hooyman, N., & St. Peter, S. (2007). Creating aging-enriched social work education: A process of curricular and organizational change. In C. J. Tompkins & A. L. Rosen (Eds.), *Fostering social work gerontology competence* (pp. 9–29). New York, NY: Haworth Press.

Hope, T., Savulescu, J., & Hendrick, J. (2008). *Medical ethics and law: The core curriculum* (Vol. 2). Edinburgh, UK: Churchill Livingstone Elsevier.

Hughes, J., & Baldwin, C. (2006). *Ethical issues in dementia care*. London, UK: Jessica Kingsley.

Iris, M., Ridings, J. W., & Conrad, K. J. (2010). The development of a conceptual model for understanding elder self-neglect. *The Gerontologist, 50*(3), 303–315. doi:10.1093/geront/gnp125

Kalish, R. (1979). The new ageism and the failure models: A polemic. *The Gerontologist, 19*, 398–402.

Knight, B. (1986). *Psychotherapy with older adults*. Beverly Hills, CA: Sage.

Laidlaw, K., Thompson, L., Dick-Siskin, L., & Gallagher-Thompson, D. (2003). *Cognitive behavior therapy with older people*. Hoboken, NJ: John Wiley & Sons.

Lyons, N. (2010). The ethical dimensions of reflective practice. In N. Lyons (Ed.), *Handbook of reflection and reflective inquiry* (pp. 519–526). New York, NY: Springer Publishing.

Mahoney, K., McGaffigan, E., Sciegaj, M., Zgoda, K., & Mahoney, E. (2017). Approaches to empowering individuals and communities. In D. Kaplan & B. Berkman (Eds.), *The Oxford handbook of social work in health and aging* (2nd ed., pp. 85–90). New York, NY: Oxford University Press.

McInnis-Dittrich, K. (2014). *Social work with older adults* (4th ed.). Boston, MA: Pearson.

Merriam, S., & Caffarella, R. (1999). *Learning in adulthood* (2nd ed.). San Francisco, CA: Jossey-Bass.

Owens, N., Padula, C., & Hume, A. (2002). Developing and using interdisciplinary case studies in teaching geriatrics to practicing health care professionals. *Educational Gerontology, 28*, 473–489. doi:10.1080/03601270290081407

Pavlou, M., & Lachs, M. (2006). Could self-neglect in older adults be a geriatric syndrome? *Journal of the American Geriatrics Society, 54*(5), 831–842. doi:10.1111/j.1532-5415.2006.00661.x

Phillips, J., Ray, M., & Marshall, M. (2006). *Social work with older people*. Houndmills, UK: Palgrave.

Sheldon, B., & MacDonald, G. (2009). *A textbook of social work* (1st ed.). Abingdon, UK: Routledge.

Sibley, J., & Ostafichuk, P. (2014). *Getting started with team-based learning*. Sterling, VA: Stylus.

Sung, K.-T., & Dunkle, R. E. (2009). How social workers demonstrate respect for elderly clients. *Journal of Gerontological Social Work, 52*, 250–260.

Taylor, J. A., & McLendon, T. (2013). Using elements of team-based learning in an introductory social work course. *Journal of Baccalaureate Social Work, 18*, 235–240.

Thompson, N. (2006). *Anti-discriminatory practice*. Houndmills, UK: Palgrave.

Wacker, R., & Roberto, K. (2014). *Community resources for older adults* (4th ed.). Los Angeles, CA: Sage.

World Health Organization. (2011). *European report on preventing elder maltreatment*. Copenhagen, Denmark: The Regional Office for Europe of the World Health Organization. Retrieved from http://www.euro.who.int/__data/assets/pdf_file/0010/144676/e95110.pdf

CHAPTER 24

A SELF-NEGLECTING CASE DILEMMA: APPLYING AN ETHICAL DECISION-MAKING TOOL

Mary Rose Day and Joan McCarthy

Globally, self-neglect is recognized as a serious and complex public health issue. Self-neglect can vary in presentation and severity and is mainly characterized by profound environmental neglect and cumulative diverse behaviors that may threaten a person's ability to live safely and independently in the community. Supporting people who self-neglect can give rise to significant ethical, professional, and personal challenges. The purpose of this chapter is to examine ethical decision making pertaining to self-neglect. An ethical decision-making tool is described and applied to a case example of self-neglect. The tool provides a step-by-step framework of actions and responsibilities to critically reflect on and respond to an ethically challenging self-neglecting individual. The tool highlights the key components of the ethical decision-making process and may contribute to building ethical capacity and confidence among health and social care professionals. Ethical frameworks have the potential to improve care and outcomes for self-neglecting clients.

Self-neglect is a complex multidimensional phenomenon that involves serious inattention (intended or not) to personal, physical, emotional, and/or social needs with the potential for serious consequences to the health and well-being of the individual who is self-neglecting and, possibly, the community in which he or she resides (Gibbons, Lauder, & Ludwick, 2006; National Centre on Elder Abuse, 2014; Pavlou & Lachs, 2006).

Although first identified in the 1950s, self-neglect continues to be poorly understood and under-researched (Lauder, Roxburg, Harris, & Law, 2009). Self-neglect has been associated with early onset and progression over the course of an individual's life (Lauder et al., 2009) and it is related to life history and coping skills (Band-Winterstein, Doron, & Naim, 2012; Day, Leahy-Warren, & McCarthy, 2013; Gibbons, 2009). For example, Lien et al. (2016) reported on a sample of 69 self-neglecting participants who had intact cognition based on the Mini-Mental State Examination. The life stories and narratives illustrated traumatic loss, victimization, or sexual abuse, and lifetime pattern of behaviors included substantial financial instability, mental illness, mistrust of people or paranoia, distrust and avoidance of the medical establishment, and substance abuse. Individuals who self-neglect may not see any immediate problems with their behaviors and some see it as normal as they strive to maintain their physical function and independence (Band-Winterstein et al., 2012; Bozinovski, 2000; Kutame, 2008). They may feel threatened and distrustful when people try to interfere.

A small proportion of people who self-neglect may hoard animals (Arluke et al., 2002) or neglect to care for their pets. Animal hoarding describes circumstances in which the number of animals as domestic pets exceeds the limits and the ability of the person to provide the animals with adequate housing and adequate standards of care while at the same time believing proper care is being provided (Holmberg, 2014). The presence of numerous animals may give rise to squalor and the smell and noise can lead to disagreement with neighbors and communities (Rasmussen, Steketee, Frost, Tolin, & Brown, 2014; Saldarriaga-Cantillo & Rivas Nieto, 2015). The hoarding of animals and neglect of pets is a complex public health issue that impacts on individuals' and animals' health (Castrodale et al., 2010) and creates social and environmental issues.

Adverse outcomes associated with self-neglect include increased hospitalization (Dong & Simon, 2013b, 2014; Dong, Simon, & Evans, 2012a), increased emergency department visits (Dong, Simon, & Evans, 2012c), hospice care (Dong & Simon, 2013a), nursing home placement (Lachs, Williams, O'Brien, & Pillemer, 2002), caregiver neglect (Dong, Simon, & Evans, 2013), emotional and financial abuse (Mardan, Jaehnichen, & Hamid, 2014), and significantly increased mortality (Dong et al., 2009; Reyes-Ortiz, Burnett, Flores, Halphen, & Dyer, 2014).

Self-neglect is associated with younger and older adult populations, but prevalence is much higher in older adults (Dong & Simon, 2015; Dong, Simon, & Evans, 2012b; Lauder et al., 2009). The harmful effects of self-neglect and animal hoarding and encounters with individuals who self-neglect can give rise to significant ethical, personal, and professional challenges.

ETHICAL ISSUES

Self-neglecting behaviors can cause ethical issues for multidisciplinary team (MDT) members. Ethical concerns can relate to refusal of treatment, services, and interventions offered; disagreement with neighbors and family members; and capacity for decision making (Leuter, Petrucci, Mattei, Tabassi, & Lancia, 2013; Mousqueda & Dong, 2011). Intervening in cases of self-neglect can be fraught with ethical ambiguity and uncertainty.

The right of autonomy (to refuse state interference in one's personal and private life) is deeply embedded in and protected by national and international legal instruments such as the European Convention on Human Rights (Article 8 and 5) and the Council of Europe (2014). It follows that when a person chooses to live in a particular way, if it is the person's choice and the person has capacity, there are only limited circumstances in which the law can intervene (Assisted Decision-Making [Capacity] Act, 2015). Irish and international legislation also protects and promotes other rights such as human life, timely and fair access to health and social care services, and confidentiality (Assisted Decision-Making [Capacity] Act, 2015; Data

Protection Act, 2003; Health Information & Quality Authority, 2016; Health Service Executive [HSE], 2014a; United Nations, 2006). The ethical principles endorsed by the Irish Health Service Executive in the safeguarding of vulnerable adults include human rights, person-centeredness, advocacy, confidentiality, empowerment, and collaboration (HSE, 2014b). All of these principles are also embraced in the professional codes of community nurses, social workers, and physicians (American Nurses Association, 2015; Irish Association of Social Workers, 2016; Irish Medical Council, 2016; Nursing and Midwifery Board of Ireland, 2014) and these codes, in turn, are used to protect and safeguard the welfare of the public against substandard care. However, these professional codes of conduct provide limited guidance on resolving ethical dilemmas when, for example, health and social care professionals must negotiate between the seemingly competing obligations of respecting individual autonomy, on the one hand, and keeping people safe on the other.

In the case of self-neglect then, the difficulty is not the absence of ethical, legal, and professional principles to guide professional conduct, it is the challenge of identifying which principles are at stake in any given situation and what to do in cases in which these principles seem to give rise to conflicting obligations. The challenge is finding the balance: promoting the independence and autonomy of individuals by not interfering and, at the same time, acting responsibly to promote the health and safety of individuals and striving to attain positive outcomes (Day, Leahy-Warren, & McCarthy, 2016).

In short, it is important that health and social care professionals know how to address the ethical issues they confront in everyday practice. Yet ethical decision making in general, and specifically, using ethical frameworks to examine ethical dilemmas, are minimally discussed in the self-neglect literature (Band-Winterstein, 2016; Day et al., 2016). To remedy this, the following section presents an ethical decision-making tool and then applies it to a self-neglect case that represents a typical situation faced by the health and social care professionals.

AN ETHICAL DECISION-MAKING TOOL

A range of models and frameworks for ethical decision making are available and each shares similar steps and components (Bartholdson, Pergert, & Helgesson, 2014; Campbell & McCarthy, 2017, in press; Jonson, Siegler, & Winslade, 2010; Kanoti, 2000; McCarthy, Campbell, Dalton-O'Connor, Andrews, & McLoughlin, 2016; Nelson, 2015). We have identified the ethical decision-making tool developed for end-of-life decision making by Campbell and McCarthy (2017, in press) as a useful tool for our purpose. This decision-making tool provides steps that can be used by health and social care professionals to reflect on the ethical dimensions of their cases and consider and evaluate possible courses of action. The actions are (1) identify the ethical problem(s) and relevant facts; (2) identify stakeholders' interests, needs, and values; (3) weigh the merits and demerits of available courses of action; (4) select the action that can best be supported by ethical principles; and (5) review (see Table 24.1). In the following section, we use the tool to analyze the situation of Mary Dobson, an individual who self-neglects.

TABLE 24.1 Decision-Making Tool

Actions	Responsibilities
1. Articulate the ethical problem(s) and identify relevant facts	Be ethically sensitive and communicate clearly
2. Identify stakeholders' interests, needs, values	Be respectful and inclusive
3. Weigh the merits and demerits of available courses of action	Be informed and fair
4. Select the action that can best be supported by ethical principles	Be impartial and transparent
5. Review	Check: Have I been sensitive, clear, respectful, inclusive, informed, fair, impartial, and transparent?

Source: Campbell and McCarthy (2017, in press).

CASE STUDY 1: Mary Dobson

Mary Dobson is an 80-year-old widowed woman who is living alone in a three-bedroom terraced house that she owns. She has good mobility, but she is undernourished, has a history of alcoholism, diabetes, cardiovascular disease, and currently has a leg ulcer that needs regular dressing. Mary sees her general practitioner (GP) periodically, but she is a very private person and over the years has had little to no contact with neighbors, her wider family, or community. Agnes Murphy, Mary's neighbor, puts in a telephone request for a public health nurse (PHN) to conduct a home visit as she has not seen Mary for a week. Agnes describes Mary as a neighbor who is severely neglecting herself, is eccentric, reclusive, and a loner. Agnes complains that "the neglected state of Mary's home will reduce the tone of the neighborhood and value of the property."

On receiving the report of concern about Mary Dobson, the PHN, Joan Richards, conducts a home visit. Mary introduces her to her 20 cats by their individual names. They appear to be well cared for and numerous empty and full cans of cat food are in the house. Joan observes that Mary's living conditions are unhygienic; there is a strong odor from cat feces, the house is cold, there is an accumulation of items (waste, empty beer bottles, etc.), access to the equipment such as sink for washing and rooms is poor, many utilities such as stove, sink, and phone are absent or in poor repair. Mary is evasive about her self-care, there is a noticeable smell of alcohol about her and she is unable to articulate her medication regimen. Joan is concerned about Mary's ability to maintain her home environment, self-care, physical function, care of leg ulcer, and cooking, shopping, and so on. Mary spends most of the day in bed with her cats. Joan leaves Mary with a heavy heart. She is seriously concerned about Mary's state of health and her safety. However, she is also anxious to respect Mary's expressed wish to remain in her own home. She is not sure how to proceed.

USING THE TOOL

Action 1. Articulate the Ethical Problem(s) and Identify Relevant Facts

The key ethical issue that arises is that Mary has clearly articulated her wishes—to continue living in her own home. However, Mary's health, well-being, and safety are at serious risk and her living conditions seem to be having a negative impact on her wider community. The concept of risk is a complex issue, which can mean different things to different people. A decision needs to be made about Mary's future treatment and care and this includes a decision about where and how Mary will receive this care.

Clinical facts include Mary's medical history of diabetes, cardiovascular disease, and a leg ulcer that is in need of clinical attention. Related facts include Mary's state of mental health, alcohol intake, and ability to self-care and cope with everyday living. It is significant that Mary's capacity for decision making seem uncertain—it is not clear whether Mary understands the consequences for her if she continues to live as she is doing now. Finally, the absence of a social network of family and friends, the unhygienic and cold home environment, and the presence of numerous animals giving rise to squalor must be part of any deliberation about Mary.

Action 2. Identify Stakeholders' Interests, Needs, and Values

Inclusiveness is a vital part of good decision making, so no person affected by the decision should be excluded from the decision-making process without adequate justification. Those who are affected by the decision must have an opportunity to give voice to what is important to them.

Mary

Mary's beliefs, values, preferences, knowledge of her situation, and understanding of the consequences of her behavior should be a central focus in the decision-making process. Mary's capacity for decision making needs to be assessed. Mary may have different levels of capacity for each of the decisions that need to be made. For example, Mary may have a very good understanding of the consequences of staying in her own home without support, but she may need some help to understand what may happen if the dressings on her leg ulcer are not changed regularly.

Mary's well-being as she understands it also needs to be considered. She appears content and relatively well considering her home living environment and poor social networks, anxiety, and so forth. Medically, her well-being is served if blood screening and medication review are conducted (diabetes, cardiovascular disease, nutrition) and if the leg ulcer is treated with a dressing regimen and antibiotics. Mary also has a close relationship with her 20 cats, with whom she spends a great deal of her time. In effect, they are part of her family and contribute to her overall well-being. Unfortunately, they may also be a threat to her health as Mary's ability to cope and care for this number of cats could be questioned due to the strong odor of cat feces.

Neighbors/Community

Agnes and other neighbors are frustrated and express concern about Mary's care, eccentricity, and health and safety. They view the cats as a nuisance and the outward appearance of the house could impact on sales of homes in the neighborhood. They are anxious and concerned that the situation will worsen; Mary will have a fall or she will be found dead. They believe that health and social care professionals have a moral duty to transfer Mary to a hospital or a nursing home to safeguard her and they want a quick response and action.

Family

Mary has no contact with family members. However, there may be family members whom Mary has alienated and who may want some involvement in her life.

Health and Social Care Professionals

Joan and any other health and allied professionals or multidisciplinary team members caring for Mary may not easily reach a consensus about what is best for her. Some members of staff may be reluctant to try to transfer Mary to hospital or residential care against her express wishes. On the other hand, if the status quo is maintained and Mary continues to live in squalor, some professionals may feel distressed if they believe that they have abandoned Mary. In either case, the professionals involved may experience moral distress because they have acted in a way that is contrary to their own moral values and personal integrity.

Some members of the team may also be experiencing conflict balancing their duty of care and their perceived obligations under law, and they may believe the situation warrants intervention (Day et al., 2016). Professionals need to be informed and knowledgeable on definitions of self-neglect, policy, legislation, reporting laws, and service approaches within their jurisdiction as they can vary across countries and states. In Ireland, the policy document "Safeguarding Vulnerable Adults at Risk of Abuse" (HSE, 2014b) recognizes serious and extreme self-neglect under safeguarding approaches.

Action 3. Weigh the Merits and Demerits of Available Courses of Action

Assess Mary and Refer Her to a Safeguarding and Protection Team

Merits

Planning a home visit and holistic assessment (physical, psychosocial, and environmental) of Mary's needs provides a comprehensive and more objective picture of Mary's situation and level of risk. Standardized self-neglect assessment and observation measurement tools, such as the 25-item Short-Form Elder Self-Neglect Assessment (SF-ESNA; Iris, Conrad, & Ridings, 2014) and the Self-Neglect Assessment Measure (SN-37; Day & McCarthy, 2016) include indicators of self-neglect across a continuum (mild to severe). The SF-ESNA has 12 items in the behavioral category and 13 items in the environmental category. The SN-37 has five factors: environment, social networks, emotional and behavioral liability, health avoidance, and self-determinism.

Case referral to the Senior Case Workers' Safeguarding Team could facilitate a multidisciplinary and multiagency response. Interdisciplinary collaboration fosters a culture of sharing, professional discussion, and safety planning that focuses on safeguarding the health, safety, and well-being of Mary, as well as her neighbors and the welfare of her animals.

An MDT meeting/case conference could be arranged under safeguarding procedures. This would enable communication and the sharing of information to consider the assessment of Mary's needs; her wishes and views; and the risk(s), merits, and demerits of nonintervention. All of these must be considered before an action plan is agreed and a lead person or agency is appointed. This approach could lead to short- and long-term benefits and better outcomes.

Demerits

Gaining Mary's permission to share information about herself, even with other health professionals, may be viewed with suspicion by her and undermine any prospects of building a relationship of trust between Mary and the health and social care professionals. In turn, getting agreement from the MDT and agencies can be a challenge. Organizational culture (i.e., team and agency culture) can influence professionals' choices and responses to self-neglect. Procedural guidelines and policy on self-neglect are not always followed by professionals and may not provide specific guidance and help to work through ethical dilemmas.

Intervene: Transfer Mary to Hospital as an Emergency Measure

Merits
Institutionalization is sometimes seen as a solution by health and social services as means of protecting vulnerable older adults (Wolf, 2003). Mary's nonadherence to medication, diabetes mellitus, cardiovascular disease, and her leg ulcer are pivotal issues that can lead to acute health problems. These medical issues might be strategically used as justification for an acute hospital admission.

In addition, some team members may see hospitalization as a means of protection for Mary from a range of health and safety risk factors, for example, isolation, environmental neglect, alcohol misuse, and infection. Hospitalization may also be seen as a quick means to access a geriatrician and have a comprehensive assessment that includes a capacity assessment. Transferring Mary to a hospital or a nursing home will also move her responsibility to acute or long-term care services. This course of action might be welcomed by neighbors.

Demerits
Mary was clear about not wishing to leave her home or change her situation. There is a chance that Mary will refuse hospitalization. Ignoring Mary's expressed preferences overrides her right of autonomy and will impact on her relationship with health and social care professionals. This approach could lead to grave distress and suffering for Mary as well as serious adverse outcomes, such as ill health, poor quality of life, and transfer to a hospital or nursing home may hasten death.

Respect Mary's Refusal of Interventions and Supports

Merits
Assuming that Mary has the capacity to make decisions about her treatment and care, then respect of Mary's refusal of interventions and supports from MDT demonstrates respect for her autonomy, preferences, and privacy. In ethics and law, if a person is assessed as having the capacity to make specific decisions for himself or herself, he or she is free to make what health professionals may believe to be unwise decisions as long as it does not place others at risk of serious harm (MacLeod & Douthit, 2015, p. 18).

Demerits
If things do not change, there remains a risk that Mary could fall or be found dead. Poor home environment, clutter, and alcohol consumption increase risk of falls and are a primary cause of accidental or unintentional injury and deaths (Lee, Burnett, & Dyer, 2016; World Health Organization, 2007). Mary's refusal to accept assistance and support places a burden on professionals and some may struggle with uncertainty as to their ethical obligations and duty of care for Mary and may feel that they have abandoned her. The neighbors may also be offended by what they see as inaction by the MDT.

Action 4. Select the Action That Can Best be Supported by Ethical Principles

A combination of two courses of action: (a) assess and refer to Safeguarding and Protection Team and (b) respect Mary's refusal of intervention and support fulfills health and social care professionals' ethical obligations under the key ethical principles of autonomy, avoiding harm and doing good, and solidarity. Briefly, these principles can be understood in the following way.

Autonomy

Autonomy is the capacity for self-determination—a person's ability to make choices about his or her own life based on his or her values and beliefs about what is important. The principle of respect for autonomy recognizes the unique values, priorities, and preferences of individuals and supports the individual in participating as fully as possible in decisions about his or her care.

Health professionals should begin by assuming that the person they are providing care for has the capacity to make his or her own decisions. They should not presume that an individual lacks capacity because of age, appearance, disability, behavior, medical condition (e.g,. mental illness or dementia), beliefs, or communication difficulties. Importantly, health professionals should not assume that a person lacks capacity because, in their view, he or she is making a decision that is unwise. What is important is that the person understands what is entailed in the decision (Assisted Decision-Making [Capacity] Act, 2015).

Avoiding Harm and Doing Good

Any action or intervention should be aimed at minimizing a person's suffering and maximizing health and well-being. Professionals should aim to improve a person's overall well-being, for example, paying attention to pain management and the avoidance of unnecessary suffering as well as the creation of opportunities for positive experiences and joy.

Solidarity

Our interdependence as human beings means that we are "fellow travelers" who have faced, or will at some point face, dependency in our lives. This understanding prompts an empathic response: The quality of care provided should reflect the standard of care we would expect for ourselves and the people we love.

This interconnectedness is reflected in the relationship between the individual who is ill and/or in need and his or her caregivers and health professionals, all of whose interests should be considered. On this view, our dependency on each other is the norm, not the exception.

MDT team members have an obligation to communicate with Mary in a way that builds rapport, pays attention to her beliefs and values, and ensures that Mary has accurate, complete, and understandable information on which to base her decisions. Health and social care professionals supporting Mary are obligated to communicate honestly with her in relation to their clinical concerns, the impact of self-neglecting behaviors and associated health and safety risks, and the possible impact of service refusal and decisions on her living situation. In doing so, they respect Mary's autonomy as well as preserve her life and maintain its quality as far as possible.

However, if individual team members assess risk in different ways and have different beliefs about what interventions and approaches are warranted they may need an opportunity to explore the rationale underlying their own perspectives. The conversation among the members of the care team should focus on devising appropriate goals of care for Mary, in the context of her own wishes, her illness, and current clinical status.

A short-term goal could be to seek agreement and engagement from Mary for Joan to conduct regular scheduled home visits. Listening to Mary's narratives and story while building a relationship can facilitate real understanding of the factors and life issues that may have impacted her life course and her reluctance to receive help.

Consultation by Joan with the MDT and an assessment will enable a team approach to work through the health and safety issues and possible responses and courses of actions in the safeguarding and protection of Mary. Mary's well-being and dignity and her health and safety should be monitored at regular intervals as well as the risk of her self-neglect to others.

Asking Mary to identify her most important and least important needs and preferences in relation to changing her situation and asking her to come up with possible actions and solutions is vital. For example, one important action might be to plan with Mary to seek new homes for some of her cats and arrange for neutering of the remaining cats. This approach is sensitive to Mary's attachment to her cats and her emotional isolation. This action will improve Mary's home environment and may also address some of the concerns of Mary's neighbors.

Action 5. Review Decision Making

The process described previously incorporates each element of responsible and ethical decision making. First, the key ethical concerns that arise and the values that are at risk in Mary's case have been clearly identified and articulated. Second, the collaborative approach taken is respectful and inclusive of the perspective and interests of all involved, for example, Mary, Joan, neighbors, family, and health and social professionals. Third, the decision making is informed by relevant ethical, legal, clinical, and regulatory standards of best practices and the approach taken is careful to avoid bias. Finally, the perspective taken is non judgmental and even-handed and the suggested steps are clearly outlined.

CONCLUSION

Self-neglect is a serious and complex public health issue. Because each self-neglecting situation is unique and fluid there is rarely a single solution or quick fix and ongoing evaluation and reassessment are needed. Significant ethical, personal, and professional challenges arise when the health and social care professionals encounter people who self-neglect, and intervening in these situations can be fraught with ethical ambiguity and uncertainty. In the absence of other models of ethical decision making in the self-neglect literature, and to illustrate how this ambiguity and uncertainty might be addressed, this chapter applied an ethical decision-making tool to a case example of self-neglect. The tool offers a means of examining each situation in a way that brings its ethical dimensions to the fore and highlights the key components of ethical decision making. It also provides a step-by-step framework of actions and responsibilities that can be used by the health and social care professionals to critically reflect on and respond to ethically challenging self-neglecting situations. It is to be hoped that, the use of this tool will contribute to building ethical capacity and confidence among the health and social care professionals who must negotiate these challenging and often fraught situations in the course of their professional practice.

IMPLICATIONS FOR RESEARCH AND PRACTICE

- The ethical decision-making tool presented in this chapter provides a framework to critically examine and evaluate choices and actions made by the health and social care professionals.
- Ethical decision making is a process that can be refined and used in addressing any ethical dilemma.
- The ethical decision-making tool has the potential to build capacity and confidence among the health and social care professionals and enable them to confront challenging situations in the absence of any dedicated support structure.
- Ethics and the use of the ethical decision-making framework must be integrated into the training and education of health and social care professionals.
- Research is needed on the perspectives of the health and social care professionals on ethical issues encountered in self-neglect practice.

REFERENCES

American Nurses Association. (2015). *Code of ethics for nurses with interpretive statements.* Silver Spring, MD: Author.

Assisted Decision-Making (Capacity) Act. (2015). House of the Oireachtas, Ireland. Retrieved from http://www.irishstatutebook.ie/eli/2015/act/64/enacted/en/html

Band-Winterstein, T. (2016). Nurses' encounters with older adults engaged in self-neglectful behaviors in the community: A qualitative study. *Journal of Applied Gerontology.* Advance online publication. doi:101177/0733464816665206. Retrieved from http://jag.sagepub.com/content/early/2016/08/26/0733464816665206.full.pdf+html

Band-Winterstein, T., Doron, I. I., & Naim, S. (2012). Elder self-neglect: A geriatric syndrome or a life course story? *Journal of Aging Studies, 26*(2), 109–118.

Bartholdson, C., Pergert, P., & Helgesson, G. (2014). Procedures for clinical ethics case reflections: An example from childhood cancer care. *Clinical Ethics, 9*(2–3), 87–95.

Bozinovski, S. D. (2000). Older self-neglecters: Interpersonal problems and the maintenance of self-continuity. *Journal of Elder Abuse & Neglect, 12*(1), 37–56.

Campbell, L., & McCarthy, J. (2017, in press). A decision-making tool for building clinical ethics capacity among Irish health professionals. *Clinical Ethics.*

Castrodale, L., Bellay, Y. M., Brown, C. M., Cantor, F. L., Gibbins, J. D., Headrick, M. L., . . . Yu, D. T. (2010). General public health considerations for responding to animal hoarding cases. *Journal of Environmental Health, 72*(7), 14–18.

Council of Europe. (2014). *Recommendation on the promotion of human rights of older persons.* Recommendation CM/Rec (2014)2. Retrieved from http://www.coe.int/t/dghl/standardsetting/hrpolicy/other_committees/cddhage/default_EN.asp

Data Protection (Amendment) Act. (2003). Retrieved from http://www.dataprotection.ie/viewdoc.asp?DocID=796

Day, M. R., Leahy-Warren, P., & McCarthy, G. (2013). Perceptions and views of self-neglect: A client-centered perspective. *Journal of Elder Abuse & Neglect, 33*(2), 145–156.

Day, M. R., Leahy-Warren, P., & McCarthy, G. (2016). Self-neglect: Ethical considerations. *Annual Review of Nursing Research, 34*(1), 89–107.

Day, M. R., & McCarthy, G. (2016). Self-neglect: Development and evaluation of a self-neglect (SN-37) measurement instrument *Archives of Psychiatric Nursing, 30*(4), 480–485.

Dong, X., & Simon, M. A. (2013a). Association between elder self-neglect and hospice utilization in a community population. *Archives of Gerontology and Geriatrics, 56*(1), 192–198.

Dong, X., & Simon, M. A. (2013b). Elder abuse as a risk factor for hospitalization in older persons. *Journal of the American Medical Association Internal Medicine, 173*(10), 911–917.

Dong, X., & Simon, M. A. (2014). Elder self-neglect is associated with an increased rate of 30-day hospital readmission: Findings from the Chicago Health and Aging Project. *Gerontology, 61*(1), 41–50.

Dong, X., & Simon, M. (2015). Prevalence of elder self-neglect in a Chicago Chinese population: The role of cognitive physical and mental health. *Geriatrics & Gerontology International, 16*(9), 1051–1062.

Dong, X., Simon, M. A., & Evans, D. (2012a). Elder self-neglect and hospitalization: Findings from the Chicago Health and Aging Project. *Journal of the American Geriatrics Society, 60*(2), 202–209.

Dong, X., Simon, M., & Evans, D. A. (2012b). Prevalence of self-neglect across gender, race, and socio-economic status: Findings from the Chicago Health and Aging Project. *Gerontology, 58*, 258–268.

Dong, X., Simon, M. A., & Evans, D. A. (2012c). Prospective study of the elder self-neglect and ED use in a community population. *American Journal of Emergency Medicine, 30*(4), 553–561.

Dong, X., Simon, M., A., & Evans, D. A. (2013). Elder self-neglect is associated with increased risk for elder abuse in a community-dwelling population: Findings from the Chicago Health and Aging Project. *Journal of Aging and Health, 25*(1), 80–96.

Dong, X., Simon, M., Mendes de Leon, C., Fulmer, T., Beck, T., Hebert, L., . . . Evans, D. (2009). Elder self-neglect and abuse and mortality risk in a community-dwelling population. *Journal of the American Medical Association, 302*(5), 517–526.

Gibbons, S. (2009). Theory synthesis for self-neglect: A health and social phenomenon. *Nursing Research, 58*(3), 194–200.

Gibbons, S., Lauder, W., & Ludwick, R. (2006). Self-neglect: A proposed new NANDA diagnosis. *International Journal of Nursing Terminologies and Classifications, 17*(1), 10–18.

Health Information & Quality Authority. (2016). *Supporting people's autonomy: A guidance document.* Dublin, Ireland: Author.

Health Service Executive. (2014a). *National Consent Policy.* Dublin, Ireland: Author.

Health Service Executive. (2014b). *Safeguarding vulnerable persons at risk of abuse: National policy and procedures.* Dublin, Ireland: HSE, Social Care Division.

Holmberg, T. (2014). Sensuous governance: Assessing urban animal hoarding. *Housing, Theory and Society, 31*(4), 464–479. doi:10.1080/14036096.2014.928650

Iris, M., Conrad, K. J., & Ridings, J. (2014). Observational measure of elder self-neglect. *Journal of Elder Abuse & Neglect, 26*, 1–33.

Irish Association of Social Workers. (2016). *Code of practice for Irish Association of Social Workers' members.* Retrieved from https://www.iasw.ie/attachments/2eb7f6f6-ca51-4f38-b869-df7e0b411e91.PDF

Irish Medical Council. (2016). *Guide to professional conduct and ethics for registered medical practitioner* (8th ed.). Dublin, Ireland: Irish Medical Council. Retrieved from http://www.medicalcouncil.ie

Jonson, A. R., Siegler, M., & Winslade, W. J. (2010). *Clinical ethics: A practical approach to ethical decisions in clinical medicine* (7th ed.). New York, NY: McGraw-Hill.

Kanoti, G. A. (2000). *Ethical dilemmas: A values guide for medical students.* London, UK: Sage.

Kutame, M. M. (2008). *Understanding self-neglect from the older person's perspective.* ProQuest Information & Learning, US. Retrieved from http://search.ebscohost.com/login.aspx? direct=true&db=psyh&AN=2008-99011-293&site=ehost-live.

Lachs, M. S., Williams, C. S., O'Brien, S., & Pillemer, K. A. (2002). Adult protective service use and nursing home placement. *The Gerontologist, 42*(6), 734–739.

Lauder, W., Roxburgh, M., Harris, J., & Law, J. (2009). Developing self-neglect theory: Analysis of related and atypical cases of people identified as self-neglecting. *Journal of Psychiatric and Mental Health Nursing, 16*(5), 447–454.

Lee, J. L., Burnett, J., & Dyer, C. B. (2016). Frailty in self-neglecting older adults: A secondary analysis. *Journal of Elder Abuse & Neglect, 28*(3), 152–162. doi:10.1080/08946566.2016.1185986

Lien, C., Rosen, T., Bloemen, E. M., Abrams, R. C., Pavlou, M., & Lachs, M. S. (2016). Narratives of self-neglect: Patterns of traumatic personal experiences and maladaptive behaviors in cognitively intact older adults. *Journal of the American Geriatrics Society, 64*(11), e195–e200. doi:10.1111/jgs.14524

MacLeod, M. Z. K., & Douthit, K. Z. (2015). Etiology and management of elder self-neglect. *Adultspan Journal, 14*, 11–23. doi:10.1002/j.2161-0029

Mardan, H., Jaehnichen, G., & Hamid, T. A. (2014). Is self-neglect associated with the emotional and financial abuse in community-dwelling? *IOSR Journal of Nursing and Health Science, 3*(3), 51–56.

McCarthy, J., Campbell, L., Dalton-O'Connor, C., Andrews, T., & McLoughlin, K. (2016). *Palliative care for the person with dementia. Guidance document 6: Ethical decision making in end-of-life care and the person with dementia.* Dublin, Ireland: Irish Hospice Foundation.

National Centre on Elder Abuse. (2014). Elder abuse prevalence and incidence fact sheet. Washington, DC: National Association of State Units on Aging.

Nelson, W. A. (2015, July/August). Making ethical decisions. *Healthcare Executive,* 46–48.

Nursing and Midwifery Board of Ireland. (2014). *Code of professional conduct and ethics for registered nurses and midwives.* Thousand Oaks, CA: Sage Publications. Retrieved from https://www.nmbi.ie/NMBI/media/NMBI/Code-of-Professional-Conduct-and-Ethics-Dec-2014_1.pdf

Pavlou, M., & Lachs, M. (2006). Could self-neglect in older adults be a geriatric syndrome? *Journal of the American Geriatrics Society, 54*(5), 831–842.

Rasmussen, J. L., Steketee, G., Frost, R. O., Tolin, D. F., & Brown, T. A. (2014). Assessing squalor in hoarding: The Home Environment Index. *Community Mental Health Journal, 50*(5), 591–596. doi:10.1007/s10597-013-9665-8

Reyes-Ortiz, C. A., Burnett, J., Flores, D. V., Halphen, J. M., & Dyer, C. B. (2014). Medical implications of elder abuse: Self-neglect. *Clinics in Geriatric Medicine, 30*(4), 807–823.

Saldarriaga-Cantillo, A., & Rivas Nieto, J. C. (2015). Noah Syndrome: A variant of Diogenes syndrome accompanied by animal hoarding practices. *Journal of Elder Abuse & Neglect, 27*(3), 270–275. doi:1 0.1080/08946566.2014.978518

World Health Organization. (2007). *WHO global report on falls prevention in older age.* Geneva, Switzerland: Author. Retrieved from http://www.who.int/ageing/publications/Falls_prevention7March.pdf

CHAPTER 25

SUMMARY AND CONCLUSION

Geraldine McCarthy, Joyce J. Fitzpatrick,
and Mary Rose Day

This book was designed to provide information to health and social care professionals on self-neglect in older adults and the associated challenges for health and social care providers. In this chapter, we summarize the main components of the content and draw conclusions based on the implications for practice and research.

Self-neglect has been described as a serious public health issue. It can be classified as serious inattention to health and hygiene (intentional or nonintentional) with potential for serious consequences to health and well-being of the individual, and possibly even the community (Gibbons, Lauder, & Ludwick, 2006; Pavlou & Lachs, 2008). Self-neglect can present along a continuum of severity, as external manifestations within the environment (filthy environment, hoarding, poor access to appliances, etc.), and as a diverse spectrum of behaviors (noncompliance with health care regimens, refusing services, as well as being angry, sad, fearful, etc.). Lustbader commented at a self-neglect symposium (National Committee for the Prevention of Elder Abuse, 2008) that the penchant for self-destruction and self-neglect is a human ailment, which is part of the life cycle. She went on to state that a variety of reasons may give rise to self-neglect, such as ignorance/denial, anxiety, alcoholism, grief, depression, and exercising the right to commit slow suicide.

It is estimated that the number of people aged 60 or older will increase from 841 million in 2015 to over 1.4 trillion by the year 2030 and 2.1 trillion by 2050 globally (United Nations, 2013). Predictions suggest that figures could rise to 3.2 trillion by 2100 (World Health Organization Health Assembly, 2016). This demographic shift with the aging of the world's population will inevitably be accompanied by an increase in the number of people living alone with multiple comorbidities, such as depression and dementia, and will increase the prevalence risk and vulnerability for self-neglect. It is evident from the chapters in this book that self-neglect is a complex multifactorial public health issue requiring responses that include a multidisciplinary and multiagency approach.

Older adults are particularly vulnerable to self-neglect, and older African Americans (85+ years) are more at risk of self-neglect (10.1%; Dong et al., 2011; Dong, Simon, & Evans, 2012). Furthermore, the prevalence of risk is higher for people with less education and lower income (Dong, Simon, & Evans, 2010). Older adults with poorer cognition and poorer physical and psychological health are more likely to report elder self-neglect (Dong & Simon, 2015). Depression arising in late life can lead to greater self-neglect (Fiske, Wetherwee, & Gatz, 2009). Adults who self-neglect have significantly higher risks of morbidity and mortality (Dong, Simon, Beck, & Evans, 2010).

Hence, self-neglect is a worldwide issue that has the potential to impact the lives of a growing number of people.

Definitions of self-neglect and services and legislative approaches to self-neglect can vary across jurisdictions. Some countries, states, and services have specific definitions of self-neglect and specific services for people who self-neglect. Self-neglect is the most reported and substantiated form of elder abuse, and approximately1.2 million self-neglect cases are referred to adult protective services (APS) in the United States annually (O'Brien, 2011). The inclusion of self-neglect (older people failing to meet basic needs) within the authority of the APS in some U.S. states can mistakenly confound practice and research on elder abuse and mistreatment. It is important that self-neglect is separated from elder abuse.

Self-neglect needs to be considered as a human issue. Knowing and understanding the life story of the self-neglecting person is very important. This can take considerable time and patience for health and social care professionals. There is strong evidence of the value of negotiated interventions based on consensus and persuasion rather than imposed measures. Self-neglect can have a major lifetime impact on children and families of people who self-neglect, including sadness and dilemmas as they struggle to be respectful and try to find quick-fix solutions to situations in which interventions are unwanted by the self-neglecting older person. Self-neglect can also have an impact on neighbors and communities; many cases are reported by the community members as concern grows for the individual or the environment.

Conceptualization of self-neglect has evolved since the 1950s. There is, however, no universally accepted definition of self-neglect and no one theory that can fully explain self-neglect. Lack of clarity on conceptualizations of self-neglect has affected practice and research.

Self-neglect is a serious public health issue, with associated factors that include depression, dementia, anxiety, delirium, hoarding (compulsive and animal), environmental neglect, and polypharmacy. A greater awareness and understanding of these issues have the potential to improve the way professionals and agencies intervene and respond.

Many authors in this book claim that assessment of self-neglecting clients should include separate assessments of self-neglect, capacity, and environment. A comprehensive geriatric assessment process by a provider with specialized preparation in geriatrics working with a multidisciplinary team is proposed as the appropriate evaluation structure for an older person with suspected self-neglecting behavior.

However, there is evidence that in practice an objective assessment of self-neglect is often absent. Three assessment measures are included in the book. The Short Form-Elder Self-Neglect Assessment (SF-ESNA) is described, and its use by practitioners is outlined. The findings present evidence for thinking about elder self-neglect as a continuum of decline, from a position of well-being (good self-care and an adequate home environment) to a situation of increasing severity of deficits with respect to self-care practices and environmental conditions. The development of the 37-item self-neglect measurement instrument, the SN-37, addressed a gap in the literature; this can be used by health and social care professionals. The SN-37 instrument has five subscales: environment, social networks, emotional and behavioral liability, and self-determinism. The third instrument described, **Making and Executing Decisions for Safe and Independent Living** (MEDSAIL), can be used with minimal training by health and social service professionals. It is recommended that persons with lower MEDSAIL scores are referred for formal comprehensive capacity testing. Although the instruments, noted previously, are useful to practitioners, the decision-making capacity of those who self-neglect is a separate issue for assessment purposes. This is especially true when health and social care professionals are making judgments and responding to self-neglect. The outcome of capacity assessment informs the level of protection required while preserving and augmenting remaining capabilities (Falk & Hoffman, 2014).

Many of the authors made recommendations for education and research. Recommendations that have transcended a number of chapters are related to self-neglect as a complex and multidimensional phenomenon that requires multidisciplinary staff training. Training should include the use of an objective assessment measure. Assessment of individuals who self-neglect must be conducted by multidisciplinary team members who are experienced and knowledgeable health and social careprofessionals. Interventions need to be guided by the legislative and policy context of jurisdiction. Good governance structures, as well as multidisciplinary and multiagency responses, are required in cases of self-neglect.

Recommendations include research on self-neglect that compares the perspectives of nurses, other health and social care professionals, and their clients. Longitudinal research to examine relationship between self-neglect, mental health, and cognitive impairment. In addition, research is needed to better understand the association between medication use and self-neglect. Furthermore, research on self-neglect will need to focus on specific interventions and associated outcomes. Evidence is needed to determine whether executive dysfunction is a cause or a result of elder self-neglect.

In conclusion, the comprehensive treatment of self-neglect, including conceptualizations and measurement challenges and professional practice applications, will be useful to practitioners, educators, and researchers across agencies and services. Inherent opportunities exist for advancing health and welfare of the most vulnerable group, older adults, at the same time protecting the rights and freedom of those who are served.

REFERENCES

Dong, X., & Simon, M. A. (2015). Elder self-neglect is associated with an increased rate of 30-day hospital readmission: Findings from the Chicago Health and Aging Project. *Gerontology, 61*(1), 41–50.

Dong, X., Simon, M., Beck, T., & Evans, D. (2010). A cross-sectional population based study of elder self-neglect and psychological, health, and social factors in a biracial community. *Aging and Mental Health, 14*(1), 74–84.

Dong, X., Simon, M. A., & Evans, D. (2010). Cross-sectional study of the characteristics of reported elder self-neglect in a community-dwelling population: Findings from a population-based cohort. *Gerontology, 56*(3), 325–334. doi:10.1159/000243164

Dong, X., Simon, M. A., & Evans, D. A. (2012). Prevalence of self-neglect across gender, race, and socioeconomic status: Findings from the Chicago Health and Aging Project. *Gerontology, 58*(3), 258–268. doi:10.1159/000334256

Dong, X., Simon, M. A., Fulmer, T., Mendes de Leon, C. F., Hebert, L. E., Beck, T., . . . Evans, D. A. (2011). A prospective population-based study of differences in elder self-neglect and mortality between black and white older adults. *Journals of Gerontology, Series A: Biological Sciences and Medical Sciences, 66A*(6), 695–704. doi:10.1093/gerona/glr053

Falk, E., & Hoffman, N. (2014). The role of capacity assessments in elder abuse investigations and guardianships. *Clinics in Geriatric Medicine, 30*(4), 851–868. doi:10.1016/j.cger.2014.08.009

Fiske, A., Wetherwee, J. L., & Gatz, M. (2009). Depression in old age. *Annual Review of Clinical Psychology, 5*, 363–389.

Gibbons, S., Lauder, W., & Ludwick, R. (2006). Self-neglect: A proposed new NANDA diagnosis. *International Journal of Nursing Terminologies and Classifications, 17*(1), 10–18.

National Committee for the Prevention of Elder Abuse. (2008). *Symposium on self-neglect: Building a coordinated response.* Washington, DC: NCEA. Retrieved from http:// www.preventelderabuse.org/new/ReportontheNCPEASelf-NeglectSymposium.doc

O'Brien, J. G. (2011). Self-neglect in old age. *Aging Health, 7*(4), 573–581.

Pavlou, M. P., & Lachs, M. S. (2008). Self-neglect in older adults: A primer for clinicians. *Journal of General Internal Medicine, 23*, 1841–1846.

United Nations. (2013). *World population ageing 2013.* Department of Economic and Social Affairs Population Division. Retrieved from http://www.un.org/en/development/desa/population/publications/pdf/ageing/WorldPopulationAgeing2013.pdf

World Health Organization Health Assembly. (2016). *Multisectoral action for a life course approach to healthy ageing: Draft global strategy and plan of action on ageing and health A69/17.* Geneva, Switzerland: World Health Organization. Retrieved from http://who.int/ageing/global-strategy/en

INDEX

Printed in the United States
By Bookmasters